Essentials of Nursing Leadership and Management

Essentials of Nursing Leadership and Management
Third Edition

Ruth M. Tappen, EdD, RN, FAAN
Christine E. Lynn Eminent Scholar and Professor
Florida Atlantic University College of Nursing
Boca Raton, FL

Sally A. Weiss, RN, EdD
Program Coordinator Nursing Department
Nova Southeastern University
College of Allied Health and Nursing
Fort Lauderdale, FL

Diane K. Whitehead, EdD, RN
Chairperson, Nursing Department
Nova Southeastern University
College of Allied Health and Nursing
Fort Lauderdale, FL

 F. A. Davis • Philadelphia

F. A. Davis Company
1915 Arch Street
Philadelphia, PA 19103
www.fadavis.com

Copyright © 2004 by F. A. Davis Company

Printed in the United States of America

Last digit indicates print number: 10 9 8 7 6 5 4 3 2

Acquisitions Editor: Joanne Patzek DaCunha, RN, MSN
Developmental Editor: Kristen Kern
Cover Designer: Louis J. Forgione

As new scientific information becomes available through basic and clinical research, recommended treatments and drug therapies undergo changes. The author(s) and publisher have done everything possible to make this book accurate, up to date, and in accord with accepted standards at the time of publication. The author(s), editors, and publisher are not responsible for errors or omissions or for consequences from application of the book, and make no warranty, expressed or implied, in regard to the contents of the book. Any practice described in this book should be applied by the reader in accordance with professional standards of care used in regard to the unique circumstances that may apply in each situation. The reader is advised always to check product information (package inserts) for changes and new information regarding dose and contraindications before administering any drug. Caution is especially urged when using new or infrequently ordered drugs.

ISBN 0–8036–1124–2

To our students, colleagues, and mentors
who continue to enrich our lives.
To our families for the joy
they bring to our lives.

Preface

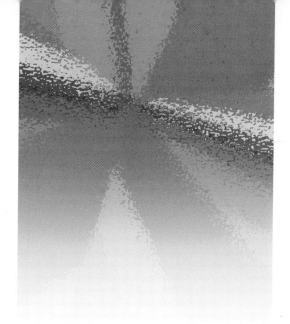

We are delighted to bring our readers this third edition of *Essentials of Nursing Leadership and Management*. We designed this textbook to help the new graduate make the transition to professional nursing practice. Its focus is on the staff nurse as a vital staff member of the health care team and manager of patient care. As a manager of care, the staff nurse must have the knowledge and skills necessary to make decisions related to setting priorities, delegating responsibilities, improving quality, understanding the legal parameters of nursing practice, and knowing the ethical issues confronting nursing today.

Based on input from students, faculty members, and reviewers, we have added information about followership and emotional intelligence to the first chapter. We also updated the chapters on historical leaders and ethics and added information about electronic communication. The legal chapter now includes actual cases pertaining to current nursing issues.

This book also provides comprehensive, practical information for developing a nursing career. Workplace issues such as change, conflict management, safety, stress, burnout, and cultural diversity are addressed in an easy-to-understand style. We increased the information provided about the NCLEX and the discussion of current issues directly affecting nursing such as the critical nursing shortage and changes in health care delivery systems.

It is our hope that this textbook will assist new graduates in developing their professional roles in the ever-changing health care environment.

We would like to thank the people at F.A. Davis for their assistance and the reviewers for their helpful suggestions.

Ruth M. Tappen

Sally A. Weiss

Diane K. Whitehead

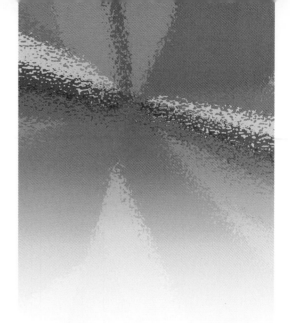

Reviewers

Cheryl L. Becker, MN, RN
Program Chair
Associate Degree Nursing
Bellevue Community College
Bellevue, WA

Leah M. Magee, RN, MSN
Professional Nurse Educator
Jameson Memorial Hospital School
  of Nursing
New Castle, PA

Hope M. Moon, RN, MSN, CNS
Program Director
Associate Degree Nursing
Lorain County Community College
Elyria, NY

Patricia L. Newland, RN, MS
Professor of Nursing
Broome Community College
Binghamton, NY

Heather Peters, RN, MS, MBA
Director of Nursing
Kishwaukee College
Malta, IL

Contents

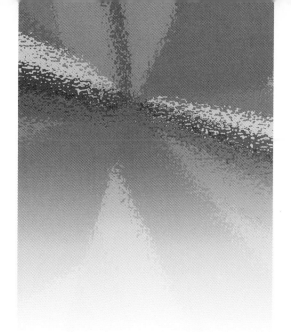

UNIT I

Leading and Managing   **1**

CHAPTER 1
Keys to Effective Leadership and Management 3

CHAPTER 2
Getting People to Work Together 19

CHAPTER 3
Giving and Receiving Feedback 33

CHAPTER 4
Dealing with Problems and Conflicts 47

CHAPTER 5
People and the Process of Change 61

UNIT II

Working Within the Organization   **73**

CHAPTER 6
Organizations, Power, and Empowerment 75

CHAPTER 7
Delegation of Client Care 91

CHAPTER 8
Managing Client Care 107

CHAPTER 9
Time Management 137

CHAPTER 10
Work-Related Stress and Burnout 151

CHAPTER 11
The Workplace 175

UNIT III

Professional Issues   **205**

CHAPTER 12
Nursing Practice and the Law 207

CHAPTER 13
Questions of Values and Ethics 223

CHAPTER 14
Historic Leaders in Nursing 241

CHAPTER 15
Your Nursing Career 257

CHAPTER 16
Nursing Today 283

CHAPTER 17
Looking to the Future 311

APPENDICES

1 Code of Ethics for Nurses 327
2 Standards Published by American Nurses Association 331
3 National Organization for Associate Degree Nursing (N-OADN)
  Resolution: Differentiated Nursing Practice 333
4 Guidelines for the Registered Nurse in Giving, Accepting or Rejecting
  a Work Assignment 335
INDEX 343

UNIT I

Leading and Managing

1 Keys to Effective Leadership and Management
2 Getting People to Work Together
3 Giving and Receiving Feedback
4 Dealing with Problems and Conflicts
5 People and the Process of Change

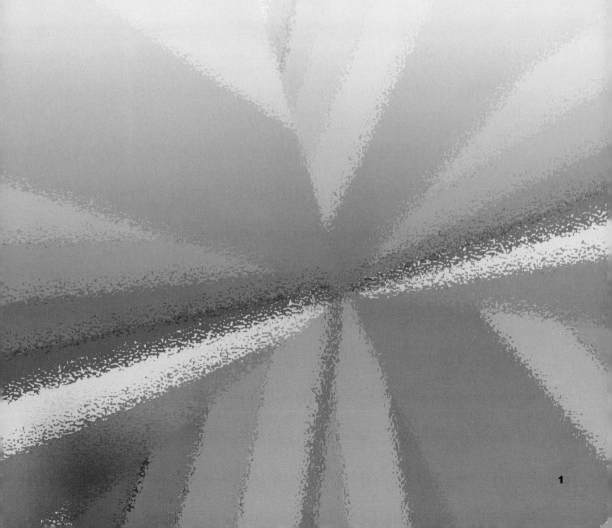

CHAPTER 1

Keys to Effective Leadership and Management

OBJECTIVES

After reading this chapter, the student should be able to:

- Define the terms *leadership, followership,* and *management.*

- Distinguish among leadership, followership, and management.

- Discuss the qualities and behaviors that contribute to effective leadership and followership.

- Discuss the qualities and behaviors that contribute to effective management.

OUTLINE

Leadership
Are You Ready to Be a Leader?
Leadership Defined

Followership
Followership Defined
Becoming a Better Follower

Management
Are You Ready to Be a Manager?
Management Defined

Comparison of Leadership and Management

What Makes a Person a Leader?
Leadership Theories
  Trait Theories
  Behavioral Theories
  Task Relationship
  Emotional Intelligence
  Situational Theories
Transformational Leadership
Qualities of an Effective Leader
Behaviors of an Effective Leader

What Makes a Person a Manager?
Management Theories
  Scientific Management
  Human Relations–Oriented Management
Qualities of an Effective Manager
Behaviors of an Effective Manager
  Interpersonal
  Decisional
  Informational

Conclusion

CHAPTER 1 SELF ASSESSMENT
Are You Ready to Be a Leader?

Before you read this chapter, evaluate your current Leadership Quotient. How often do you ...

1. Critically analyze new information or opinions you encounter:
   Never _____ Every once in a while _____ Sometimes _____ Often _____

2. Provide positive feedback to classmates, colleagues, coworkers:
   Never _____ Every once in a while _____ Sometimes _____ Often _____

3. Provide negative feedback to classmates, colleagues, coworkers:
   Never _____ Every once in a while _____ Sometimes _____ Often _____

4. Talk about your vision for the future:
   Never _____ Every once in a while _____ Sometimes _____ Often _____

5. Initiate discussion of a problem or misunderstanding:
   Never _____ Every once in a while _____ Sometimes _____ Often _____

6. Pursue new learning opportunities:
   Never _____ Every once in a while _____ Sometimes _____ Often _____

You will read about each of the above leadership actions and more in this chapter.

Nurses work with an extraordinary variety of professional and nonprofessional personnel: physicians, therapists, social workers, psychologists, technicians, aides, unit managers, and housekeepers, to name just a few, as well as patients, clients, and clients' families.

The study of leadership and management is essentially the study of how to work effectively with other people. In this chapter, we define *leadership, followership,* and *management* and the relationships among them. We then discuss the characteristics and behaviors that make nurses effective leaders, followers, and managers. These characteristics and behaviors are your keys to effective leadership and management.

Leadership

Are You Ready to Be a Leader?

You may be thinking, "I'm just beginning my career in nursing. How can you expect me to be a leader now?" This is an important question. New nurses do need time to learn how to function in a work environment and to refine their clinical skills. But they can begin to assume some leadership within these new nursing roles. Consider the following example:

Billie Blair Thomas is a new staff nurse at Green Valley Nursing Care Center. After orientation, she was assigned to a very active rehabilitation unit with high admission and discharge rates. Billie noticed that the assignment of resident admissions and discharges was rather haphazard. Anyone who was "free" at the moment was directed to handle them. Sometimes unlicensed assistive personnel were assigned to admit or discharge residents. Billie felt that using aides was inappropriate because they have no training in discharge planning and their assessment skills are limited.

Billie thought there was a better way to handle admissions and discharges but was not sure that she should mention it because she was so new. "Maybe they've already thought of this," she said to a former classmate. "It's such an obvious solution." They began to talk about what they had learned in their leadership course before graduation. "I just keep hearing our instructor saying, 'There's only one manager, but anyone can be a leader if they act on their good ideas.'"

"If you want to be a leader, you have to act on your idea," her friend said.

"Maybe I will," Billie replied.

Billie decided to speak with her nurse manager, an experienced rehab nurse who seemed not only approachable but also open to new ideas. "I have been so busy getting our new computer system in place before the surveyors come that I wasn't paying attention to that," the nurse manager told her. "I'm really happy you brought it to my attention."

Billie's nurse manager raised the issue at the next executive meeting, giving credit to Billie for having brought it to her attention. The other nurse managers had the same response. "We were so focused on the new computer system that we overlooked that. We need to take care of this situation as soon as possible. That Billie Blair Thomas has leadership potential."

Leadership Defined

The essence of leadership is the ability to influence other people. Effective leaders enable people to move "in the same direction, toward the same destination, at the same speed, not because they have been forced to, but because they want to" (Lansdale, 2002, p. 63). The three primary tasks of a leader are to help people develop a sense of direction and purpose, to build the group's commitment to its goals, and to face the numerous challenges that arise in a health care setting (Drath, 2001):

1 Set direction: mission, goals, vision, purpose

2 Build commitment: motivation, spirit, teamwork

3 Confront challenges: innovation, change, turbulence

Effective nurse leaders are those who, through their integrity, sense of possibility, and willingness to take risks, engage others to work together effectively in pursuit of a shared goal (Byrne 2003). That goal may be providing excellent patient care, designing a cost-saving procedure, or challenging the ethics of a new policy.

◘ Followership

Followership and leadership are separate but reciprocal roles. Without followers, one cannot be a leader; conversely, one cannot be a follower without a leader, either (Lyons, 2002).

Being an effective follower is as important to the new nurse as is being an effective leader. In fact, most of the time most of us are followers: members of a team, attendees at a meeting, staff of a care nursing care unit, and so forth.

Followership Defined

Followership is not a passive, unthinking role. On the contrary, the most valuable follower (team member, staff nurse, etc.) is a skilled, self-directed employee, one who participates actively in setting the group's direction, invests his or her time and energy in the work of the group, thinks critically, and advocates for new ideas (Grossman & Valiga, 2000). Imagine working on a patient care unit where all staff members, from the unit secretary to the assistant nurse manager, willingly took on extra tasks without being asked (Spreitzer & Quinn, 2001), came back early from coffee breaks, completed their charting on time, suggested ways to improve patient care, and were proud of the high quality care they provide. Wouldn't it be wonderful to be a part of that team?

Becoming a Better Follower

There are a number of things you can do to become a better follower:

• If you discover a problem, inform your team leader or manager right away. Even better, include a suggestion for solving the problem in your report.

• Freely invest your interest and energy in your work.

• Be supportive of new ideas and new directions suggested by others.

• When you disagree, explain why you do not support an idea or suggestion.

• Listen carefully and reflect on what your leader or manager says.

• Continue to learn as much as you can about your specialty area.

• Share what you learn with others.

Being an effective follower will not only make you a more valuable employee but also can increase the meaning and satisfaction you get from your work.

Management

Are You Ready to Be a Manager?

For most new nurses, the answer is *no,* you should not assume managerial responsibility. The breadth and depth of your experience are insufficient; you should focus your energies toward developing your own skills before you begin supervising others.

Management Defined

Effective managers, according to Covey, are able to elicit from each employee "creativity, consistent excellent productivity, and maximum potential contribution toward . . . continuous improvement of process, product, and service" (1992, p. 276). Translated into terms that are more relevant to nursing, the effective nurse manager is responsible for ensuring not only that patient care is given but also that it is given in the most effective and efficient manner possible.

In 1916, Henri Fayol defined *management* as planning, organizing, commanding, coordinating, and controlling the work of a given set of employees (Wren, 1972). This definition has influenced thinking in management, including nursing management, for years. However, Mintzberg (1989) said that Fayol's list of management functions does not really describe what managers do. Instead, the manager's function is to do whatever is necessary to make sure that employees do their work and do it well. According to Lombardi (2001), managers spend two thirds of their time on people management. The remainder is taken up by budget work, meetings, preparing reports, and other "administrivia" that comes with most management positions.

Comparison of Leadership and Management

The terms *leadership* and *management* are often used interchangeably, although the differences between them are straightforward. Managers (1) have *formal authority* to direct the work of a given set of employees, and (2) are *formally responsible* for the quality of that work and what it costs to do it. Neither of these conditions is necessary to be a leader.

Leadership is an essential part of effective management, but the reverse is not true: you do not have to be a manager to be a leader but you do need to be a good leader to be an effective manager (Table 1–1). You can be the youngest, the newest, or even the least experienced nurse yet still have opportunities to be a leader, as Billie Blair Thomas did. These opportunities will increase as your experience increases and so will your readiness to assume managerial responsibility.

TABLE 1–1

Differences Between Leadership and Management

Leadership	Management
Based on influence and shared meaning	Based on authority and influence
An informal role	A formally designated role
An achieved position	An assigned position
Part of every nurse's responsibility	Usually responsible for budgets, hiring and firing people
Initiative	
Independent thinking	Improved by the use of effective leadership skills

What Makes a Person a Leader?

Leadership Theories

Different theories about how a person becomes a leader and what type of leader is most effective have been proposed and tested. Although much research has been done on this subject, no theory has emerged as the clear winner. The reason for this may be that different qualities and behaviors are most important in different situations faced by leaders. The result is that we do not yet have the single best answer to the question: What makes a person a leader? In nursing, for example, some situations require quick thinking and fast action. Others require some time to figure out the best solution to a complicated problem. Different leadership qualities and behaviors are needed in these two different situations.

Let's look now at some of the best-known leadership theories and the many qualities and behaviors that have been identified as those of the effective nurse leader (Pavitt, 1999; Tappen, 2001).

Trait Theories

At one time or another, you've probably heard someone say, "Leaders are born, not made." In other words, some of us are natural leaders but others of us are not. In reality, leadership may come more easily to some of us than to others, but every one of us can be a leader if we develop the necessary knowledge and skill.

Many of the early research studies on leadership were done in an attempt to identify the qualities, or *traits*, that distinguish a leader from a nonleader. The traits most often identified are:

- Intelligence
- Initiative

Other qualities that were found to be associated with leadership are:

- Excellent interpersonal skills
- High self-esteem
- Creativity
- Willingness to take risks
- Ability to tolerate the consequences of taking risks

Behavioral Theories

The *trait theories* were concerned with what a leader *is*; the *behavior theories* are concerned with what the leader *does*. One of the most influential of these behavioral theories is concerned with leadership style (White & Lippitt, 1960) (Table 1–2). The three styles are:

- **Authoritarian leadership** (also called *autocratic, directive, controlling*). The authoritarian leader gives orders, makes decisions for the group as a whole, and

TABLE 1–2
Comparison of Authoritarian, Democratic, and Laissez-Faire Theories

	Authoritarian	Democratic	Laissez-Faire
Degree of freedom	Little freedom	Moderate freedom	Much freedom
Degree of control	High control	Moderate control	Little control
Decision making	By the leader	Leader and group together	By the group or by no one
Leader activity level	High	High	Minimal
Assumption of responsibility	Leader	Shared	Abdicated
Output of the group	High quantity, good quality	Creative, high quality	Variable, may be poor quality
Efficiency	Very efficient	Less efficient than authoritarian	Inefficient

Source: Adapted from White, R.K., & Lippitt, R. (1960). *Autocracy and Democracy: An Experimental Inquiry.* New York: Harper & Row.

bears most of the responsibility for the outcomes. For example, when a decision needs to be made, an authoritarian leader would say, "I've given this a great deal of thought and decided that this is the way we're going to solve our problem." Although this is an efficient way to run things, it usually stifles creativity and may inhibit motivation. Authoritarian leadership may be either punitive or benign.

- **Democratic leadership** (also called *participative*). In contrast to the authoritarian leader, the democratic leader shares the planning, decision-making, and responsibility for outcomes with other members of the group. Although this is often a less efficient way to run things, it is more flexible and more likely to foster motivation and creativity. Democratic leadership is characterized by guidance rather than control.

- **Laissez-faire leadership** (also called *permissive, nondirective*). The laissez-faire ("let it alone") leader does very little planning or decision-making and fails to encourage others to participate, either. In fact, laissez-faire leadership is really a lack of leadership. For example, when a decision needs to be made, a laissez-faire leader may postpone making the decision or never make the decision at all. In most instances, the laissez-faire leader leaves people feeling confused and frustrated because there is no goal, no guidance, and no direction. Some very mature individuals thrive under laissez-faire leadership because they need little guidance. Most people, however, flounder under this kind of leadership.

Pavitt summed up the difference among these three styles nicely: a democratic leader tries to move the group toward its goals, an autocratic leader tries to move the group toward the leader's goals, and a laissez-faire leader makes no attempt to move the group (1999, p. 330ff).

Task Relationship

Another important distinction in leadership style is the one between a *task* focus and a *re-*

lationship focus (Blake, Mouton, & Tapper, 1981). Some leaders emphasize the tasks (e.g., reducing medication errors, completing patient records) and fail to realize that interpersonal relationships (e.g., attitude of physicians toward nursing staff, treatment of housekeeping staff by nurses) have considerable impact on the morale and productivity of employees. Others focus on the interpersonal aspects and ignore the quality of the job being done as long as people get along with each other. The most effective leader is able to balance the two, attending to both the task and the relationship aspects of working together.

Emotional Intelligence

The importance of the relationship aspects of leadership has been brought to our attention recently by the work on emotional intelligence by Goleman and colleagues (2002). Consciously addressing the effect of people's feelings on the team's emotional reality is what distinguishes ordinary leaders from "stars." How is this done?

First, be attuned to your own emotions and learn how to manage them, channel them, and stay calm and clear-headed in the face of problems and crises. The emotionally intelligent leader welcomes constructive criticism, asks for help when needed, can juggle multiple demands without losing focus, and can turn problems into opportunities.

Second, the emotionally intelligent leader listens attentively to others, picks up unspoken concerns, acknowledges others' perspectives, and brings people together in an atmosphere of respect, cooperation, collegiality, and helpfulness so that they can direct their energies toward achieving the team's goals (Fig. 1–1). "The enthusiastic, caring, and supportive leader generates those same feelings throughout the team," wrote Porter-O'Grady of the emotionally intelligent leader (2003, p. 109). Whatever it is called, the ability to connect with people is a fundamental leadership skill (Ang & Fong, 2003).

Situational Theories

It has become increasingly clear that people and leadership situations are far more com-

---

Competencies of the Emotionally Intelligent Leader

- **Self Awareness**
  Attuned to own emotional state

- **Social Awareness**
  Attuned to others' emotional state

- **Self Management**
  Able to stay calm, clear-headed

- **Relationship Management**
  Redirects emotional energies toward shared objectives

Figure 1–1   Based on Goleman, D., Boyatzes, R., & McKee, A. (2002). *Primal Leadership: Realizing the Power of Emotional Intelligence.* Boston: Harvard Business School Press.

plex than the early theories recognized. Furthermore, situations may change rapidly, requiring even more complex theory to explain people's responses (Bennis, Spreitzer, & Cummings, 2001). In recognition of this, less simplistic theories have evolved to replace the trait and behavioral theories.

Adaptability is the key to the situational approach (McNichol, 2000). Instead of assuming that one particular approach works in all situations, situational theories recognize the complexity of work situations and encourage the leader to consider many factors when deciding what action to take.

The following is an illustration of how just one factor can affect people's response to an organizational change.

Two nurse managers were talking before the nursing administration council meeting began. "How did your staff react to the new 6 A.M. to 2 P.M. hours for the day tour?" Jennifer Chinn asked her friend Esther Cabriollo.

"They love it," said Esther.

"Really?" said Jennifer. "My staff is so upset. They said it was an inhumane schedule and that they have to be at work before the birds get up in the morning. You should hear their complaints."

"Most of my staff thinks it's just the opposite," said Esther. "Many have young children. With this new schedule, their spouses can take the children to school in the morning, and they can be home in time to meet the school bus. They said it's the most humane change the administration has ever made."

"That explains it," said Jennifer. "Most of my staff have older children who have a lot of activities in the evening, and they're all having trouble getting up an hour earlier in the morning. Their situation is entirely different."

Every situation is different. A change that is welcomed by one group of people may be hated by another group. Similarly, the type of leadership approach that is being used may affect people's responses. Another important situational factor is the type of organization in which the leader works (see Chap. 6). Situational theories emphasize the importance of understanding all of the factors that affect a particular group of people in a particular environment.

Transformational Leadership

Although the situational theories were an improvement over earlier theories in recognizing how complex the process of influencing others really is, there was still something missing; meaning, inspiration, and vision were still not given enough attention (Tappen, 2001). Although not the only factors addressed in transformational leadership theory, they are the distinguishing features of transformational leadership theory.

According to the transformational theory of leadership, people need a sense of mission that goes beyond good interpersonal relationships or the appropriate reward for a job well done (Bass & Avolio, 1993). This is especially true in nursing. Caring for people, sick or well, is the goal of our profession, not manufacturing widgets. Most of us chose nursing to do something for the good of humankind: this is our vision. One goal of nursing leadership is to guide us toward achievement of that vision.

Transformational leaders can communicate their vision in a manner that is so meaningful and exciting that it inspires commitment in the people with whom they work (Trofino, 1995). If successful, the goals of the leader and staff will "become fused, creating unity, wholeness, and a collective purpose" (Barker, 1992, p. 42). The qualities and behaviors associated with transformational leadership are included in the next two sections.

Qualities of an Effective Leader

Effective leadership is defined as the accomplishment of the goals shared by leader and followers. Integrity, courage, initiative, energy, optimism, perseverance, balance, ability to handle stress, and self-awareness are qualities of effective leaders in nursing (Fig. 1–2).

- **Integrity.** Integrity is expected of health care professionals. Clients, colleagues, and employers all expect nurses to be honest, law-abiding, and trustworthy. Adherence to both a code of personal ethics and a code of professional ethics (Appendix 1, American Nurses Association Code for Nurses) is expected of every nurse.

Would-be leaders who do not exhibit these characteristics cannot expect them of their followers either.

- **Courage.** Sometimes, being a leader means taking some risks. In the story of Billie Blair Thomas, for example, Billie needed some courage to speak to her nurse manager about a problem she had observed.

- **Initiative.** Good ideas are not enough. To be a leader, you must act on those good ideas. This requires initiative on your part.

- **Energy.** Leadership also requires energy. Both leadership and management are hard but satisfying endeavors that require effort on your part. It is also important that you use your energy wisely.

- **Optimism.** When the work is difficult and one crisis seems to follow another in rapid succession, it is easy to become discouraged. However, it is important not to let discouragement keep you and your coworkers from seeking ways to resolve your difficulties. In fact, the ability to see a problem as an opportunity is part of the optimism that makes a person an effective leader. Like energy, optimism is "catching." An optimistic leader can remotivate a discouraged group. Holman (1995) called this being a *winner* instead of a *whiner* (Table 1–3).

- **Perseverance.** Effective leaders do not give up easily. Instead, they persist, con-

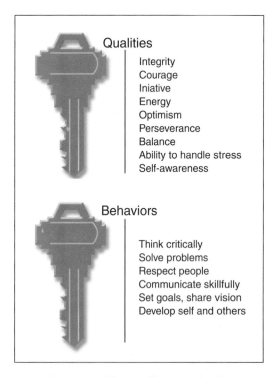

Qualities

Integrity
Courage
Iniative
Energy
Optimism
Perseverance
Balance
Ability to handle stress
Self-awareness

Behaviors

Think critically
Solve problems
Respect people
Communicate skillfully
Set goals, share vision
Develop self and others

Figure 1–2   Keys to effective leadership.

TABLE 1–3
Winner or Whiner—Which Are You?

A winner says . . .	A whiner says . . .
We have a real challenge here.	This is really a problem. Do I have to?
I'll give it my best.	That's nice, I guess.
That's great!	Impossible. It can't be done.
We can do it.	
Yes!	Maybe . . .

Source: Adapted from Holman, L. (1995). *Eleven Lessons in Self-leadership: Insights for Personal and Professional Success.* Lexington, Ky.: A Lessons in Leadership Book.

tinuing their efforts when others are tempted to give up the struggle. This persistence often pays off.

• **Balance.** In our effort to become the best nurses we can be, we may forget that other aspects of life are equally important. As important as our clients and colleagues are to us, family and friends are important too. Although school and work are meaningful activities, cultural, social, recreational, and spiritual activities also have meaning. The most effective leaders have found a balance between work and play.

• **Ability to handle stress.** There is some stress in almost every job. Coping with stress in as positive and healthy a manner as possible helps you conserve your energy and be a model for others. We review more about maintaining balance and handling stress in Chapter 10.

• **Self-awareness.** People who do not understand themselves are limited in their ability to understand the motivations of other people. They are also far more likely to fool themselves than are people who are self-aware. For example, it is much easier to be fair with a coworker you like than with one you do not like. Recognizing that you like some people more than others is the first step in preventing unfair treatment based on personal likes and dislikes.

Behaviors of an Effective Leader

As mentioned earlier, leadership requires action. The effective leader not only takes action but also chooses the action carefully. Important leadership actions include thinking critically, solving problems, respecting people, communicating skillfully, setting specific goals/communicating a vision for the future, and developing oneself and others:

• **Thinking critically.** Critical thinking is the careful, deliberate use of reasoned analysis to reach a decision about what to believe or what to do (Feldman, 2002). The essence of critical thinking is questioning and analyzing ideas, suggestions, habits, routines, common practices, and policies before deciding to accept or reject them. To avoid falling prey to the assumptions and biases of oneself and others, ask yourself frequently, "Why do I believe that?" (Ulrich & Glendon, 1999).

• **Solving problems.** Client problems, paperwork problems, staff problems: these and others occur frequently and need to be solved. The effective leader helps people to identify problems and to work through the problem-solving process to find a reasonable solution.

• **Respecting the individual.** Although we all have much in common, each of us has different wants and needs and has had different life experiences. For example, some people really value the psychological rewards of helping others; other people are more concerned about earning a decent salary. There is nothing wrong with either of these points of view; they are simply different. The effective leader recognizes these differences in people and helps them find the rewards in their work that mean the most to them.

Skillful communication includes the following:

• **Listening to others.** We have separated listening from communicating with other people just to emphasize that communication involves both giving and receiving information, not just giving out information. The only way to find out people's individual wants and needs is to watch what they do and to listen to what they tell you. It is amazing how often leaders fail simply because they did not listen to what other people were trying to tell them.

• **Encouraging the exchange of information.** Many misunderstandings and mistakes occur because people failed to share enough information with each other. The leader's role is to make sure that the channels of communication remain open and that people use them.

- **Providing feedback.** Everyone needs some information about the effectiveness of his or her performance. Frequent feedback, both positive and negative, is needed so that people can continually improve their performance:

Some nurse leaders find it difficult to give negative feedback because they fear that they will upset the other person. How else can a person know where improvement is needed? Negative feedback can be given in a manner that is neither hurtful nor resented by the individual receiving it. In fact, it is often appreciated.

Other nurse leaders fail to give positive feedback, assuming that coworkers will know when they are doing a good job. This is also a mistake because everyone appreciates positive feedback. In fact, for some people, it is the most important reward they get from their jobs.

- **Setting specific goals/communicating a vision for the future.** Just as each one of us is unique in terms of our experiences, needs, and wants, we are also likely to have unique goals for ourselves. An important leadership task is to find the common thread in all of those goals and to help the group reach a consensus about its goals. This may require considerable discussion before it is achieved.

The effective leader also has a vision for the future. Communicating this vision to the group and involving everyone in working toward that vision create the inspiration that keeps people going when things become difficult. Even better, involving people in creating the vision is not only more satisfying for employees but also has the potential for the most creative and innovative outcomes (Kerfott, 2000). It is this vision that helps make our work meaningful.

- **Developing oneself and others.** Learning does not end with leaving school. In fact, experienced nurses will tell you that school is just the beginning, that it only prepares you to continue learning throughout your career. As new and better ways to care for clients are discovered, it is your responsibility as a professional to critically analyze these new approaches and decide whether they would be better for your clients than current approaches to care.

Effective leaders not only continue to learn but also encourage others to do the same. Sometimes leaders function as teachers. At other times, their role is primarily to encourage and guide others to seek more knowledge. Observant, reflective, analytical practitioners know that learning takes place every day if one is open to it (Kaagan, 1999).

▢ What Makes a Person a Manager?

Management Theories

Although there are many management theories, it is most important to be familiar with the two major but opposing schools of thought in management: the human relations approach to management and scientific management. As you will see, one emphasizes the relationship aspects of managing people, and the other emphasizes the task aspects of management.

Scientific Management

Almost 100 years ago, Frederick Taylor argued that most jobs could be done more efficiently if they were thoroughly analyzed (Lee, 1980; Locke, 1982). Given a properly designed task and sufficient incentive to get the work done, workers would be more productive. For example, Taylor encouraged paying people by the piece; that is, by the number of "widgets" made (in health care, the equivalent would be by the number of clients bathed or monitored), rather than by the number of hours worked. This would be an incentive to get the most work done in the least amount of time, Taylor postulated.

The work itself was also analyzed to improve efficiency. In health care, for example, there has been a lot of discussion about the time it takes to bring patients to radiology or

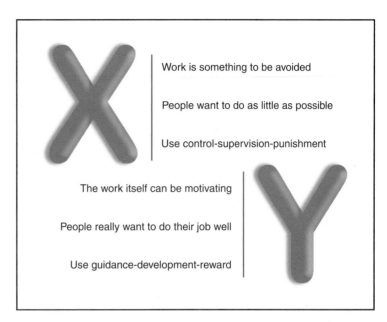

Figure 1–3   Theory X versus theory Y.

Work is something to be avoided

People want to do as little as possible

Use control-supervision-punishment

The work itself can be motivating

People really want to do their job well

Use guidance-development-reward

to physical therapy versus bringing the radiographer or therapist to the patient. An emphasis on eliminating excess staff and increasing the productivity of remaining employees is based on this kind of thinking.

Nurse managers who use the principles of scientific management emphasize the task aspects of providing health care. They pay particular attention to the type of assessments and procedures done on the unit, the equipment needed to provide this care efficiently, and the strategies that would facilitate efficient accomplishment of these tasks. These nurse managers keep careful records of the amount of work accomplished and reward those who accomplish the most.

Human Relations–Oriented Management

McGregor's theory X and theory Y provide a good example of the difference between scientific management and human relations–oriented management. *Theory X*, said McGregor (1960), reflects a common attitude among managers that most people really do not want to work very hard and that the manager's job is to make sure that they do work hard. According to theory X, a manager needs to employ strict rules, constant supervision, and the threat of punishment (reprimands, withheld raises, and threats of

job loss) to create industrious, conscientious workers.

Theory Y, which McGregor preferred, is the opposite viewpoint. Theory Y managers believe that the work itself can be motivating and that people will work hard if their managers provide a supportive atmosphere. A theory Y manager emphasizes guidance rather than control, development rather than close supervision, and reward rather than punishment (Fig. 1–3).

A human relations–oriented nurse manager is concerned with keeping employee morale as high as possible, assuming that satisfied, motivated employees will do the best work. Employees' attitudes, opinions, hopes, and fears are important to this type of nurse manager. Considerable effort is expended to work out conflicts and promote mutual understanding among the staff to provide an atmosphere in which people can do their best work.

Qualities of an Effective Manager

The effective nurse manager possesses a combination of qualities: leadership, clinical expertise, and business sense. None of these alone is enough; it is the combination that prepares an individual for the complex task of managing a group or team of health care providers. Let's look at each of these briefly:

- **Leadership.** All of the people skills of the leader are essential to the effective manager. They are the core skills needed to function as a manager.

- **Clinical expertise.** It is very difficult to either help others develop their skills or evaluate how well they have done this without possessing clinical expertise oneself. It probably is not necessary (or even possible) to know everything all other professionals on the team know, but it is important to be able to assess the effectiveness of their work in terms of patient outcomes.

- **Business sense.** Nurse managers also need to be concerned with the bottom line; that is, with the cost of providing the care that is given, especially in comparison with the benefit received from that care. In other words, nurse managers need to be able to analyze how much time is spent to provide a given amount of client care and how effective that client care has been. These are complex tasks that require knowledge of budgeting, understanding of staffing, and measurement of patient outcomes, much of which is beyond the scope of this textbook.

There is some controversy over the amount of clinical expertise versus business sense that is needed to be an effective nurse manager. Some argue that a person can be a "generic" manager, that the job of managing people is the same no matter what tasks they perform. Others argue that the manager must understand the tasks better than anyone else in the work group. Our position is that both are needed, along with excellent leadership skills.

Behaviors of an Effective Manager

Mintzberg (1989) divided the manager's activities into three categories: interpersonal, decisional, and informational. We will use these categories but have taken some liber-

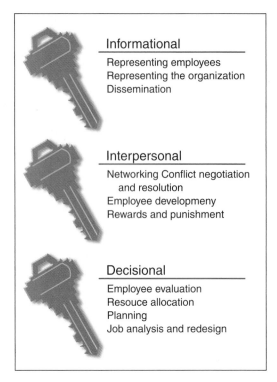

Informational

Representing employees
Representing the organization
Dissemination

Interpersonal

Networking Conflict negotiation
    and resolution
Employee developmeny
Rewards and punishment

Decisional

Employee evaluation
Resouce allocation
Planning
Job analysis and redesign

Figure 1–4   Keys to effective management.

ties with them and added some activities suggested by other authors (Dunham-Taylor, 1995; Montebello, 1994) and by our own observations of nurse managers (Fig. 1–4).

Interpersonal

The interpersonal area is one in which leaders and managers have overlapping responsibilities. However, the manager has some additional responsibilities that are seldom given to leaders. The following are interpersonal skills that nurse managers need in addition to those of a nurse leader:

- **Networking.** The position of nurse managers in the hierarchy provides them with many opportunities to develop positive working relationships with other disciplines, departments, and units within the organization.

- **Conflict negotiation and resolution.** Managers often find themselves resolving conflicts between employees, between clients and staff members, and between staff members and administration.

- **Employee development.** Providing for the continuing learning and upgrading of the skills of employees is a managerial responsibility that overlaps with managers' informational responsibilities.

- **Rewards and punishments.** Managers are in a position to provide both tangible (e.g., salary increases, time off) and intangible (e.g., praise, recognition) rewards as well as punishments.

Decisional

Nurse managers are also responsible for making many, often difficult, decisions:

- **Employee evaluation.** Managers are responsible for conducting formal performance appraisals of their staff members.

- **Resource allocation.** In decentralized organizations, nurse managers are often given a set amount of money for running their units or departments and must allocate these resources wisely, especially when they are very limited.

- **Hiring and firing employees.** Most nurse managers participate in or carry out themselves the employment and termination of staff for their units or departments.

- **Planning for the future.** Even though the day-to-day operation of most units is a sufficiently complex and time-consuming responsibility, nurse managers must also look ahead and prepare themselves and their units for future changes in budgets, organizational priorities, and patient populations.

- **Job analysis and redesign.** In a time of extreme cost consciousness, nurse managers are frequently being called on to analyze and redesign the work of their units or departments to make them as efficient and cost-effective as possible.

Informational

Nurse managers often find themselves in positions within the organizational hierarchy in which they acquire much information that is not available to their staff. They also have much information about their staff that is not readily available to the administration, placing them in a strategic position within the information web of any organization. The effective manager uses this position for the benefit of both the staff and the organization. The following are some examples:

- **Spokesperson.** Managers often speak for administration when relaying information to their staff members. Likewise, they often speak for staff members when relaying information to administration. In addition, they frequently represent their work group or department at various meetings and discussions.

- **Monitoring.** Effective nurse managers purposely spend much of their day out of their offices, with their staff (Hardesty, 2002). Nurse managers monitor the activities of their units or departments. This may include the number of clients seen, average length of stay, infection rates, and so forth. They also monitor the staff (e.g., absentee rates, tardiness, unproductive time) and the budget (e.g., money spent, money left to spend in comparison with money needed to operate the unit).

- **Dissemination.** Nurse managers share information with their clients, staff members, and employers. This information may be related to the results of their monitoring efforts, new developments in health care, policy changes, and so forth.

As you can see, nurse managers have very complex, responsible positions within health care organizations. Ineffective managers may do harm to their employees and to the organization, but effective managers can help their staff members grow and develop as health care professionals while providing the highest quality care to their clients.

Conclusion

The key elements of leadership, followership, and management have been discussed in this chapter. Every registered nurse needs leadership and followership skills to be effective as a practitioner and colleague. Many of the leadership qualities and behaviors mentioned here are discussed in more detail in later chapters. Nurses who assume management positions need leadership skills as well as an additional set of management qualities and behaviors.

Study Questions

1   What are the differences between leadership and management? In what ways are they alike?

2   Why are effective followers as important as effective leaders?

3   Compare and contrast the authoritarian, democratic, and laissez-faire styles of leadership. List alternative names for each of these styles. What effect does each of these leadership styles have on followers?

4   Why do nurse managers need business sense? Under what circumstances would clinical expertise be more important than business sense? When would it be less important?

5   Select an individual whose leadership skills you particularly admire. What are some qualities and behaviors that this individual displays? In what ways could you emulate this person?

6   Describe the ideal nurse manager.

Critical Thinking Exercise

Joe Garcia has been an operating room nurse for 5 years. He was often on call on Saturday and Sunday, but he enjoyed his work and knew that he would not be called unless he was really needed. When a large health care corporation bought the hospital he worked for, Joe was initially pleased because he thought that this would increase his opportunities for advancement.

A multicar accident on a nearby interstate highway occurred on the second weekend after the hospital had been purchased. Most of the accident victims were taken to the city-owned hospital, but two were brought to the emergency room of the hospital where Joe worked. One was critically injured; the other had minor cuts and bruises. Joe was called in to prepare for emergency surgery. When he arrived, he was told that the patient had died.

As usual, Joe requested payment for the time spent traveling to and from the hospital on the emergency call. Joe was not paid for this time on his next paycheck. When he asked about it, his nurse manager told him that he would not be paid because he did not do any work. "That's not fair," he said, "I'm going to speak with the director about this."

"The last person who complained to the director was fired," the nurse manager warned him.

"I can't believe that," said Joe. "The director has always been fair with all of us."

"No more," replied the nurse manager. "The director has been replaced. This is no longer the fair, employee-centered organization we used to work for. With this new management, your protest, however justified it is, will be harshly received and you might regret having raised the issue. The choice is up to you."

Joe decided that he did not want to work in such an institution. With his 5 years of operating room experience, he quickly found another operating room position in an organization that utilized a more humanistically oriented approach to management.

1 What style of leadership and school of management thought seem to be preferred by Joe Garcia's employer?

2 What style of leadership and school of management were preferred by Joe?

3 What effect did the change in approach have on Joe?

4 Which of the listed qualities of leaders and managers did the nurse manager display? Which behaviors? Which ones did the nurse manager not display?

5 If you were Joe, what would you have done? If you were the nurse manager, what would you have done? Why?

REFERENCES

Ang, R., & Fong, C.F. (First Quarter 2003). Nursing leadership: The Singapore experience. *Reflections on Nursing Leadership*. 26–28.

Barker, A.M. (1992). *Transformational Nursing Leadership: A Vision for the Future*. New York: National League for Nursing Press.

Bass, B.M., & Avolio, B.J. (1993). Transformational leadership: A response to critiques. In Chemers, M.M., & Ayman, R. (eds.). *Leadership Theory and Research: Perspectives and Direction*. San Diego: Academic Press.

Bennis, W., Spreitzer, G.M., & Cummings T.G. (2001). *The Future of Leadership*. San Francisco: Jossey-Bass.

Blake, R.R., et al. (1981). *Grid Approaches for Managerial Leadership in Nursing*. St. Louis, Mo.: C.V. Mosby.

Byrne, J.A. (February 17, 2003). Leaders are made, not born. *Business Week*, 16.

Covey, S.R. (1992). *Principle-Centered Leadership*. New York: Simon & Schuster.

Drath, W. (2001). *The Deep Blue Sea*. San Francisco: Jossey-Bass.

Dunham-Taylor, J. (1995). Identifying the best in nurse executive leadership. *Journal of Nursing Administration*, 25(7/8), 24–31.

Feldman, D.A. (2002). *Critical Thinking: Strategies for Decision Making*. Menlo Park, Calif.: Crisp Publications.

Goleman, D., Boyatzes, R., & McKee, A. (2002). *Primal Leadership: Realizing the Power of Emotional Intelligence*. Boston: Harvard Business School Press.

Grossman, S., & Valiga, T.M. (2000). *The New Leadership Challenge: Creating the Future of Nursing*. Philadelphia: F.A. Davis.

Hardesty, P. (2002). Full circle. *Nursing Spectrum*, 12 (12): 3.

Holman, L. (1995). *Eleven Lessons in Self-leadership: Insights for Personal and Professional Success*. Lexington, Ky.: A Lessons in Leadership Book.

Kaagan, S.S. (1999). *Leadership Games: Experiential Learning for Organizational Development*. Thousand Oaks, Calif.: Sage Publications.

Kerfott, K. (2000). Leadership: Creating a shared destiny. *Dermatologic Nursing*, 12(5), 363–364.

Lansdale, B.M. (2002). *Cultivating Inspired Leaders*. West Hartford, Conn.: Kumarian Press.

Lee, J.A. (1980). *The Gold and the Garbage in Management Theories and Prescriptions*. Athens, Ohio: Ohio University Press.

Locke, E.A. (1982). The ideas of Frederick Taylor: An evaluation. *Academy of Management Review*, 7(1), 14.

Lombardi, D.N. (2001). *Handbook for the New Health Care Manager*. San Francisco: Jossey-Bass/AHA Press.

Lyons, M.F. (2002). Leadership and followership. *The Physician Executive*, Jan/Feb, 91–93.

McGregor, D. (1960). *The Human Side of Enterprise*. New York: McGraw-Hill.

McNichol, E. (2000). How to be a model leader. *Nursing Standard*, 14(45), 24.

Mintzberg, H. (1989). *Mintzberg on Management: Inside Our Strange World of Organizations*. New York: Free Press.

Montebello, A. (1994). *Work Teams That Work*. Minneapolis: Best Sellers Publishing.

Pavitt, C. (1999). Theorizing about the group communication-leadership relationship. In Frey, L.R. (ed.). *The Handbook of Group Communication Theory and Research*. Thousand Oaks, Calif.: Sage Publications.

Porter-O'Grady, T. (2003). A different age for leadership,

part II. *Journal of Nursing Administration,* 33(2): 105–110.

Spreitzer, G.M., & Quinn, R.E. (2001). *A Company of Leaders: Five Disciplines for Unleashing the Power in Your Workforce.* San Francisco: Jossey-Bass.

Tappen, R.M. (2001). *Nursing Leadership and Management: Concepts and Practice.* Philadelphia: F.A. Davis.

Trofino, J. (1995). Transformational leadership in health care. *Nursing Management,* 26(8), 42–47.

Ulrich, D.L., & Glendon, K.J. (1999). *Interactive Group Learning: Strategies for Nurse Educators.* New York: Springer Publishing.

White, R.K., & Lippitt, R. (1960). *Autocracy and Democracy: An Experimental Inquiry.* New York: Harper & Row.

Wren, D.A. (1972). *The Evolution of Management Thought.* New York: Ronald Press.

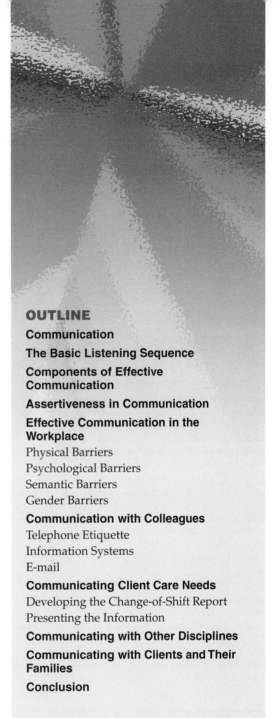

CHAPTER 2

Getting People to Work Together

OBJECTIVES

After reading this chapter, the student should be able to:

- Describe various forms of communication.
- Define the basic listening sequence.
- Analyze factors influencing communication.
- Discuss the importance of effective communication.
- Use assertive communication.
- Discuss technology as a form of communication.
- Deliver an effective and informative change-of-shift report.

OUTLINE

Communication
The Basic Listening Sequence
Components of Effective Communication
Assertiveness in Communication
Effective Communication in the Workplace
Physical Barriers
Psychological Barriers
Semantic Barriers
Gender Barriers
Communication with Colleagues
Telephone Etiquette
Information Systems
E-mail
Communicating Client Care Needs
Developing the Change-of-Shift Report
Presenting the Information
Communicating with Other Disciplines
Communicating with Clients and Their Families
Conclusion

CHAPTER 2 SELF ASSESSMENT
Communication

1. Think about the way you communicate. How do you ask for what you want?

2. What type of communicator are you?

3. Do your nonverbal communication styles contradict your verbal communication styles?

4. When confronting another person, do you use "I" statements or "You" statements?

5. What makes you uncomfortable during verbal interactions?

Claude has been working on a busy oncology floor for several years. He usually has a caseload of six to eight clients on his shift, and he believes that he provides safe, competent care to his clients.

While Claude was on his way to medicate a client suffering from cancer of the bone, a colleague called to him, "Claude, come with me, please." Claude responded, "I need to medicate Mr. J. in Room 203. I will come right after that. Where will you be?" "Never mind!" his colleague answered. "I'll find someone who's more helpful. Don't ask me for help in the future."

This was not the response Claude had expected. He thought he had expressed both an interest in his client and a willingness to help his colleague. What was the problem?

After Claude gave Mr. J. his pain medication, he went back to his colleague. "Sonja, what's the matter?" he asked. Sonja replied, "Mrs. V. fell in the bathroom. I needed someone to stay with her while I got her walker." "Why didn't you tell me it was urgent?" asked Claude. "I was so upset about Mrs. V. that I wasn't thinking about what else you were doing," answered Sonja. Claude said, "And I didn't ask you why you needed me. I guess we need to work on our communication, don't we?"

In the busy and sometimes chaotic world of nursing practice, nurses work continuously with all sorts of people. This variety makes the job dynamic and challenging. Just when it appears that things have settled down, something else happens that requires immediate attention. All of these busy people need to communicate effectively with each other. They also must responsibly delegate tasks to others or the workload will be insurmountable. This chapter helps new nurses communicate more effectively with their colleagues, work with people of all kinds, and share the workload equitably, even in situations that are filled with multiple demands and constant change.

■ Communication

Communication is the core of leadership. It is the method through which leadership is achieved. Leadership occurs through relationships with other people, and communication is the means used to engage and support these relationships (Mulholland, 1991).

The process of communication between two people historically has been viewed as consisting of five elements (Berlo, 1960):

1 The encoder, or sender

2 The message, or the information that needs to be conveyed

3 The sensory channel, or the method of sending the communication

4 The decoder, who receives the message

5 The feedback, or return; the feedback to the sender indicates the degree of understanding of the message

A more contemporary model of comunication views the process as a circular one that is affected by many factors. Communication in this model has both content and a relationship context. This means the activity is continuous, mutually interdependent, and influenced by the behaviors of each communicator. Cultural influences, gender, communication abilities, values, needs, goals, and previous experiences all affect the content of the communication (Arnold & Boggs, 1995; Blais, Hayes, Kozier, & Erb, 2002; Fontaine & Fletcher, 2002) (Fig. 2–1).

People often assume that communication is simply giving information to another person. Communication involves the spoken word and also the nonverbal message, the emotional state of people involved, and the cultural background that affects their interpretation of the message (Fontaine & Fletcher, 2002). Active listening is necessary to pick up all three levels of meaning in a communication. Surface listening, or inattention, often causes misinterpretation of the message. An individual's attitude also influences what is heard and how the message is interpreted.

The two basic channels of communication are verbal and nonverbal:

• *Verbal.* Verbal communication uses words to communicate messages. Writing or speaking in a code or language that is mutually understood achieves communication. Talking is the verbal or spoken mode. Written communication translates a thought or spoken word into printed form.

• *Nonverbal.* Nonverbal communication is a set of behaviors that conveys messages without words. It often supplements verbal communication. Most nonverbal communication is done unconsciously and is more difficult to control than verbal communication. Discrepancies often exist between verbal and

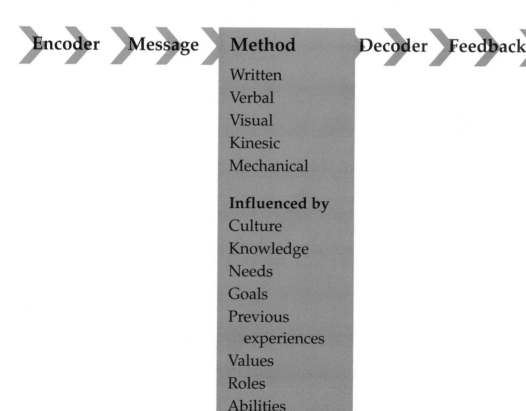

Figure 2–1 Understanding the message.

nonverbal communication. What is stated is not necessarily felt or believed. It is important for nurses to observe nonverbal behavior when communicating with colleagues and clients and to try to make their own nonverbal behavior congruent with their verbal communications. Telling people you understand their problem when you appear thoroughly confused or inattentive is an example of incongruence between verbal and nonverbal communication. The way people move their bodies or parts of their bodies while communicating is called *body language.* People use body language as a way of presenting themselves to the world (Varcarolis, 2001).

• *Paralanguage* is the nonverbal component of spoken language. Paralanguage includes speech rhythm, pitch, stress, intonation, rate, and volume (Fontaine & Fletcher, 2002), all of which affect the interpretation of the message being communicated.

◼ The Basic Listening Sequence

Listening is the most critical of all communication skills. You indicate to another person that you are listening through attending behaviors, such as eye contact, attentive body language, vocal qualities, and verbal tracking.

Eye contact requires the listener to look at the speaker. This indicates interest in the information being conveyed. Although expected in American culture, direct eye contact is considered disrespectful in some other cultures. Members of some cultures look away when they are being spoken to, yet look directly at the other individual and make direct eye contact only when they are speaking. During interactions with colleagues or clients who are culturally different, these behaviors need to be understood and not misinterpreted as disinterest or rudeness on the part of the other person.

Attentive body language conveys interest and openness. Leaning forward, having open arms, and maintaining an interested facial expression indicate that the listener is actively involved in the interaction and open to the other person's ideas. Sitting back, folding the arms across the chest, and looking away indicate disinterest in what is occurring or unwillingness to accept what the other person is saying.

Vocal qualities include pitch, volume, and rapidity of speech. When people are hurried, annoyed, angry, anxious, or distracted by other thoughts or activities, their vocal qualities change. Their speech may become rapid and choppy or slow and halting. The pitch, or highness, of the voice may change; this occurs when a person is surprised or anxious. Volumes change when individuals are annoyed or angry. A listener needs to be aware of changing pitch and volume when responding during communication.

Verbal tracking is paying attention to what is being said. To verbal track accurately, one must actively listen to what is being said. Often, summarizing and paraphrasing parts of the conversation indicate to the speaker that what is being said has been heard (Box 2–1).

◼ Components of Effective Communication

To communicate effectively with others, consider the following seven principles (Table 2–1).

1 Information giving alone is not communication. As stated earlier, communication requires the sharing of information. Sharing information means that the person receiving it understands the content of the message,

BOX 2–1
Basic Listening Sequence

• Listening
• Eye contact
• Attentive body language
• Vocal qualities
• Verbal tracking

TABLE 2–1
Seven Principles of Communication

Principle One:	Information giving is not communication.
Principle Two:	The sender is responsible for clarity.
Principle Three:	Use simple and exact language.
Principle Four:	Encourage feedback.
Principle Five:	The sender must have credibility.
Principle Six:	Acknowledging the contributions of others is essential.
Principle Seven:	Direct channels of communication are best.

Source: Tappen, R.M. (1995). *Nursing Leadership and Management Concept and Practice* (ed. 3). Philadelphia: F.A. Davis, with permission.

the feelings communicated in the message, or both.

2 The sender is responsible for clarity. Making messages clear to the others involved in the communication decreases frustration and confusion. It is up to the sender to be sure that the message is understood. Asking for feedback from the receiver helps to clarify any confusion. Help the sender to communicate more effectively by bringing focus to the interaction. Repeating key words or phrases as questions or using open-ended questions can accomplish this. For example: "You have been telling me that Susan is not providing safe care to her patients. Can you tell me specifically what you have identified as unsafe care?"

3 Use simple and exact language. Clearly and concisely state both written and spoken messages in language that is easily understood by all involved.

4 Encourage feedback. This is the best way to help people understand each other and work together better. Remember that feedback may not be complimentary and that the ideas of the receiver and sender may be in conflict. It is important to always evaluate feedback and deal with it in a constructive manner.

5 The sender must have credibility. The personal and the professional credibility of the sender are both important. If the receiver does not perceive the sender as credible, it is not likely that the message will be given importance.

6 Acknowledging the contributions of others is essential. It may sometimes be difficult to do this, but everyone wants to feel that he or she has worth.

7 Direct channels of communication are best. The greater the number of individuals involved in filtering a message, the less likely the message is to be received correctly. Just as in the game Whisper Down the Lane, messages sent through a variety of senders become distorted. Most of the time, face-to-face communication is preferable to telephone or written communication because people can see nonverbal behaviors and ask for immediate clarification. Information that is controversial or that may elicit negative responses should definitely be delivered so that the receiver can ask questions or receive further clarification. A memo delivered "To all nursing staff" in which cutbacks in staffing are discussed will deliver a different message from a meeting in which all staff members are allowed to talk about their feelings and ask questions.

■ Assertiveness in Communication

Assertive behaviors allow people to stand up for themselves and their rights without violating the rights of others. Several authors have stated that nurses lack assertiveness, claiming that nurses would rather work to maintain harmony than voice opinions that may result in confrontation (Tappen, 2001). Assertiveness is different from aggressiveness (Tappen, Weiss, & Whitehead, 2001). People use aggressive behaviors to force their wishes or ideas on others. In assertive communication, an individual's position is stated clearly and firmly using "I" statements. For example:

The nurse manager noticed that Steve's charting has been of lower quality than expected during the past few weeks. She rescheduled her lunch break to have some time to speak with him. After her break, the nurse manager said to Steve, "JCAHO surveyors are coming in several months. I have been reviewing records and noticed that on several of your charts some pertinent information is missing. I have scheduled time today and tomorrow from 1:00 to 2:00 in the afternoon for us to review the charts. This allows you time to make the necessary corrections and return the charts to me."

By using "I" statements, the nurse manager is confronting the issue without being accusatory. Assertive communication always requires congruence between verbal and nonverbal messages. If she shook her finger close to Steve's face or used a loud voice, the nurse manager might think she was being assertive when in reality her manner was aggressive.

Many misconceptions exist regarding assertive communication. The first is that all communication is either aggressive or passive. Actually, communication may be passive, aggressive, passive-aggressive, or assertive. *Passive communication* happens when someone does not voice opinions about an issue. Aggressive individuals express their opinions in a direct and often hostile manner that infringes on others' rights. These people think that they must be the "winner" in all communications. Passive-aggressive communication is aggressive communication presented in a passive way. During passive-aggressive communication, little verbal communication takes place and the verbal and nonverbal behaviors are not congruent.

The second misconception is that people who communicate assertively always get what they want. Being assertive involves both rights and responsibilities. Assertive communicators have the right to speak up, but they also must be prepared to listen to the response.

The third misconception about assertiveness is that it is unfeminine. This misconception is based on the false idea that all nurses are women. Women are often taught to withdraw rather than be assertive. Learning to be assertive is part of effective nursing action. Nurses who continue patterns of either nonassertive or overaggressive behaviors may have a negative impact on themselves and the nursing profession (Arnold & Boggs, 2002). During the 1990s, more men entered the nursing profession than in previous

years. Although this trend has continued, the profession remains predominantly female.

The fourth misconception is that assertiveness and aggressiveness are synonymous, but to be assertive is not the same as being aggressive. Assertiveness does not force agreement between participants but permits them to disagree while promoting clarification of each position. Developing assertive behavior may decrease stress as individuals respond in a manner and at a time that is appropriate.

◻ Effective Communication in the Workplace

People often are unwilling or unable to accept responsibility or to perform a specific task because they do not fully understand what is expected of them. Professional nurses are required to communicate client information to other members of the nursing team. Although this may sound easy, there are potential barriers to communication. These barriers may be physical, psychological, or semantic.

Physical Barriers

Physical barriers to communication include extraneous noise, too much activity in the area where the communication is taking place, or physical separation of the people trying to engage in verbal interaction.

Psychological Barriers

Psychological "noise" such as increased anxiety may interfere with the ability to pay attention to the other speaker. Social values, emotions, judgments, and cultural influences also impede communication. Previous life experiences and preconceived ideas about other cultures also influence how we communicate.

Semantic Barriers

Semantic refers to the meaning of words. Sometimes, no matter how great the effort, the message just does not get across. For example, words such as *neat, cool,* and *bad* may convey meanings other than those intended. Many individuals have learned English as a second language and therefore understand only literal translations of certain words. For example, to many people, *cool* means interesting, unique, clever, or even sharp (e.g., "This is a cool way to find the vein"). To someone for whom the word *cool* refers only to temperature (e.g., "It is cool outside"), the preceding statement would make very little sense.

Gender Barriers

Men and women develop dissimilar communication skills and are inclined to communicate differently. Often, they give different meanings to conveyed information or feelings. This may be related to psychosocial development. Boys learn to use communication as a way to negotiate and to develop independence, whereas girls use communication to confirm, minimize disparities, and create or strengthen closeness (Blais, Hayes, Kozier, Erb, 2002).

◼ Communication with Colleagues

Members of the nursing team include administrators, directors of nursing, supervisors, clinical specialists, nurse managers, ancillary personnel, and nursing students. Each of these individuals is involved with client care in different ways.

Promoting trust and sincerity enhances communication among team members. Congruency between your words and your deeds promotes trust. If team members feel that you are trustworthy and sincere, they will be more likely to ask questions and seek clarification if they are uncertain of something. Box 2–2 gives guidelines for facilitating communication among team members.

To manage client care effectively, it is important to keep the lines of communication open on all levels. Using active listening skills and assertive behavior supports clear communication.

BOX 2–2
Guidelines for Facilitating Good Communication

- Practice active listening.
- Communicate genuine interest and concern.
- Provide adequate information.
- Use the team members' ideas in the plan of action.
- Maximize feelings of self-respect.
- Focus on the team members' ability to help themselves.
- Do not minimize the value of time allowed to learn.
- Praise competent performance.
- State expectations clearly and identify key points.
- Be willing to look at alternatives that others may feel are important.
- Demonstrate respect for the values and dignity of all team members.
- Depersonalize potential conflict situations.

Telephone Etiquette

Nurses spend a significant amount of time gathering and relating information by telephone. Using telephone etiquette takes into account the needs of both senders and receivers. The courtesy and clarification that you would use in a face-to-face contact are just as important in a telephone contact.

Information Systems

Communication through the use of computer technology is rapidly growing in nursing practice. A study conducted by KPMG-Peat Marwick of health care systems that were using bedside terminals found that medication errors and use of client call bells decreased and nurse productivity increased. The use of computerized patient records allows health care providers to retrieve and distribute patient information precisely and quickly. Decisions regarding client care can be made more efficiently with less waiting time. Additional benefits of computerized systems for health care applications are listed in Box 2–3 (Arnold & Pearson, 1992; Hebda, Czar, & Mascara, 1998).

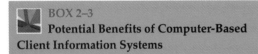

BOX 2–3
Potential Benefits of Computer-Based Client Information Systems

- Increased hours for direct patient care
- Patient data accessible at bedside
- Improved accuracy and legibility of data
- Immediate availability of all data to all members of the team
- Increased safety related to positive patient identification, improved standardization, and improved quality
- Decreased medication errors
- Increased staff satisfaction

Source: Adapted from Arnold, J., & Pearson, G. (eds.). (1992). Computer Applications in Nursing Education and Practice. New York: National League for Nursing.

E-mail

Today, most institutions use e-mail. Using e-mail competently and effectively requires writing skills; the same communication principles apply to both e-mail and letter writing. When communicating via e-mail, you are not only making a first impression but also leaving a written record (Shea, 2000).

The rules for using e-mail in the workplace are somewhat different than for using e-mail among friends. Much of the humor and wit found in personal e-mail is not appropriate for the work setting. Professional e-mail may remain informal; however, the message must be clear, concise, and courteous. Think about what you need to say before you write it. Then write it, read it, and re-read it. Once you are satisfied that the message is clear and concise, then send it.

Many executives read their own e-mail, which means that it is often possible to contact them directly. Many systems make it easy to send e-mail out to everyone at the health care institution. For this reason, it is important to keep e-mail professional. Remember the "chain of command": always go through the proper channels, even when using e-mail.

The fact that you have the capability to send e-mail instantly to large groups of people does not necessarily make it a good idea. You need to be careful if you have access to an all-company mailing list. It is easy to accidentally send e-mail through the system without meaning for this to happen. Consider the following example:

A respiratory therapist and a department administrator at a large health care institution—both involved other people—were engaged in relationship. They started sending each other personal notes over the company e-mail system. One day, one of them accidentally sent one of these notes to all the employees at the health care institution.

Both were fired. The moral of this story is simple: Don't send anything over e-mail that you would not want published on the front page of a national newspaper or magazine or reported on the national news.

Although voice tone cannot be "heard" via e-mail, the use of certain words and writing styles indicate emotion. A rude tone of mail may provoke extreme reactions.

Follow the "rules of netiquette" (Shea, 2000) when communicating through e-mail. Some of these rules are listed in Box 2–4.

▢ Communicating Client Care Needs

Developing the Change-of-Shift Report

It is important to understand exactly how your day at work will begin. Regardless of

BOX 2–4
Rules of Netiquette

1. If you were face-to-face, would you say this?
2. Follow the same rules of behavior online that you follow when dealing with individuals in the real world.
3. Only send copies of information to those individuals who need the information.
4. Avoid flaming; that is, sending remarks intended to cause a negative reaction.
5. Do not write in all capital letters; this indicates anger.
6. Respect other people's privacy.
7. Do not abuse the power of your position.
8. Proofread your e-mail before sending it.

Adapted from Shea, V. (2000). *Netiquette.* San Rafael, Calif.: Albion.

which shift an individual works, some things never change. Nurses traditionally give one another "the report." The change-of-shift report has become the accepted method of communicating client care needs from one nurse to another. During the report, pertinent information related to events that occurred is given to the individuals responsible for providing continuity of care (Box 2–5). Although historically the report has been given face-to-face, there are also newer ways to share information. Many health care institutions use audiotape and computer printouts as mechanisms for information-sharing. These mechanisms allow the nurses from the previous shift to complete their tasks and those coming on duty to make inquiries for clarification as necessary.

The report should be organized, concise, and complete, with relevant details. Not every unit uses the same system for giving a change-of-shift report. The system is easily modified according to the pattern of nursing care delivery and the types of clients serviced. For example, many intensive care units, because of their small size and the more acute needs of their clients, use walking rounds as a mechanism for giving the report. This system allows nurses to discuss the current client status and to set goals for care for the next several hours. Together, the nurses gather objective data as one ends a shift and the other begins. This way, there is no confusion as to the client's status at shift change. This same system is often used in emergency departments and labor and delivery units. Larger client care units may find the walking report time-consuming and an inefficient use of resources.

It is helpful to take notes or create a worksheet while listening to the report. A worksheet helps organize the work for the day (Fig. 2–2). As specific tasks are mentioned, the nurse coming on duty makes a note of the activity in the appropriate time slot. Medications and treatments can also be added. Any changes from the previous day are noted, particularly when the nurse is familiar with the client. Recording changes counteracts the tendency to remember what was done the day before and repeat it, often without checking for new orders. During the day, the worksheet acts as a reminder of the tasks that have been completed and those that still need to be done.

Presenting the Information

Reporting skills improve with practice. When presenting information in a report, certain things must be included. Begin the report by identifying the client and the

---

BOX 2–5
Information for Change-of-Shift Report

- Identify the client, including the room and bed numbers.
- Include the client diagnosis.
- Account for the presence of the client on the unit. If the client has left the unit for a diagnostic test, surgery, or just to wander, it is important for the oncoming staff members to know the client is off the unit.
- Provide the treatment plan that specifies the goals of treatment. Note the goals and the critical pathway steps either achieved or in progress. Personalized approaches can be developed during this time and client readiness for those approaches evaluated. It is helpful to mention the client's primary care physician. Include new orders and medications and treatments currently prescribed.
- Document client responses to current treatments. Is the treatment plan working? Present evidence for or against this. Include pertinent lab values as well as any untoward reactions to medications or treatments. Note any comments the client has made regarding the hospitalization or treatment plan that the oncoming staff members need to address.
- Omit personal opinions and value judgments about clients as well as personal/confidential information not pertinent to providing client care. If you are using computerized information systems, make sure that you are knowledgeable in how to present the material accurately and concisely.

Name_____ **Room #** _____ **Allergies**_____

0700	0800	0900	1000	1100	1200	1300	1400	1500	1600	1700	1800

Name_____ **Room #** _____ **Allergies**_____

0700	0800	0900	1000	1100	1200	1300	1400	1500	1600	1700	1800

Name_____ **Room #** _____ **Allergies**_____

0700	0800	0900	1000	1100	1200	1300	1400	1500	1600	1700	1800

Figure 2–2   Organization and time management schedule for client care.

admitting as well as current diagnoses. Include the expected treatment plan and the client's responses to the treatment. For example, if the client has had multiple antibiotics and a reaction occurred, this information is important to relay to the next nurse. Value judgments and personal opinions about the client are not pertinent to the report (Fig. 2–3).

All individuals involved in client care share information through verbal and written communication in an interdisciplinary team conference. The team conference begins by stating the client's name, age, and diagnoses. Each member of the interdisciplinary team then explains the goal of his or her discipline, the interventions, and the outcome. Effectiveness of treatment, development of new interventions, and setting of new goals are then discussed. The key to a successful interdisciplinary conference is

ROOM # _____ PATIENT NAME_____ DIAGNOSES_____

DIET_____ ACTIVITY_____

1900	0100
2000	0200
2100	0300
2200	0400
2300	0500
2400	0600

Figure 2–3 Client information report.

presenting the information in a clear and concise manner.

◼ Communicating with Other Disciplines

In many settings, nurses are the client care managers. Integration, coordination, and communication among all disciplines deliv-

ering care to a specific client ultimately are the responsibility of the nurse care manager. Nurses spend time with the client on a day-to-day basis and therefore are in a particularly advantageous position to observe the client's responses to treatments. For example:

Mr. Richards is a 75-year-old man who was in a motor vehicle accident. He had right-sided weakness and dysphagia. The speech therapy, physical therapy, and social services departments were called in to see Mr. Richards. A speech therapist was working with Mr. Richards to assist him with swallowing. He was to receive pureed foods for the second day. The RN assigned an LPN to feed Mr. Richards. The LPN reported that although Mr. Richards had done well the previous day, he had difficulty swallowing today. The RN immediately notified the speech therapist, and a new treatment plan was developed.

The role of professional nurses in relation to their clients' physicians is to communicate changes in the client's condition, share other pertinent information, discuss modifications of the treatment plan if necessary, and clarify physician orders. This can be stressful for a new graduate who still has some role insecurity. Using good communication skills and having the necessary information at hand are helpful when discussing client needs.

Before calling a physician, make sure that all the information you need is available. The physician may want more clarification. If you are calling to report a drop in a client's blood pressure, be sure to have at hand the list of the client's medications, vital signs, and blood pressure trends, together with a general assessment of the client's present status.

Sometimes when a nurse calls a physician, the physician does not return the call. It is important to document all physician contacts in the client's record. Many units keep physician calling logs. In the log, enter the physician's name, the date, the time, and the reason for the call. Also enter the time the physician returns the call.

Professional nurses are responsible for accepting, transcribing, and implementing physicians' orders. The two main types of orders are *written* and *verbal*. *Written orders* are dated and placed on the appropriate institutional form. *Verbal orders* are given from the physician directly to the nurse, either by telephone or face-to-face. A verbal order needs to be written on the appropriate institutional form, the time and date noted, and the form signed as a verbal order by the nurse. Most institutions require the physician to co-sign the order within 24 hours. When receiving a verbal order, repeat it back to the physician for confirmation. If the physician is speaking too rapidly, ask him or her to speak more slowly. Then repeat the information for confirmation.

Professionalism and a courteous attitude by all parties are necessary ingredients to maintain collegial relationships with physicians and other health care professionals.

◼ Communicating with Clients and Their Families

Communicating with clients and their families occupies a major portion of the nurse's day. Nurses teach clients and their families about medications and the client's condition, clarify the physician's treatment plan, and explain procedures. To do this effectively, nurses need to use communication skills and recognize the barriers to communication.

Today's health care environment requires nurses to be creative and effective when communicating with clients and their families. The health care consumer, often confronted by the bureaucracy of the managed care environment, may enter the setting in a highly charged emotional state. Nurses need to recognize the signs of the anxious or angry client and promptly intervene to defuse the situation before it escalates. Practicing good listening skills and showing interest in the client often help.

Early morning admissions on the day of surgery and short-term stays make client teaching a challenge. The nurse must complete the admission requirements, surgical checklists, and preoperative teaching within a short period of time. Time for postoperative teaching is also shortened. It is important for the nurse to communicate clearly and concisely what will be done and what is expected of the client. Allow time for questions and clarifications. For many clients, a written preoperative and/or postoperative teaching guide helps to clarify the instructions.

◼ Conclusion

The responsibility for delivering and coordinating client care is an important part of the role of the professional nurse. To accomplish this, nurses need good communication skills. Being assertive without being aggressive and conducting interactions in a professional manner enhance the relationships nurses develop with colleagues, physicians, and other members of the interdisciplinary team.

Perhaps if Claude and his colleague had known more about communication, especially how to ask for help, their day would not have been so difficult. Staying calm and using good communication skills demonstrates professionalism and an ability to work with others.

Study Questions

1 Role-play a situation between a client and a nurse. Have a third student make a list of the different attending skills you used with the client during the interaction. (Some examples for role-play: Teaching a client about compliance with a medication regimen; showing a client how to self-administer insulin; coping with a client who says, "I hate it here.")

2 This is your first position as an RN, and you are working with an LPN who has been on the unit for 20 years. Your first day on the job she says to you, "The only difference between you and me is the size of the paycheck." Demonstrate how you would respond to this statement using assertive communication techniques.

3 A physician orders, "Vit K 10 mg. IV." You realize that this is a dangerous order. How would you approach the physician?

4 A client is admitted to the same-day surgical center for a breast biopsy. She is accompanied by her significant other, who has just had an altercation with an admissions secretary about the managed care criteria for payment. The client is required to wait for 30 minutes after her designated arrival time. The nurse comes out to call the client back to the holding area and the significant other turns and says loudly, "What is wrong with you people? Can't you ever get anything straight? If you can't get the insurance right and you can't get the time right, how can we expect you to get the surgery right?" As the nurse, how would you diffuse the situation?

Critical Thinking Exercise

Eric worked the evening shift. Every day when he got the report from Yvonne, he heard how difficult the day had been, what a "pain" certain patients were, and excuses as to why so many things had been left for him to do. Eric quietly listened to this and continued to pick up after Yvonne. He did not discuss the situation with anyone but felt very anxious because he was always behind before he could begin. One afternoon Eric became annoyed and yelled, "What is your problem? Everything is left for me to do, and all you give me are excuses. Besides complaining, what do you do all day?"

1 What type of communicator is Eric?

2 Identify the behavior Eric exhibited that enabled Yvonne to continue her behavior.

3 How could Eric have handled this situation with Yvonne in a more constructive manner?

4 If you were the team leader, how would you handle this situation?

Student Activities

1. While working in your clinical setting, critique a communication between a staff nurse and a physician. Identify the communication techniques used by both individuals. Write your answer in the space provided.

2. Conversation is an essential nursing tool. If you had 30 minutes to spend with each of the following clients while performing a nursing activity that allowed you to communicate freely, what would you discuss? Give your rationale in the space provided.

   a. A 36-year-old amputee who has been in a rehab hospital for 3 weeks following a motorcycle accident.

   b. The family of an unconscious client who suffered a traumatic brain injury and is in the intensive care unit.

REFERENCES

Arnold, E., & Boggs, K. (2002). *Professional Communication Skills for Nurses, 4th* ed. Philadelphia: W.B. Saunders.

Arnold, J., & Pearson, G. (eds.). (1992). *Computer Applications in Nursing Education and Practice.* New York: National League for Nursing.

Berlo, D.K. (1960). *The Process of Communication.* San Francisco: Reinhart Press.

Blais, K.B., Hayes, J.S., Kozier, B., & Erb, G. (2002). *Professional Nursing Practice: Concepts and Perspectives,* 4th ed. Upper Saddle River, N.J.: Prentice-Hall.

Fontaine, K.L., & Fletcher, J.S. (2002). *Mental Health Nursing,* 5th ed. Redwood City, Calif.: Prentice-Hall

Hebda, T., Czar, P., & Mascara, C. (1998). *Handbook of Informatics for Nurses and Health Care Professionals.* Menlo Park, Calif.: Addison-Wesley.

Mulholland, J. (1991). *The Language of Negotiation: A Handbook of Practical Strategies.* London: Rutledge.

Shea, V. (2000). *Netiquette.* San Rafael, Calif.: Albion.

Tappen, R.M. (1995). *Nursing Leadership and Management: Concepts and Practice,* 3rd ed. Philadelphia: F.A. Davis.

Tappen, R.M. (2001). *Nursing Leadership and Management: Concepts and Practice,* 4th ed. Philadelphia: F.A. Davis.

Tappen, R.M., Weiss, S.A., & Whitehead, D.K. (2001). *Essentials of Nursing Leadership and Management,* 2nd ed. Philadelphia: F.A. Davis.

Varcarolis, E.M. (2001). *Foundations of Psychiatric–Mental Health Nursing,* 4th ed. Philadelphia: W.B. Saunders.

CHAPTER 3

Giving and Receiving Feedback

OBJECTIVES

After reading this chapter, the student should be able to:

- Provide positive and negative feedback in a constructive manner.

- Respond to feedback in a constructive manner.

- Evaluate the conduct of performance appraisals.

- Participate in formal peer review.

OUTLINE

Feedback Is Essential

Guidelines for Providing Feedback
Provide Both Positive and Negative Feedback
Give Immediate Feedback
Provide Frequent Feedback
Give Negative Feedback Privately
Be Objective
Base Feedback on Observable Behavior
Accept Feedback in Return
Include Suggestions for Change
Communicate in a Nonthreatening Manner

Seeking Evaluative Feedback
When Is Evaluative Feedback Needed?
Responding to Evaluative Feedback

Performance Appraisal
Procedure
Standards for Evaluation

Peer Review
Fundamentals of Peer Review
A Comprehensive Peer Review System

Conclusion

CHAPTER 3 SELF ASSESSMENT
Do You Know How to Provide Feedback?

Indicate whether you think each of the following recommendations for providing feedback is correct. Then check your answers.

1. It is more important to correct people than to praise them.
   True_____ False_____

2. Always allow yourself to "cool off" before correcting someone.
   True_____ False_____

3. It is preferable to correct someone in private rather than in front of others.
   True_____ False_____

4. General statements are preferable to descriptions of specific incidents when providing feedback. True_____ False_____

5. Seek feedback on your performance from others, including your patients.
   True_____ False_____

6. Include suggestions for improvement when giving negative feedback.
   True_____ False_____

7. Save your corrective comments for the annual formal evaluation sessions.
   True_____ False_____

Answers: 1. F, 2. F, 3. T, 4. F, 5. T, 6. T, 7. F

In good weather, Herbert usually played basketball with his kids after dinner. Yesterday, however, he told them he was too tired. This evening, he said the same thing. When they urged him to play anyway, he snapped at them and told them to leave him alone.

"Herbert!" his wife exclaimed, "Why did you do that?"

"I don't know," he responded. "I'm just so uptight these days. My annual review was supposed to be today, but my nurse manager was out sick. I have no idea what she is going to say. I can't think about anything else."

If Herbert's nurse manager had been providing informal feedback to staff on a regular basis, Herbert would have known where he stood. He would have had a good idea about what his strengths and weaknesses were and would not be afraid of an unpleasant surprise during the review. He would also be looking forward to the opportunity to review his accomplishments and make plans with his manager for further developing his skills. He still would have been disappointed that she was unavailable, but he would not have been as distressed by it.

The process of giving and receiving evaluative feedback is an essential leadership responsibility. Done well, it is very helpful, promoting growth and increasing employee satisfaction. Done poorly, as in Herbert's case, it can be stressful, even injurious. In this chapter, we consider the do's and don'ts of giving and receiving feedback, how to share positive and negative evaluative comments with your coworkers, and how to respond constructively when you are on the receiving end of such comments.

◙ Feedback Is Essential

Why Do People Need Feedback?

We all need feedback because it is difficult for us to see ourselves as others see us. Furthermore, competent people generally underestimate their ability and focus on their shortcomings and incompetent people generally fail to recognize their incompetence (Channer & Hope, 2001). The following are just a few of the reasons that evaluative feedback is such an important leadership responsibility. Effective, evaluative feedback:

- **Reinforces constructive behavior.** Positive feedback lets people know which behaviors are the most productive and encourages continuation of these behaviors.

- **Discourages unproductive behavior.** Correction of inappropriate actions begins with provision of negative feedback.

- **Provides recognition.** The power of praise (positive feedback) to motivate people is often underestimated.

- **Develops employee skills.** Feedback helps people to identify their strengths and weaknesses and guides them in seeking opportunities to further develop their strengths and manage their weaknesses (Rosen, 1996).

◙ Guidelines for Providing Feedback

Done well, evaluative feedback can reinforce motivation, strengthen teamwork, and improve the quality of care given. When poorly done, evaluation can reinforce poor work habits, increase insecurity, and destroy motivation and morale (Table 3–1).

Evaluation involves making judgments and communicating these judgments to others. People make judgments all the time about all types of things. Unfortunately, these judgments are often based on opinions, preferences, and inaccurate or partial information.

Subjective, biased judgment offered as objective feedback has given evaluation a bad name. Poorly communicated feedback has

TABLE 3–1

Do's and Don'ts of Providing Feedback

Do . . .	Don't . . .
Include positive comments	Focus only on the negative
Be objective	Let personalities intrude
Be specific when correcting someone	Be vague
Treat everyone the same	Play favorites
Correct people in private	Correct people in front of others

Source: Adapted from Gabor, D. (1994). *Speaking Your Mind in 101 Difficult Situations.* New York: Stonesong Press (Simon & Schuster).

an equally negative effect. You will find that many people who are uncomfortable with evaluation have been recipients of subjective, biased, or poorly communicated evaluations in the past.

Evaluative feedback is most effective when it is given immediately, frequently, and privately. To be constructive, it must be objective, based on observed behavior, and skillfully communicated. The feedback message should include the reasons that a behavior has been judged satisfactory or unsatisfactory. If the message is negative, it should be nonthreatening and include both suggestions and support for change and improvement (Box 3–1).

Provide Both Positive and Negative Feedback

Leaders and managers often neglect to provide positive feedback. If questioned, people

BOX 3–1
Tips for Providing Helpful Feedback

- Provide both positive and negative feedback.
- Give immediate feedback.
- Provide frequent feedback.
- Give negative feedback privately.
- Base feedback on observable behavior.
- Communicate effectively.
- Include suggestions for change.

who do not give positive feedback often respond, "If I don't say anything, that means everything is okay." Unfortunately, they do not realize that some people assume that everything is *not* okay when they receive no feedback. Others assume that no one is aware of how much effort they have made unless it is acknowledged with positive feedback.

Most people want to do their work well. They also want to know that their efforts are recognized and appreciated. Kron (1981) called positive feedback a "psychological paycheck." She pointed out that it is almost as important to people as their actual paychecks. It is a real pleasure, not only for staff members but also for their leaders and managers, to be able to share the satisfaction of a job well done with someone else. Leaders and managers should do everything they can to reward and retain their best staff members (Bowers & Lapziger, 2001).

Some say that nurses do not do enough to support each other as colleagues and that they avoid sharing direct feedback with coworkers (DeMarco, 1998). Whether that is true or not, giving positive feedback is an important way to support your colleagues and reinforce constructive behavior.

Providing negative feedback is just as necessary as providing positive feedback but probably more difficult to do well. Too often, negative feedback is critical rather than helpful. Simply telling someone that something has gone wrong or could have been done better is easier than making the feedback a learning experience for the receiver by suggesting ways to make the needed changes or by working together to develop a strategy for improvement. It is also easier to make broad, critical comments (e.g., "You're too slow") than it is to describe the specific behavior that needs improvement (e.g., "Waiting in Mr. D.'s room while he brushes his teeth takes up too much of your time") and then add a suggestion for change (e.g., "You could get your bath supplies together while he finishes").

Providing no negative feedback at all is the easiest but least effective solution to the problem of being too critical. Unsatisfactory work must be acknowledged and discussed with the people involved. Too many managers are "wishy washy, not wanting to hurt people's feelings" (Watson & Harris, 1999, p. 172). Tolerating poor work encourages its continuation and undermines the motivation of the whole team.

Give Immediate Feedback

The most helpful feedback, positive or negative, is given as soon as possible after the behavior has occurred. There are several reasons for this. Immediate feedback is more meaningful to the person receiving it. Also, if feedback is delayed too long, the person may have forgotten the incident altogether or assumed that your silence indicated approval.

Problems that are ignored often get worse. At the same time, a lot of frustration and anger can build up in the leader and others affected by the problems. When feedback is given as soon as possible, there is no time for this buildup.

Provide Frequent Feedback

Feedback should be not only immediate but also frequent. Frequent constructive feedback keeps motivation and awareness levels high and avoids the possibility that problems will grow larger and more serious before they are confronted. It also becomes easier with practice. If giving and receiving feedback are frequent and integral parts of team functioning, feedback will be easier to give and it will be less threatening to most people. It becomes an ordinary, everyday occurrence, one that happens spontaneously and is familiar to everyone on the team.

Give Negative Feedback Privately

Giving negative feedback privately rather than in front of others prevents unnecessary embarrassment. It also avoids the possibility that those who overhear the discussion may misunderstand it and draw erroneous conclusions from it. A good manager praises staff in public but punishes (corrects) them in private (Matejka, Ashworth, & Dodd-McCue, 1986).

Be Objective

Being objective when giving feedback to others can be very difficult. First, evaluate people on the basis of job expectations and the results of their efforts (Fonville, Killian, & Tranberger, 1998). Do not compare them, favorably or unfavorably, with other staff members (Gellerman & Hodgson, 1988).

Another way to increase objectivity is to always give a reason that you have judged a behavior as good or poor. Be sure you consider the effect or outcome of the behavior in forming your conclusion. Give reasons for both positive and negative messages. For example, if you tell a coworker, "That was a good patient interview," you have told that person nothing except that the interview pleased you. However, when you add, ". . . because you asked open-ended questions that encouraged the client to explore personal feelings," you have identified the specific behavior that made your evaluation positive and reinforced this specific behavior.

Finally, use broad and generally accepted standards for making judgments as much as possible, rather than basing evaluation on your personal likes and dislikes. Objectivity can be increased by using standards that reflect the consensus of the team, the organization, the community, or the nursing profession. Formal evaluation is based on agreed-on, written standards of what is acceptable behavior. Informal evaluation, however, is based on unwritten standards. If these unwritten standards are based on personal preferences, the evaluation will be highly subjective. The following are some examples:

- A team leader who describes a female social worker as having a professional appearance because she wears muted suits instead of bright dresses to work is using a personal standard to evaluate that social worker.

- A supervisor who asks an employee to stop wearing jewelry that could get caught in the equipment used at work is applying a standard for safety in making the evaluative statement.

- A nursing home administrator who insists that staff members include every resident in the weekly birthday party is applying a narrower and more personal standard than the administrator who insists that staff members offer every resident the opportunity to participate in social activities.

Base Feedback on Observable Behavior

An evaluative statement should describe observed performance; it is not a self-report or your interpretation of another's behavior. Observation is much more likely to be factual and less likely to evoke a defensive response. For example, saying, "You were impatient with Mrs. G. today" is an interpretive comment. Saying, "You interrupted Mrs. G. before she finished explaining her problem" is based on observable behavior. The second statement is more specific and may be more accurate because the caregiver may have been trying to redirect the conversation to more immediate concerns rather than feeling impatient. The latter statement is also more likely to evoke an explanation than a defensive response.

Lombardi (2001) suggested keeping a performance logbook to record your observations of staff behavior. If you do this, be sure to record specific dates, events, and any follow-up discussion with the staff member. Also make sure that the logbook serves as a chronicle of the entire scope of each person's job and that it does not become a finger-pointing exercise or a source of intimidation for staff.

Accept Feedback in Return

An evaluative statement is a form of confrontation. Any message that contains a statement about the behavior of a staff member is confronting that staff member with his or her behavior. The leader who gives evaluative feedback needs to be prepared to receive feedback in return and to engage in active listening. Active listening is especially important because the person receiving the evaluation may respond with high emotion. The following is an example of what may happen:

You point out to Mr. S. that his patients need to be monitored more frequently. Mr. S. emotionally responds that he is doing everything possible for the patients and does not have a free moment all day for one extra thing. In fact, Mr. S. tells you, he never even takes a lunch break and goes home exhausted. Active listening and problem solving aimed at relieving his overloaded time schedule are a must in this situation.

When you give negative feedback, allow time for the individuals to express their feelings and for problem solving to find ways to improve a situation. This is particularly important if the problem has been ignored long enough to become serious (Box 3–2).

Include Suggestions for Change

When you give feedback that indicates that some kind of change in behavior is needed, it is helpful to suggest alternative behaviors. This is easier to do when the change is a simple one.

BOX 3–2
Tactful Guidelines for Providing Negative Feedback

T	=	Think before you speak.
A	=	Apologize quickly if you've made a mistake.
C	=	Converse, don't be patronizing or sarcastic.
T	=	Time your comments carefully.
F	=	Focus on behavior, not on personality.
U	=	Uncover hidden feelings.
L	=	Listen for feedback.

Source: Gabor, D. (1994). *Speaking Your Mind in 101 Difficult Situations.* New York: Stonesong Press (Simon & Schuster)

When complex change is needed (as with Mr. S.), you may find that the person is aware of the problem but does not know how to solve it. In such a case, oversimplified solutions are inappropriate, but an offer to engage in searching for the solution is appropriate. A willingness to listen to the other person's side of the story and assist in finding a solution indicates that your purpose is to help rather than just to criticize the individual.

Communicate in a Nonthreatening Manner

Threatening messages reduce motivation and inhibit learning by diverting people's energies into activities aimed at reducing the threat and hiding future mistakes instead of reporting them. Staff members who make a mistake often face questions about their competency and find considerable guilt and blame placed on them (Hemman, 2002). Although a small degree of anxiety may increase learning, too much fear immobilizes people. The ultimate purpose for providing informal evaluation is, after all, to improve the function of the team and its individual members. An error that is reported immediately can often be corrected. Calm discussion of its cause and prevention of future errors can be a learning experience for the entire team.

Negative feedback may contain hints of dire consequences, probably in the mistaken belief that it will increase the person's motivation to change. The following are some common examples:

- "You're not going to last long if you keep doing that."

- "People who want to do well here make sure their assignments are done on time."

- "Don't argue with the doctors; they'll report you to the nursing office."

When a person's behavior actually does threaten his or her job security, however, a formal evaluation stating this fact directly and specifying needed changes is appropriate.

You may have assumed that people in the ranks above you (e.g., manager, head nurse, supervisor, director) could not be threatened by feedback from you. This is not true. They are all human and as susceptible to feeling threatened as you are. You need to follow the same guidelines in giving feedback to people above you in the organization as you do with people below you in the hierarchy.

Seeking Evaluative Feedback

It is equally important to be able to accept constructive criticism (Kelly & Aiken, 1999). The reasons for seeking feedback are the same as those for giving it to others. The criteria for evaluating the feedback you receive are also the same.

When Is Evaluative Feedback Needed?

There are a number of different situations in which you need to seek feedback (Box 3–3). For example, you may find yourself in a work situation in which you receive very little feedback, or you may be getting only positive and no negative comments (or vice versa).

You also need to look for feedback when you feel uncertain about how well you are doing or whether you have correctly interpreted the expectations of the job. The following are examples of these situations:

- You have been told that good client care is the highest priority but feel totally frustrated by never having enough staff members to give good care.

- You thought you were expected to do case finding and health teaching in your community but receive the most recognition for the number of home visits made and the completeness of your records.

Another instance in which you should request feedback is when you feel that your needs for recognition and job satisfaction have not been met adequately.

Request feedback in the form of "I" messages. If you have received only negative comments, ask, "In what ways have I done well?" If you receive only positive comments, you can ask, "In what areas do I need to improve?" Or, if you are seeking feedback from a client, you could ask, "How can I be of more help to you?"

Responding to Evaluative Feedback

Sometimes, it is appropriate to critically analyze the feedback you are getting. If the feedback seems totally negative or you feel threatened by receiving it, ask for further explanation. You may have misunderstood what the person meant to say.

It is hard to avoid responding defensively to negative feedback that is subjective or laced with threats and blame. If you are the recipient of such a poorly done evaluation, however, it may help both you and your supervisor to try to guide the discussion into more constructive areas. You can ask for reasons why the evaluation was negative, on what standard it was based, what the person's expectations were, and what the person suggests as alternative behavior.

When the feedback is positive but nonspecific, you may also want to ask for some clarification so that you can learn what that person's expectations really are. Do not hesitate to seek that psychological paycheck. Tell other people about your successes; most are happy to share the satisfaction of a successful outcome or positive development in a client's care.

BOX 3–3
Situations in Which to Ask for Feedback

- When you do not know how well you are doing
- When you receive only positive comments
- When you receive only negative comments
- When you believe that your accomplishments have not been recognized

◘ Performance Appraisal

Performance appraisal is the formal evaluation of an employee by a superior, usually a manager or supervisor. To prepare an appraisal, the employee's behavior is compared with his or her job description and the standard describing how the employee is expected to perform (Hayes, 2002). Employees need to know what has to be done, how much has to be done, and when it has to be done. Evaluate actual performance, not good intentions.

Procedure

In the ideal situation, the performance appraisal begins when the employee is hired. Based on the written job description, the employee and manager discuss performance expectations and then write a set of objectives that they think the employee can reasonably accomplish within a given time. The objectives should be written at a level of performance that demonstrates that some learning, refinement of skill, or advancement toward some long-range objective has taken place. The following are examples of objectives a new staff nurse could accomplish in the first 6 months of employment:

- Complete the staff nurse orientation program successfully.

- Master the basic skills necessary to function as a staff nurse on the assigned unit.

- Supervise the unlicensed assistive personnel assigned to his or her patients.

Monthly reviews of progress toward these goals help keep the new staff member on track and provide opportunities to identify needs for further orientation or extended training (Hayes, 2002; Lombardi, 2001). Six months later, the staff nurse and nurse manager sit down again and evaluate the staff nurse's performance in terms of the previously set goals. The evaluation is based on both the staff nurse's self-evaluation and the nurse manager's observation of specific behaviors. New objectives for the next 6 months and plans for achieving them may be agreed on at the time of the appraisal or at a separate meeting (Beer, 1981). A copy of the performance appraisal and the new goals must be available to employees so that they can refer back to them and check on their progress.

It is important to set aside adequate time for feedback and goal-setting processes. Both the staff nurse and the nurse manager bring data for use at this session. These data include a self-evaluation by the staff nurse and observations by the evaluator of the employee's activities and their outcomes. Data may also be obtained from peers and clients. Some organizations use surveys for getting this information from clients.

Most of the guidelines for providing informal evaluative feedback discussed earlier apply to the conduct of performance appraisals. Although not as frequent or immediate as informal feedback, formal evaluation should be just as objective, private, nonthreatening, skillfully communicated, and growth promoting.

Standards for Evaluation

Unfortunately, many organizations' employee evaluation procedures are far from ideal. Their procedures may be inconsistent, subjective, and even unknown to the employee in some cases. The following is a list of standards for a fair and objective employee evaluation procedure that you can use to judge your employer's procedures:

- Standards are clear, objective, and known in advance.

- Criteria for pay raises and promotions are clearly spelled out and uniformly applied.

- Conditions under which employment may be terminated are known.

- Appraisals are part of the employee's permanent record and have space for employee comments.

- Employees may inspect their own personnel file.

- Employees may request and be given a reasonable explanation of any rating and may appeal the rating if they do not agree with it.

- Employees are given a reasonable amount of time to correct any serious deficiencies before other action is taken, unless the safety of self or others is immediately threatened.

In some organizations, collective bargaining agreements are used to enforce adherence to fair and objective performance appraisals. However, collective bargaining agreements may emphasize seniority (length of service) over merit, a situation that does not promote growth and change.

◘ Peer Review

Peer review is the evaluation of an individual's practice by his or her colleagues (peers) who have similar education, experience, and occupational status. Its purpose is to provide the individual with feedback from those who are best acquainted with the requirements and demands of that individual's position, colleagues. Peer review is directed to both *actions* (process) and the *outcomes* of actions. It also encompasses decision-making (critical thinking), technical, and interpersonal skills (Mustard, 2002).

Professionals frequently observe and judge their colleagues' performance. Many feel uncomfortable telling colleagues directly what they think of their colleagues' performance, however, so they don't share their thoughts with the individual practitioner unless informal feedback is shared regularly or a formal system of peer review is established (Katzenbach & Smith, 2003). Whenever staff members meet to audit records or otherwise evaluate the quality of care they have given, they are engaging in a kind of peer review. Formal peer review programs are often one of the last formal evaluation procedures to be implemented in a health care organization.

Fundamentals of Peer Review

There are many possible variations in the peer review process. The observations may be shared only with the person being reviewed, with the person's supervisor, or with a review committee. The evaluation report may be written by the reviewer, or it may come from the review committee. The use of a committee defeats the purpose of peer review if the committee members are not truly peers of the individual being reviewed.

A Comprehensive Peer Review System

Peer review systems can simply be informal feedback regularly shared among colleagues, or they may be comprehensive systems that are fully integrated into the formal evaluation structure of a health care organization. When a peer review system is fully integrated, the evaluative feedback from one's peers is joined with the performance appraisals done by the nurse manager and both are used to determine pay raises and promotions for individual staff nurses. This is a far more collegial approach than the hierarchical one typically used, in which employees are evaluated only by their manager.

A comprehensive peer review system begins with the development of job descriptions (Boxes 3–4 & 3–5) and performance standards (Table 3–2) for each level within the nursing staff. When you compare Box 3–4, Box 3–5, and Table 3–2, you will see that the job description is a very general statement, whereas the standards are specific behaviors that can be observed and recorded.

In a participative environment, the standards are developed by committees having representatives from different units and from each staff level, from the new staff nurse to top-level management. In some instances, they are very specific, quantifiable criteria, but others are likely to require professional judgment as to the quality of the care provided (Chang et al., 2002).

> **BOX 3–4**
> **Sample Job Description: Clinical Nurse I (CN I)**
>
> The CN I supports the philosophy of primary nursing by planning and coordinating nursing care for a group of patients within his or her district.
>
> It is the CN I's responsibility to direct auxiliary personnel to fully implement the care plan.
>
> The CN I supports the management of the unit and uses resource persons and/or materials when need arises. He or she has satisfactorily mastered the basic skills required to work on the assigned unit.
>
> The CN I's scope of nursing practice is focused on an assigned group of patients and does not extend into the administration aspects of the unit at large.

In some organizations, the standards may be considered the minimal qualifications for each level. In this case, additional activities and professional development are expected before promotion to the next level. The candidate for promotion to an advanced-level position prepares a promotion portfolio for review (Schultz, 1993). The promotion portfolio may include a self-assessment, peer reviews, patient surveys, a management performance appraisal, and evidence of professional growth. Evidence of professional growth can be based on participating in the quality improvement program, evaluating a new product or procedure, serving as a translator or disaster volunteer, making postdischarge visits to clients from the unit, or taking courses related to nursing.

Writing useful job descriptions and measurable standards of performance is an arduous but rewarding task. It requires clarification and explication of the work nurses actually do and goes beyond the usual generalizations about what nursing is and what nurses do. Under effective group leadership and with strong administrative support for this process, it can be a challenging and stimulating experience. Without their support and guidance, however, the committee work can be frustrating when the group gets bogged down in details and disagreements.

When the job descriptions and performance standards for each level have been developed and agreed on, a procedure for their use must also be worked out. This can be done in several ways. In some organizations, an evaluation form that lists the performance standards can be completed by one or two colleagues selected by the individual staff member. In some organizations, the information from these forms is then used along with

> **BOX 3–5**
> **Sample Job Description: Clinical Nurse IV (CN IV)—Unit Clinician**
>
> The CN IV is an advanced clinical nurse who supports the practice of primary nursing on the unit, as well as hospital-wide. He or she is recognized within the specialty area and throughout the hospital as being proficient in the delivery of complicated nursing care.
>
> The CN IV has mastered the many facets of nursing care required at the CN II and CN III levels. This qualification is validated through the acquisition of national certification in the appropriate specialty area.
>
> The CN IV coordinates and directs emergency situations, seeks out learning opportunities for the unit staff, and serves as a resource for all aspects of nursing care delivery.
>
> The CN IV collaborates closely with physicians on the unit for the implementation of the care plan. This may be facilitated through assessing special equipment needs, as well as through planning multidisciplinary programs.
>
> The CN IV works closely with the nurse manager in planning unit goals and objectives and unit-specific orientation programs and assists with staff performance evaluations.
>
> The CN IV acts as a liaison between his or her unit and the Department of Nursing Education and Patient Education.

TABLE 3–2
Sample Performance Standards

Responsibility	CN I	CN II	CN III	CN IV
To Patient				
Plans care for duration of stay on clinical unit.	a. Family/social concerns are addressed in the assessment process, as evidenced by nursing care documentation. b. All admission documentation on assigned patients is recorded. c. History reflects information relevant to current hospitalization. d. Patient problem/outcome statements are current and/or designated as achieved. e. Patient teaching, transfer, and/or discharge preparation is documented.	a. through e. f. Utilizes nursing history for care planning by auditing charts for integration of problem statements. g. Assesses supplies/equipment and has them readily available for patient use. h. Initiates discharge summary sheet prior to discharge.	a. through h. i. Identifies need for and/or initiates appropriate family/social referrals with documentation. j. Assesses and documents cultural differences, patient support systems, and expectations for hospitalization. k. Documents patient's response to teaching as identified in nursing care documentation.	a. through k. l. Collaborates with the Department of Patient Education in designing and revising patient teaching materials.
To Peers				
Avails himself/herself to coworkers at all times.	a. Notifies peers when required to leave the clinical area. b. Assumes responsibility for IVs and orders of LPN on assigned patients. c. Responds promptly to all emergency situations that arise in the district.	a. through c. d. Takes initiative to offer assistance to other nurses and with assigned patients. e. Serves as preceptor to students/orientees.	a. through e. f. Acts as senior resource coordinator in absence of nurse manager.	a. through f. g. Coordinates/teaches two programs in conjunction with the Department of Nursing Education annually. h. Conducts staff conferences to evaluate clinical competencies of personnel with documentation.

Source: Adapted from Professional Nursing Advancement Program, Baptist Hospital of Miami, Florida.

the nurse manager's evaluation to determine pay raises and promotions. In others, the evaluation from one's peers is used for counseling purposes only and is not taken into consideration in determining pay raises or promotions. This second approach provides useful feedback but weakens the impact of peer review.

A different approach is the use of a professional practice committee. The committee, comprised of colleagues selected by the nursing staff, reviews the peer evaluation forms and makes its recommendations to the director of nursing or vice president for client care services, who then makes the final decision regarding the appropriate rewards (raises, promotions, commendations) or penalties (demotion, transfer, termination of employment).

Conclusion

A comprehensive evaluation system can be an effective mechanism both for increasing the quality of care by improving staff skills and morale and for reducing the costs of providing that care by increasing staff productivity. Constructive feedback demands objectivity and fairness in dealing with each other and leadership on the part of both staff members and management. Done well, it can provide many opportunities for increased professionalism and learning as well as ensure appropriate rewards for high performance levels and professionalism on the job.

Study Questions

1 Why is feedback important? Who needs to receive feedback? Who should give feedback to health care providers?

2 Describe the difference between constructive and destructive feedback.

3 Describe an ideal version of a 3-month performance appraisal of a new staff nurse. Why do nurse managers sometimes fail to meet this ideal when providing formal evaluative feedback? Can new staff nurses do anything to improve these procedures in their place of employment?

4 What is peer review? How is it different from other types of evaluation? Why is it important?

Critical Thinking Exercise

Tyrell Jones is a new unlicensed assistant who has been assigned to your acute rehabilitation unit. Tyrell is a hard worker; he comes in early and often stays late to finish his work. But Tyrell is gruff with the clients, especially with the male clients. If a client is reluctant to get out of bed, Tyrell often challenges him saying, "C'mon, man. Don't be such a wimp. Move your big butt." Today, you overheard Tyrell telling a female client who said she didn't feel well, "You're just a phony. You like being waited on, but that's not why you're here." The woman started to cry.

1 You are the newest staff nurse on this unit. How would you handle this situation? What would happen if you ignored it?

2 If you decided that you should not ignore it, with whom should you speak? Why? What would you say?

3 Why do you think Tyrell speaks to clients this way?

REFERENCES

Beer, M. (1981, Winter). Performance appraisal: Dilemmas and possibilities. *Organizational Dynamics, 24.*

Bowers, B., & Lapziger D. (2001). *The New York Times Management Reader.* New York: Times Books.

Chang, B.L., Lee, J.L., Pearson, M.L., Kahn, K.L., Elliott, M.N., & Rubenstein, L.L. (July/August 2002). Evaluating quality of nursing care. *Journal of Nursing Administration, 32*(7/8), 405–415.

Channer, P., & Hope, T. (2001). *Emotional Impact: Passionate Leaders and Corporate Transformation.* Hampshire, Great Britain: Palgrave.

DeMarco, R.F. (1998). Caring to confront in the workplace: An ethical perspective. *Nurse Outlook, 46,* 130–135.

Fonville, A.M., Killian, E.R., & Tranberger, R.E. (1998). Developing new nurse leaders. *Nurse Economics, 16,* 83–87.

Gabor, D. (1994). *Speaking Your Mind in 101 Difficult Situations.* New York: Stonesong Press (Simon & Schuster).

Gellerman, S.W., & Hodgson, W.G. (1988). Cyanamid's new take on performance appraisal. *Harvard Business Review, 88*(3), 36–41.

Hayes, H. (Winter 2002). Employee training and job descriptions. *Maryland Medicine, 3*(1), 39–41.

Hemman, E.A. (2002). Creating healthcare cultures of patient safety. *Journal of Nursing Administration, 32*(7/8), 419–427.

Katzenbach, J.R., & Smith, D.K. (2003). *The Wisdom of Teams.* New York: Harper Collins.

Kelly, J.A., & Aiken, E. (1999). Creating a legacy of leadership in the South. In Vance, C., & Olson, R.K. (eds.). *The Mentor Connection in Nursing* (pp. 164–167). New York: Springer.

Kron, T. (1981). *The Management of Patient Care: Putting Leadership Skills to Work.* Philadelphia: W.B. Saunders.

Lombardi, D.N. (2001). *Handbook for the New Health Care Manager.* San Francisco: Jossey-Bass.

Matejka, J.K., Ashworth, D.N., & Dodd-McCue, D. (1986). Discipline without guilt. *Supervisory Management, 31*(5), 34–36.

Mustard, L.W. (2002). Caring and competency. *JONA's Healthcare Law, Ethics and Regulation, 4*(2), 36–43.

Rosen, R.H. (1996). *Leading People: Transforming Business from the Inside Out.* New York: Viking Penguin.

Schultz, A.W. (1993). Evaluation for clinical advancement system. *Journal of Nursing Administration, 23*(2), 13–19.

Watson, T., & Harris, P. (1999). *The Emergent Manager.* London: Sage Publications.

CHAPTER 4

Dealing with Problems and Conflicts

OBJECTIVES

After reading this chapter, the student should be able to:

- Identify common sources of conflict in the workplace.

- Guide an individual or small group through the process of problem resolution.

- Participate in informal negotiations.

- Discuss the purposes of collective bargaining.

OUTLINE

Conflict

Sources of Conflict
Competition Between Groups
Increased Workload
Multiple Role Demands
Threats to Professional Identity and
  Territory
Threats to Safety and Security
Scarce Resources
Cultural Differences
Invasion of Personal Space

When Conflict Occurs

Resolving Problems and Conflicts
Win, Lose, or Draw?
Other Conflict Resolution Myths
Problem Resolution
  Identify the Problem or Issue
  Generate Possible Solutions
  Evaluate Suggested Solutions
  Choose the Best Solution
  Implement the Solution Chosen
  Is the Problem Resolved?
Negotiating an Agreement Informally
  Scope the Situation
  Set the Stage
  Conduct the Negotiation
  Agree on a Resolution of the Conflict
Formal Negotiation: Collective Bargaining
The Pros and Cons of Collective Bargaining

Conclusion

CHAPTER 4 SELF ASSESSMENT
How Do You Respond to Conflict?

Answer the following questions honestly:

1. When someone disagrees with you, do you usually
   a. Avoid the subject
   b. Try to find the basis for the disagreement
   c. Argue with the person

2. If you walked in on an argument between two nursing aides in the utility room, would you
   a. Turn around and leave
   b. Ask what the problem might be
   c. Tell them to stop arguing

3. If your paycheck were $100 less than you expected it to be, would you
   a. Wait to see if the shortfall was made up in the next pay period
   b. Call the payroll department to find out why it was short
   c. Tell payroll you want a check for the missing $100 immediately

4. If a patient told you he was going to sue the hospital after he was sent home, would you
   a. Try to be especially nice to him for the rest of his stay
   b. Find out how the hospital usually handles threats to sue
   c. Explain to him that lawsuits are one of the reasons health care is so expensive

5. If your team leader spends her day at the desk or in meetings and does not conduct patient rounds, would you
   a. Request reassignment to a better team leader
   b. Discuss the problem with the nurse manager
   c. Tell the team leader she's not setting a good example for the rest of the team

Assess Your Style

Problem Avoidance: If you selected *a* for most of your answers.

Negotiation and Resolution: If you selected *b* for most of your answers.

Direct Confrontation: If you selected *c* for most of your answers.

Each of us brings different experiences, beliefs, values, and habits with us to work. These differences are a natural part of our being unique individuals and members of different segments of our society. Various pressures and demands in the workplace also generate problems and conflicts among people at work. Any or all of these can interfere with our ability to work together. Consider Case 1, which is the first of three that will be used to illustrate how to deal with problems and conflicts.

◼ Conflict

There are no totally conflict-free work groups (Van de Vliert & Janssen, 2001). Small or large, conflicts are a daily occurrence in the life of a nurse manager (McElhaney, 1996), and they can interfere with getting the work done, as you will see in Case 1.

Unresolved conflicts have potentially harmful effects on people. Serious conflicts can be very stressful for the people involved. Stress symptoms such as difficulty concentrating, anxiety, sleep disorders, withdrawal, or other interpersonal relationship problems can occur. Bitterness, anger (Lombardi, 2001), even violence can erupt in the workplace if conflicts are not handled well.

Conflict also has a positive side, however. For example, in the process of learning how to manage conflict, people can develop more open, cooperative ways of working together (Tjosvold & Tjosvold, 1995). They can begin to see each other as people with similar needs, concerns, and dreams instead of as competitors or blocks in the way of progress.

Case 1

Team A and Team B

Team A has stopped talking to Team B. If several members of Team A are out sick, no one on Team B will help Team A with their work. Likewise, Team A members will not take telephone messages for anyone on Team B. Instead, they ask the person to call back later. When members of the two teams pass each other in the hall, they either glare at each other or turn away to avoid eye contact. Arguments erupt when members of the two teams need the same computer terminal or another piece of equipment at the same time.

When a Team A nurse reached for a pulse oximeter at the same moment as a Team B nurse did, the second nurse said, "You've been using that all morning."

"I've got a lot of patients to monitor," was the response.

"Oh, you think you're the only one with work to do?"

"We take good care of our patients."

"Are you saying we don't?"

The nurses fell silent when the nurse manager entered the room.

"Is something the matter?" she asked. Both nurses shook their heads and left quickly.

"I'm not sure what's going on here," the nurse manager thought to herself, "but something's wrong, and I need to find out what it is right away."

We will return to this case later as we discuss workplace problems and conflicts, their sources, and how to resolve them.

Being involved in successful conflict resolution can be an empowering experience (Horton-Deutsch & Wellman, 2002). Our goal in dealing with conflict is to create an environment in which conflicts are dealt with in as cooperative and constructive a manner as possible rather than in a competitive and destructive manner in order to be of greatest benefit to the people involved.

◘ Sources of Conflict

Why do conflicts occur? Health care brings people of different ages, genders, income levels, ethnic groups, educational levels, lifestyles, and professions together for the purpose of restoring or maintaining people's health. Differences of opinion over how to best accomplish this goal are a normal part of working with people of various skill levels and backgrounds (Wenckus, 1995). In addition, the workplace itself can be a generator of conflict (Box 4–1). Let's look at some of the most common reasons why conflict occurs in a workplace.

Competition Between Groups

An increase in tension between or among various groups of people within the workplace has been the subject of much interest in the media. Union–management conflicts regularly occur in some workplaces. Gender-based conflicts, including equal pay for women and sexual harassment issues, are other examples (Ehrlich, 1995).

Increased Workload

Emphasis on cost reductions has resulted in increased pressure to get as much work as possible out of each employee, sometimes more work than a person can reasonably do in a day (Trossman, 1999). This leaves many health care workers feeling that their employers are taking advantage of them (Ketter, 1994) and causes conflict if these workers believe others are not working as hard as they are.

Multiple Role Demands

Inappropriate task assignments (e.g., asking nurses to mop floors as well as nurse their clients), often the result of cost control efforts, can lead to disagreements about who does what task and who is responsible for the outcome.

Threats to Professional Identity and Territory

When role boundaries are blurred (sometimes even erased), professional identities are threatened and people may react in defense of them. Who, for example, is supposed to teach the discharged client about taking medication at home: the pharmacist, physician, nurse, or all three? If all three do this, who does what part of the teaching?

Threats to Safety and Security

When roles are blurred, cost saving is emphasized, and staff members face layoffs, individuals' economic security is threatened. This can be a source of considerable stress and tension (Qureshi, 1996; Rondeau & Wagar, 2002).

Scarce Resources

Inadequate money for pay raises, equipment, supplies, or additional help can increase competition between or among

BOX 4–1
Potential Conflict Generators

1. Competition between groups
2. Increased workload
3. Multiple role demands
4. Threats to professional identity and territory
5. Threats to safety and security
6. Scarce resources
7. Cultural differences
8. Invasion of personal space

Source: Adapted from McElhaney, R. (1996). Conflict management in nursing administration. *Nursing Management*, 27(3), 49–50.

departments and individuals as they scramble to grab their share of the little there is to distribute.

Cultural Differences

Different beliefs about how hard a person should work, what constitutes productivity, and even what it means to arrive at work "on time" can lead to problems if they are not reconciled.

Invasion of Personal Space

Crowded conditions and the constant interactions that occur at a busy nurses' station can increase interpersonal tension and lead to battles over precious work space (McElhaney, 1996).

◼ When Conflict Occurs

Conflicts can occur at any level and involve any number of people, including your boss, subordinates, peers, or patients (Sanon-Rollins, 2000). On the individual level, they can occur between two people working together on a team, between two people in different departments, or even between a staff member and a client or family member (Box 4–2). On the group level, conflict can occur between two teams (as in Case 1), two departments, or two different professional groups (e.g., nurses and social workers over who is responsible for discharge planning). On the organizational level, conflicts can occur between two organizations (e.g., when two home health agencies compete for a contract with a large hospital). Our focus in this chapter is primarily on the first two levels, between or among individuals and groups of people within a health care organization.

◼ Resolving Problems and Conflicts

Win, Lose, or Draw?

Some people think about problems and conflicts that occur at work in the same way as they think about a football game or tennis match: unless the score is tied at the end of the game, someone has to win and someone has to lose. There are some problems with this comparison to sports competition. First, our aim is to work together more effectively, not to defeat the other party. Second, the people who lose are likely to feel bad about losing. As a result, they may spend their time and energy preparing to win the next round, rather than on their work. Third, a tie (neither side wins or loses) may be just a stalemate; no one has won or lost, but the problem is also still there.

So the answer to the question "Win, lose, or draw?" is "none of the above." Instead, a win-win result in which both sides gain some benefit is the best resolution (Haslan, 2001).

Other Conflict Resolution Myths

Many people think of what can be "won" even in a win-win situation as a fixed amount: "I get half and you get half. The problem is that if I get three-quarters or all of what I wanted then you will only get one quarter or less of what you wanted." This is the *fixed pie* myth of conflict resolution (Thompson & Fox, 2001). Another erroneous assumption is called the *devaluation reaction*: "If the other side is getting what they want, that is, if what we've agreed to is good for them, then it has to be bad for us." The real

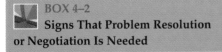

> **BOX 4–2**
> **Signs That Problem Resolution or Negotiation Is Needed**
>
> - You feel very uncomfortable in a situation.
> - Members of your team are having trouble working together.
> - Team members stop talking with each other, are withdrawing from conversation.
> - Team members begin "losing their cool," are attacking each other verbally.
>
> Source: Adapted from Patterson, K., Grenny, J., McMillan, R., & Surtzler, A. (18 March 2003). Crucial conversations: Making a difference between being healed and being seriously hurt. *Vital Signs, 13*(5), 14–15.

problem with these erroneous beliefs is that they can be serious barriers to achievement of a mutually beneficial (win-win) resolution of a conflict.

When differences and disagreements first arise, *problem solving* may be sufficient. If the situation has already developed into a full-blown conflict, however, *negotiation,* either informal or formal, of a settlement may be necessary.

Problem Resolution

The use of the problem-solving process in patient care should be familiar to you by now. The same approach can be used when staff problems occur. The goal is to find a solution to a given problem that satisfies everyone involved. The process itself, illustrated in Figure 4–1, includes identifying the issue or problem, generating possible solutions, evaluating the suggested solutions, choosing what appears to be the best solution, implementing that solution, evaluating the degree to which the problem has been resolved, and, finally, concluding either that the problem is

resolved or that it will be necessary to repeat the process to find a better solution.

Identify the Problem or Issue

Sometimes, it is easy to identify the real issue or problem. At other times, however, some discussion and exploration of the issues are necessary before the real problem emerges. "It would be nice," wrote Browne and Kelley, "if what other people were really saying was always obvious, if all their essential thoughts were clearly labeled for us . . . and if all knowledgeable people agreed about answers to important questions" (1994, p. 5). Of course, this is not what usually happens. People are often vague about what their real concern is; sometimes, they are genuinely uncertain about what the real problem is. Emotional involvement may further cloud the issue. All of this needs to be sorted out so that the problem is clearly identified and a solution can be sought.

Generate Possible Solutions

Here creativity is especially important. If you are guiding people through this process, try

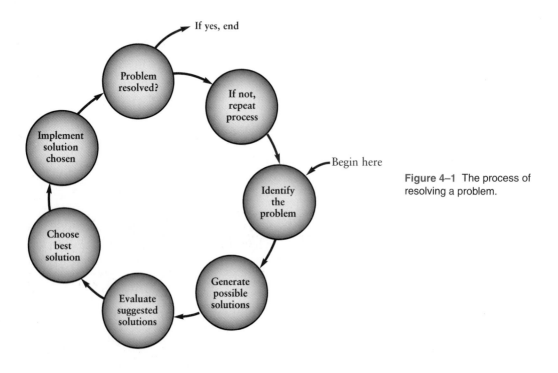

Figure 4–1 The process of resolving a problem.

to discourage them from using old solutions for new problems. It is natural for people to try to repeat something that worked well for them in the past, but solutions that were previously successful may not work in the future (Walsh, 1996). Instead, encourage people to spend some time searching for innovative solutions (Smialek, 2001).

Evaluate Suggested Solutions

An open-minded, objective evaluation of each suggestion is needed, but accomplishing this is not always easy. When a group problem solves, it is sometimes difficult to separate the suggestion from its source. For example, on an interdisciplinary team, the status of the person who made the suggestion may influence whether the suggestion is judged to be useful. Whose solution is most likely to be the best one: the physician's or the unlicensed assistant's? That depends. Judge the suggestion on its merits, not its source.

Choose the Best Solution

Which of the suggested solutions is most likely to work? A combination of suggestions is often the best solution.

Implement the Solution Chosen

The true test of any suggested solution is how well it actually works. Once a solution has been implemented, it is important to give it time to work. Impatience sometimes leads to premature abandonment of a good solution.

Is the Problem Resolved?

Not every problem is resolved successfully on the first attempt. If the problem has not been resolved, the process needs to be resumed with even greater attention to what the real problem is and how it can be successfully resolved.

Let's consider a situation in which problem solving was helpful (Case 2).

The nurse manager asked Ms. Deloitte to meet with her to discuss the problem. The following is a summary of the problem solving they did:

- **The Issue.** Ms. Deloitte wanted to take her vacation from the end of December through early January. Assuming this was all right, she had purchased nonrefundable tickets. The policy forbids vacations from December 20 to January 2nd. The

---

Case 2

The Vacation

Francine Deloitte has been a unit secretary for 10 years. She is prompt, efficient, accurate, courteous, flexible, and productive—everything a nurse manager could ask for in a unit secretary. When nursing staff members are very busy, she distributes afternoon snacks or sits with a family for, few minutes until a nurse is available. There is only one issue on which Ms. Deloitte is insistent and stubborn: taking her 2-week vacation over the Christmas and New Year holidays. This is forbidden by hospital policy, but every nurse manager has allowed her to do this because it is the only special request she ever makes and because it is the only time she visits her family during the year.

A recent reorganization of the administrative structure had eliminated several layers of nursing managers and supervisors. Each remaining nurse manager was given responsibility for two or three units. The new nurse manager for Ms. Deloitte's unit refused to grant her request for vacation time at the end of December. "I can't show favoritism," she explained. "No one else is allowed to take vacation time at the end of December." Assuming that she could have the time off as usual, Francine had already purchased a nonrefundable ticket for her visit home. When her request was denied, she threatened to quit. On hearing this, one of the nurses on Francine's unit confronted the new nurse manager saying. "You can't do this. We are going to lose the best unit secretary we've ever had if you do."

former nurse manager had not enforced this policy with Ms. Deloitte, but the new nurse manager wanted to enforce the policy with everyone, including Ms. Deloitte.

- **Possible Solutions**
  1 Ms. Deloitte resigns.
  2 Ms. Deloitte is fired.
  3 Allow Ms. Deloitte to take her vacation as planned.
  4 Allow everyone to take vacations between December 20 and January 5 as requested.
  5 Allow no one to take a vacation between December 20 and January 5.

- **Evaluate Suggested Solutions.** Ms. Deloitte preferred solutions 3 and 4. The new nurse manager preferred 5. Neither wanted 1 or 2. They could agree only that none of the solutions satisfied both of them, so they decided to try again.

- **Second List of Possible Solutions**
  1 Reimburse Ms. Deloitte for the cost of the tickets.
  2 Allow Ms. Deloitte to take one last vacation between December 20 and January 5.
  3 Allow Ms. Deloitte to take her vacation over Thanksgiving instead.
  4 Allow Ms. Deloitte to begin her vacation on December 26 so that she would work on Christmas Day but not on New Year's Day.
  5 Allow Ms. Deloitte to begin her vacation earlier in December so that she could return in time to work on New Year's Day.

- **Choose the Best Solution.** As they discussed the alternatives, Ms. Deloitte said that she could change the days of her flight without a penalty. The nurse manager said that she would allow solution 5 on the second list if Ms. Deloitte understood that she could not take vacation time between December 20 and January 5 in the future. Ms. Deloitte agreed to this.

- **Implement the Solution.** Ms. Deloitte returned on December 30 and worked both New Year's Eve and New Year's Day.

- **Evaluate the Solution.** The rest of the staff members had been watching the situation very closely. Most felt that the solution finally agreed on had been fair to them as well as to Ms. Deloitte. Ms. Deloitte felt she had been treated honestly and fairly. The nurse manager believed they had found a solution that was fair to Ms. Deloitte but still reinforced her determination to enforce the vacation policy.

- **Resolved or Resume Problem Solving?** Ms. Deloitte, staff members, and the nurse manager all felt that the problem had been solved satisfactorily.

Negotiating an Agreement Informally

When a problem has grown too big, too complex, or too heated, a more elaborate process may be required to resolve it. On evaluating Case 1, the nurse manager decided that the tensions between Team A and Team B had become so great that negotiation would be necessary.

The process of negotiation is a complex one that requires much careful thought beforehand and considerable skill in its implementation. Box 4–3 is an outline of the most essential aspects of negotiation. We will use Case 1 to illustrate how it can be done.

BOX 4–3
The Informal Negotiation Process

- Scope the situation. Ask yourself:
  - What am I trying to achieve?
  - What is the environment in which I am operating?
  - What problems am I likely to encounter?
  - What does the other side want?
- Set the stage.
- Conduct the negotiation.
  - Set the ground rules.
  - Clarify the problem.
  - Make your opening move.
  - Continue with offers and counteroffers.
- Agree on the resolution of the conflict.

Scope the Situation

To be successful, it is important to thoroughly understand the entire situation. Walker and Harris (1995) suggested asking yourself three questions:

1 What am I trying to achieve? The nurse manager in Case 1 is concerned about the tensions between Team A and Team B. She wants the members of these two teams to be able to work together in a cooperative manner, which they are not doing at the present time.

2 What is the environment in which I am operating? The members of Teams A and B were openly hostile to each other. The overall climate of the organization, however, was a benign one. The nurse manager knew that teamwork was encouraged and that her actions to resolve the conflict would be supported by administration.

3 What problems am I likely to encounter? The nurse manager knew that she had allowed the problem to go on too long. Even physicians, social workers, and visitors to the unit were getting caught up in the conflict. Team members were actively encouraging other staff to take sides, making clear they felt that "if you're not with us, you're against us." This made people from other departments very uncomfortable because they had to work with both teams. The nurse manager knew that resolution of the conflict would be a relief to many people.

It is important to ask one additional question in preparation for negotiations:

4 What does the other side want? In this situation, the nurse manager was not certain what either team really wanted. She realized that she needed this information before she could begin to negotiate.

Set the Stage

When a conflict such as the one between Teams A and B has gone on for some time, the opposing sides are often unwilling to meet to discuss the problem. If this occurs, it may be necessary to confront them with direct statements designed to open communications between the two sides and challenge them to seek resolution of the situation. At the same time, it is important to avoid any implication of blame because this provokes defensiveness rather than willingness to change.

To confront Teams A and B with their behavior toward one another, the nurse manager called them together at the end of the day shift. "I am very concerned about what I have been observing lately," she told them. "It appears to me that instead of working together, our two teams are working against each other." She continued with some examples of what she had observed, taking care not to mention individual names and not blaming anyone for the problem. She was also prepared to take responsibility for having allowed the situation to deteriorate before taking this much-needed action.

Conduct the Negotiation

As indicated earlier, conducting a negotiation requires a great deal of skill. Many conflicts become very emotional. Past experience may affect feelings about a current conflict. You or another individual involved in the conflict may have a grudge against someone who caused problems in the past (Barnes, 1998). Painful memories of previous unresolved conflicts may cause difficulty in making a clear-headed appraisal of the current situation. Recognizing the effect of these emotions is essential to negotiating effectively (Barnes, 1998). When faced with a highly emotional situation, do not respond with even more emotion. Instead, find out why emotions are high and refocus the discussion on the issues (Shapiro & Jankowski, 1998). Without effective leadership to prevent personal attacks, confrontation and negotiation can actually worsen the situation. With effective leadership, the conflict may be resolved (Box 4–4).

1 Set ground rules. Members of Teams A and B began flinging accusations at each other as soon as the nurse manager made her statement. The nurse manager stopped this quickly and said, "First, we need to set some ground rules for this discussion. Everyone

> ### BOX 4–4
> ### Tips for Leading the Discussion
>
> - Create a climate of comfort.
>   - Let others know the purpose is to resolve a problem or conflict.
>   - Freely admit to your own contribution to the problem or conflict.
>   - Begin with the presentation of facts.
>   - Recognize your own emotional response to the situation.
> - Set ground rules.
>   - Do not make personal remarks.
>   - Avoid placing blame.
>   - Allow each person an opportunity to speak.
>   - Do speak for yourself but not for others.
>   - Focus on solutions.
>   - Keep an open mind.
>
> Source: Adapted from Patterson, K., Grenny, J., McMillan, R., & Surtzler, A. (18 March 2003). Crucial conversations: Making a difference between being healed and being seriously hurt. *Vital Signs*, 13(5), 14–15.

will get a chance to speak, but not all at once. Please speak for yourself, not for others. And please do not make personal remarks or criticize your coworkers. We are here to resolve this problem, not to make it worse." She had to remind the group of these ground rules several times during the meeting. Teaching others how to negotiate often creates a more collaborative environment in which the negotiation will take place (Schwartz & Pogge, 2000).

2 Clarification of the problem. The nurse manager wrote a list of problems raised by team members on the board. As the list grew longer, she asked the group, "What do you see here? What is the real problem?" The group remained silent. Finally, someone in the back of the room said, "We don't have enough people, equipment, or supplies to get the work done." The rest of the group nodded in agreement.

3 Opening move. Once the problem is clarified, it is time to obtain everyone's agreement to discuss the matter and seek a way to resolve the conflict. In more formal negotia-

tions, you may make a statement about what you wish to achieve. For example, if you are negotiating a salary increase, you might begin by saying, "I am requesting a 10 percent increase for the following reasons . . . ." Of course, your employer will probably make a counteroffer, such as, "The best I can do is 3 percent." These are the opening moves of a negotiation.

4 Continue the negotiations. The discussion should continue in an open, nonhostile manner. Each side's concerns may be further explained and elaborated. Additional offers and counteroffers are common. As the discussion continues, it is usually helpful to emphasize areas of agreement as well as disagreement so that both parties are encouraged to continue the negotiations (Tappen, 2001).

Agree on a Resolution of the Conflict

After much testing for agreement, elaboration of each side's positions and concerns, and making of offers and counteroffers, the people involved should finally reach an agreement.

The nurse manager of Teams A and B led them through a discussion of their concerns related to working with severely limited resources. The teams soon realized that they had a common concern and that they might be able to help each other rather than compete with each other. The nurse manager agreed to become more proactive in seeking more resources for the unit. "We can simultaneously seek new resources and develop creative ways to use the resources we already have," she told the teams. Relationships between members of Team A and Team B improved remarkably after this meeting. They learned that they could accomplish more by working together than they had ever achieved separately.

Formal Negotiation: Collective Bargaining

There are many varieties of formal negotiations, from real estate transactions to international peace treaty negotiations. A formal negotiation process of special interest to nurses is collective bargaining, which is highly formalized because it is governed by law and contracts called *collective bargaining agreements.*

Collective bargaining involves a formal procedure governed by labor laws such as the National Labor Relations Act. Nonprofit health care organizations were added to the organizations covered by these laws in 1974. Once a union or professional organization has been designated as the official bargaining agent for a group of nurses, a contract defining such important matters as salary increases, benefits, time off, unfair treatment, and promotion of professional practice is drawn up. This contract then governs employee–management relations within the organization.

Case 3 is an example of how collective bargaining agreements can influence the outcome of a conflict between management and staff in a health care organization.

A collective bargaining contract is a legal document that governs the relationship between management and staff represented by the union (which, for nurses, may be the nurses' association or another health care workers' union). The contract may cover some or all of the following:

- **Economic issues.** Salaries, shift differentials, length of the workday, overtime, holidays, sick leave, breaks, health insurance, pensions, severance pay

- **Management issues.** Promotions, layoffs, transfers, reprimands, grievance procedures, hiring and firing procedures

---

Case 3

Collective Bargaining

The chief executive officer (CEO) of a large home health agency in a southwestern resort area called a general staff meeting. She reported that the agency had grown rapidly and was now the largest in the area. "Much of our success is due to the professionalism and commitment of our staff members," she said. "With growth come some problems, however. The most serious problem is the fluctuation in patient census. Our census peaks in the winter months when seasonal residents are here and troughs in the summer. In the past, when we were a small agency, we all took our vacations during the slow season. This made it possible to continue to pay everyone his or her full salary all year. However, given pressures to reduce costs and the large number of staff members we now have, we cannot continue to do this. We are very concerned about maintaining the high quality of patient care currently provided, but we have calculated that we need to reduce staff by 30 percent over the summer in order to survive financially."

The CEO then invited comments from the staff members. The majority of the nurses said they wanted and needed to work full-time all year. Most supported families and had to have a steady income all year. "My rent does not go down in the summer," said one. "Neither does my mortgage payment or the grocery bill," said another. A small number said that they would be happy to work part-time in the summer if they could be guaranteed full-time employment from October through May. "We have friends who would love this work schedule," they added.

"That's not fair," protested the nurses who needed to work full-time all year. "You can't replace us with part-time staff." The discussion grew louder and the participants more agitated. The meeting ended without a solution to the problem. Although the CEO promised to consider all points of view before making a decision, the nurses left the meeting feeling very confused and concerned about the security of their future income. Some grumbled that they probably should begin looking for new positions "before the ax falls."

The next day, the CEO received a telephone call from the nurses' union representative. "If what I heard about the meeting yesterday is correct," said the representative, "your plan is in violation of our collective bargaining contract." The CEO reviewed the contract and found that the representative was correct. A new solution to the financial problems caused by the seasonal fluctuations in patient census would have to be found.

• **Practice issues.** Adequate staffing, standards of care, code of ethics, other quality-of-care issues, staff development opportunities

Concerns over issues such as restructuring and lower levels of RN staffing have increased interest in unionization recently (Murray, 1999).

The Pros and Cons of Collective Bargaining

Some nurses think that it is unprofessional to belong to a union. Others point out that physicians and teachers are also union members and that the protections offered by a union outweigh the downside. There is no easy answer to this question.

Probably the greatest advantage of collective bargaining is protection of the right to fair treatment and the availability of a written grievance procedure that specifies both the employee's and the employer's rights and responsibilities if an issue or complaint arises that cannot be settled between employee and manager informally (Forman & Merrick, 2003). The greatest disadvantage of using collective bargaining as a way to deal with conflict is that it clearly separates management-level people from staff-level people. Any nurses who make staffing decisions may be classified as supervisors and be ineligible to join the union, separating them from the rest of their colleagues (Martin, 2001). The result is that "management" and "staff" are treated as opposing parties rather than as people who are trying to work together to provide essential services to their clients, which is our ultimate goal in dealing with problems and conflicts in the workplace. The collective bargaining contract also adds another layer of rules and regulations between staff members and their supervisors. Because management of such employee-related rules and regulations can take almost one-quarter of a manager's time (Drucker, 2002), this can become a drain on a nurse manager's time and energy.

▣ Conclusion

Conflict is inevitable within any large, diverse group of people who are trying to work together over an extended period of time. However, it does not have to be destructive, nor does it have to be a negative experience if it is handled skillfully by everyone involved. In fact, conflict can stimulate people to learn more about each other and how to work together in more effective ways. Resolution of a conflict, when it is done well, can lead to improved working relationships, more creative methods of operation, and higher productivity.

Study Questions

1   Debate the question of whether conflict is constructive or destructive. How can good leadership affect the outcome of a conflict?

2   Give an example of how each of the eight sources of conflict listed in this chapter can lead to a serious problem or conflict. Then discuss ways to prevent the occurrence of conflict from each of the eight sources.

3   What is the difference between problem resolution and negotiation? Under what circumstances would you use one or the other?

4   Identify a conflict (or potential conflict) in your clinical area and explain how either problem resolution or negotiation could be used to resolve it.

Critical Thinking Exercise

A not-for-profit hospice center in a small community received a generous gift from the grateful family of a client who had died recently. The family asked only that the money be "put to the best use possible."

Everyone in this small facility had an opinion about the best use for the money. The administrator wanted to renovate their old, run-down headquarters. The financial officer wanted to put the money in the bank "for a rainy day." The chaplain wanted to add a small chapel to the building. The nurses wanted to create a food bank to help the poorest of their clients. The social workers wanted to buy a van to transport clients to health care providers. The staff agreed that all the ideas had merit, that all of the needs identified were important ones. Unfortunately, there was only enough money to meet one of them.

The more the staff members discussed how to use this gift, the more insistent each group became that their idea was best. At their last meeting, it was evident that some were becoming frustrated and others were becoming angry. It was rumored that a shouting match between the administrator and the financial officer had occurred.

1 In your analysis of this situation, identify the sources of the conflict that are developing within this facility.

2 What kind of leadership actions are needed to prevent the escalation of this conflict?

3 If the conflict does escalate, how could it be resolved?

4 Which idea do you think has the most merit?

5 Why did you select the one you did?

6 Try role-playing a negotiation among the administrator, the financial officer, the chaplain, a representative of the nursing staff, and a representative of the social work staff. Can you suggest a creative solution?

REFERENCES

Barnes, G.P. (1998). *Successful Negotiating.* Franklin Lakes, N.J.: Career Press.

Browne, M.M., & Kelley, S.M. (1994). *Asking the Right Questions: A Guide to Critical Thinking.* Englewood Cliffs, N.J.: Prentice-Hall.

Drucker, P.F. (2002). They're not employees, they're people. *Harvard Business Review,* 80(2), 70–77, 128.

Ehrlich, H.J. (1995). Prejudice and ethnoviolence on campus. *Higher Education Extension Service Review,* 6(2), 1–3.

Forman, H., & Merrick, F. (2003). Grievances and complaints: Valuable tools for management and for staff. *Journal of Nursing Administration,* 33(3), 136–138.

Haslan, S.A. (2001). *Psychology in Organizations.* Thousand Oaks, Calif.: Sage.

Horton-Deutsch, S.L., & Wellman, D.S. (2002). Christman's principles for effective management. *Journal of Nursing Administration,* 32, 596–601.

Ketter, J. (1994). Protecting RNs with the Fair Labor Standards Act. *American Nurse,* 26(9), 1–2.

Lombardi, D.N. (2001). *Handbook for the New Health Care Manager.* San Francisco: Jossey-Bass.

Martin, R.H. (25 June 2001). Ruling may limit ability to unionize. *Advance for Nurses,* p. 9.

McElhaney, R. (1996). Conflict management in nursing administration. *Nursing Management,* 27(3), 49–50.

Murray, M.K. (1999). Is healthcare reengineering resulting in union organizing of registered nurses? *Journal of Nursing Administration,* 29(10), 4–7.

Patterson, K., Grenny, J., McMillan, R., & Surtzler, A. (18 March 2003). Crucial conversations: Making a difference between being healed and being seriously hurt. *Vital Signs,* 13(5), 14–15.

Qureshi, P. (1996). The effects of threat appraisal. *Nursing Management,* 27(3), 31–32.

Rondeau, K.V., & Wagar, T.H. (2002). Reducing the hospital workforce: What is the role of human resource management practices? *Hospital Topics, 89*(1), 12–18.

Sanon-Rollins, G. (2000). Surviving conflict on the job. *Nursing Spectrum Career Fitness Guide* (pp. 6767–6868). Barrington, Ill.: Gannett.

Schwartz, R.W., & Pogge, C. (2000). Physician leadership: Essential skills in a changing environment. *American Journal of Surgery, 180*(3), 187–192.

Shapiro, R.M., & Jankowski, M.A. (1998). *The Power of Nice.* New York: John Wiley & Sons.

Smialek, M.A. (2001). *Team Strategies for Success.* Lanham, Md.: The Scarecrow Press.

Tappen, R.M. (2001). *Nursing Leadership and Management: Concept and Practice.* Philadelphia: F.A. Davis.

Thompson, L., & Fox, C.R. (2001). Negotiation within and between groups in organizations: Levels of analysis. In M.E. Turner (ed.). *Groups at Work* (pp. 221–266). Mahwah, N.J.: Laurence Erlbaum.

Tjosvold, D., & Tjosvold, M.M. (1995). *Psychology for Leaders: Using Motivation, Conflict, and Power to Manage More Effectively.* New York: John Wiley & Sons.

Trossman, S. (1999). Stress! It's everywhere! And it can be managed. *American Nurse, 31*(4), 1–2.

Van de Vliert, E., & Janssen, O. (2001). Description, explanation and prescription of intragroup conflict behaviors. In M.E. Turner (ed.). *Groups at Work* (pp. 267–297). Mahwah, N.J.: Laurence Erlbaum.

Walker, M.A., & Harris, G.L. (1995). *Negotiations: Six Steps to Success.* Upper Saddle River, N.J.: Prentice-Hall.

Walsh, B. (3 June 1996). When past perfect isn't. *Forbes ASAP,* p. 18.

Wenckus, E. (21 February 1995). Working with an interdisciplinary team. *Nursing Spectrum,* 5, 12–14.

CHAPTER 5

People and the Process of Change

OBJECTIVES

After reading this chapter, the student should be able to:

- Describe the process of change.

- Recognize resistance to change and identify possible sources of resistance.

- Suggest strategies to reduce resistance to change.

- Assume a leadership role in implementing change.

OUTLINE

Change
A Natural Phenomenon
Macro and Micro Change
The Process of Change
The Comfort Zone
Resistance to Change
Sources of Resistance
  Technical Concerns
  Psychosocial Needs
  Position and Power
Recognizing Resistance
Lowering Resistance
  Dissemination of Information
  Disconfirmation of Currently Held Beliefs
  Provision of Psychological Safety
  Use of Command
Leading the Implementation of Change
Designing the Change
Planning the Implementation
Implementing the Change
Integrating the Change
Conclusion

CHAPTER 5 SELF-ASSESSMENT
Do You Know How to Play the Change Game?

Following is a list of "rules" for leading change. Mark each one either as a useful rule to *keep* or a rule to *delete*.

Rule 1. Squelch all dissent immediately—eliminate anyone who opposes the change.
Keep _____ Delete _____

Rule 2. Keep the pace of change high at all times.
Keep _____ Delete _____

Rule 3. Make sure everyone understands what changes will be made and why.
Keep _____ Delete _____

Rule 4. Keep everyone informed as the change progresses.
Keep _____ Delete _____

Rule 5. Don't allow any modifications once the change process is under way.
Keep _____ Delete _____

Rule 6. Demonstrate clearly why the change is a beneficial one.
Keep _____ Delete _____

Rule 7. Show people that the "old" way of doing things was not as good as the "new" way.
Keep _____ Delete _____

Keep: Rules 3, 4, 6, & 7

Delete: Rules 1, 2, & 5

When asked the theme of a recent nursing management conference, a top nursing executive thought for a moment and then replied, "Change, change, and more change." Whether we call it innovation, turbulence, or change, this theme seems to be a constant in the workplace today. For example, people working today can expect to make as many as 7 to 10 major job changes in their lifetime compared to their parents who, on average, made only 1 or 2 major job changes in their lives (Dent, 1995). In this chapter, we discuss the process of change, how people respond to change, and how leaders and managers can influence change and help people cope with change when it becomes overwhelming.

Change

A Natural Phenomenon

Change is a naturally occurring phenomenon, a part of everyone's lives. Every day, we have new experiences, meet new people, and learn something new. We grow up, leave home, graduate from college, and begin a career, perhaps a family as well. Some of these changes are milestones in our lives, ones we have prepared for and anticipated for some time. Others are entirely unexpected, sometimes welcome and sometimes not. Many are exciting, leading us to new opportunities and challenges. When change occurs too rapidly or demands too much of us, however, it can make us very uncomfortable (Bilchik, 2002).

Macro and Micro Change

The "ever-whirling wheel of change" (Dent, 1995, p. 287) in health care seems to spin faster every year. Cost reductions, managed care, Medicare and Medicaid reform, work redesign, restructuring, downsizing, and staff shortages are major concerns. Managed care alone has profoundly changed the way health care is delivered in many parts of the United States (Trinh & O'Connor, 2002). The changes sweeping through our health care system affect clients and caregivers alike. These changes are *macro level* (large scale) changes that affect virtually every health care facility. These macro-level changes are discussed in more detail in other chapters of this book.

Change anywhere in a system creates "ripples throughout the system" (Parker & Gadbois, 2000, p. 472). Every change that occurs at this macro level filters down to the *micro level* (small scale), to our teams, and to us as individuals. For better or worse, nurses, their colleagues in other disciplines, and their clients are participants in these changes. The micro level of change is the primary focus of this chapter.

◼ The Process of Change

The Comfort Zone

The basic stages of the change process are *unfreezing, change,* and *refreezing* (Lewin, 1951; Mander, Gomes, & Castle, 2002). Let's assume that a work situation is basically stable before change is introduced. Although some changes occur naturally, people are generally accustomed to each other, have a routine for doing their work, and feel that they know what to expect and how to deal with whatever problems may arise in the course of a day. In other words, they are operating within their "comfort zone" (Farrell & Broude, 1987; Lapp, 2002). A change of any magnitude is likely to move people out of this comfort zone into discomfort. This first stage in the change process is called *unfreezing* (Fig. 5–1).

Many health care institutions offer nurses the choice of weekday or weekend work on day, evening, or night shifts. Given these choices, nurses with young children are likely to find their comfort zone on weekday evening or night shifts. Imagine the discomfort they would experience if confronted with a change to alternate weekends or day shifts on call. Announcement of such a change would rapidly unfreeze their usual routine and move them into the discomfort zone. They might have to find a new babysitter or begin a search for a new child care center that is open on weekends. An alternative would be the establishment of a child care center where they work. Another alternative would be to find a new position that offers better working hours.

Whatever alternative they chose, the nurses would be challenged to find a solu-

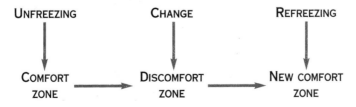

Figure 5–1 The change process. Source: Based on Farrell, K., & Broude, C. (1987). *Winning the Change Game: How to Implement Information Systems with Fewer Headaches and Bigger Paybacks.* Los Angeles: Breakthrough Enterprises; and Lewis, K. (1951). *Field Theory in Social Science: Selected Theoretical Papers.* New York: Harper & Row.

tion that allows them to move into a new comfort zone. To do this, they would have to find a consistent, dependable source of child care suited to their new schedule and to the needs of their children, in other words, find a way to move into a new comfort zone and *re-freeze* their situation. If the nurses did not find a satisfactory alternative, they could remain in an unsettled state, in a discomfort zone, caught in a conflict between their professional and personal responsibilities.

As this example illustrates, even what some people consider a small change can disturb the people involved in it. In the next section, we consider the many reasons that change is unsettling and why people resist it.

◼ Resistance to Change

People resist change for a variety of reasons, which vary from person to person and situation to situation. For example, you may find that one client care technician is delighted with an increase in responsibility and another one is upset about being given the same increase in responsibility. Some are ready to risk change; others seem to prefer the status quo (Hansten & Washburn, 1999). You may also find that one change in routine provokes a storm of protest, whereas another change is hardly noticed. Let's see why this is true.

Sources of Resistance

Resistance to change comes from three major sources: technical concerns, psychosocial needs, and threats to a person's position and power (Araujo Group).

Technical Concerns

Some resistance to change is based on concerns about whether the proposed change itself is a good idea. In some cases, these concerns are justified.

The Professional Practice Committee of a small hospital suggested replacing a commercial mouthwash with a mixture of hydrogen peroxide and water to save money. A staff nurse objected to this proposed change, saying that she had read a research study several years ago that found peroxide solutions to be an irritant to the oral mucosa (Tombes & Gallucci, 1993).

Fortunately, the chairperson of the Professional Practice Committee recognized that this objection was based on technical concerns and requested that a more thorough study of the research literature be done before instituting the change. "From now on," she told the staff nurse, "we will investigate the implications of a proposed change more thoroughly before recommending it. Thank you."

Psychosocial Needs

According to Maslow (1970), human beings have a hierarchy of needs, from basic physiological needs for oxygen, fluids, and nutrients to the higher-order needs for belonging, self-esteem, and self-actualization (Fig. 5–2). Maslow observed that the more basic needs (those lower on the hierarchy) must be at least partially met before a person is motivated to seek fulfillment of the higher-order needs.

Change can make it more difficult for a person to meet any or all of these physiolog-

EXAMPLES

Highest level	Self-actualization	Growth, development Fulfill potential
	Esteem	Self-esteem, respect Recognition
	Love and belonging	Acceptance, approval, inclusion, friendship
	Safety and security	Physical safety, trust Stability, assistance
Lowest level	Physiological needs	Air, water, food, sleep, shelter, sex, stimulation

Figure 5–2 Maslow's hierarchy of needs. Source: Based on Maslow, A.H. (1970). *Motivation and Personality.* New York: Harper & Row.

ical and psychosocial needs. For example, if a massive downsizing occurs and a person's job is eliminated, fulfillment of virtually all of these levels of needs may be threatened, from having enough money to pay for food and shelter to opportunities to fulfill one's career potential.

In other cases, the threat is subtler and may be harder for the leader or manager to anticipate. For example, an institution-wide evaluation of the effectiveness of the advanced practice role would be a great threat to a staff nurse who is working toward accomplishing a lifelong dream of becoming an advanced practice nurse in oncology. In contrast, it would have little impact on nursing aides unless an actual change in staffing occurred. A staff reorganization that involves reassigning aides to different units, however, would threaten the belonging needs of an aide who has very close friends on his or her unit but few friends outside work.

Position and Power

Status, power, and influence, once gained within an organization, are hard to give up. This applies to people anywhere in the organization, not just those at the top.

A clerk in the surgical suite had been preparing the operating room schedule for many years.

Although his supervisor really had the authority to revise the schedule, she rarely did so because the clerk was skillful in preparing realistic schedules that balanced the needs and desires of various parties, including some very demanding surgeons.

When the operating room supervisor was transferred to another facility, her replacement decided that she had to review the schedules before they were posted because they were ultimately her responsibility. The clerk became defensive. He tried to avoid the supervisor and posted the schedules without her approval whenever he could. This surprised the new supervisor. She had heard how skillful the clerk was and did not think that her review of the schedules would be threatening. She had not realized the importance of this task to the clerk.

The opportunity to tell others when and where they could operate had given this clerk a feeling of power and importance. The supervisor's insistence on reviewing his work reduced the importance of his position.

What seemed to the new supervisor to be a very small change in routine had provoked surprisingly strong resistance because it threatened the clerk's position and power within the organization.

As you will learn in Chapter 6 on power and organizations, empowerment is a source of motivation and satisfaction for most people. Although some changes empower people, others threaten their sense of empowerment, especially when they feel that the change was imposed on them and that they had no choice in the matter.

Recognizing Resistance

It is easy to recognize resistance to a change when it is expressed directly. When a person says to you, "That's not a very good idea," "I'll quit if you reassign me to the night shift," or "There's no way I'm going to do that," there is no doubt that you are encountering resistance. When resistance is less direct, however, it can be difficult to recognize unless you know what to look for.

Resistance may be *active* or *passive* (Heller, 1998). Active resistance can take the form of attacks or outright refusals to comply, such as the statements in the previous paragraph, writing "killer" memos that destroy the idea or the person who suggested it, quoting existing rules that make the change difficult or impossible to implement, or organizing resistance to the change (encouraging others to resist). Passive approaches use avoidance: canceling appointments to discuss implementation of the change, being too busy to make the change, refusing to commit to changing or agreeing to it but doing nothing to change, and simply ignoring the entire process as much as possible (Table 5–1). Once resistance has been recognized, action can be taken to lower or even eliminate it.

TABLE 5–1

Resistance to Change

Active	Passive
Attacking the idea	Avoiding discussion
Refusing to change	Ignoring the change
Arguing against the change	Refusing to commit to the change
Organizing resistance of other people	Agreeing but not acting

Lowering Resistance

A great deal can be done to lower people's resistance to change. Strategies fall into four categories: dissemination of information, disconfirmation of currently held beliefs, provision of psychological safety, and use of command (Tappen, 2001).

Dissemination of Information

Much resistance is simply the result of misunderstandings about a proposed change. Sharing information about the proposed change can be done on a one-to-one basis, in group meetings, or through written materials distributed to everyone involved using print or electronic means.

Disconfirmation of Currently Held Beliefs

Leaders can take action that provides a catalyst for change (Lichiello & Madden, 1996). For example, simply providing disconfirming information is often persuasive enough to lower resistance to change when people are reluctant to give up their current beliefs, opinions, or comfortable routines. When this happens, providing evidence that what people are doing or believing is inadequate, incorrect, or inefficient can increase their willingness to change.

Jolene was a little nervous when it was her turn to present information on a new enteral feeding procedure to the Clinical Practice Committee. Committee members were very demanding: they wanted clear, research-based information presented in a concise manner. Opinions, generalities, and vague references ("Somebody told me . . . ") were not acceptable. She had prepared thoroughly and even practiced her presentation at home until she could speak without referring to her notes.

The presentation went well. Committee members commented on the thoroughness of her presentation and the quality of the information presented. To her disappointment, however, no action was taken on her proposal to adopt the new procedure. Returning to her unit, she shared her disappointment with the nurse manager. Together, they reviewed the presentation using the unfreezing–change–refreezing process for bringing about change as a guide.

The nurse manager agreed that Jolene had thoroughly reviewed the information on enteral feeding. The problem, she explained, was that Jolene had not attended to the need to unfreeze a situation to lower resistance to change. As they talked, Jolene realized that she had not put any emphasis on the high risk of contamination and resulting gastrointestinal disturbances of the procedure currently in use. In other words, members of the committee were still feeling comfortable with the current procedure because she had not emphasized the risk involved in failing to change it.

At the next meeting, Jolene presented additional information on the risks associated with the current enteral feeding procedures. This *disconfirming evidence* was persuasive. The committee accepted her proposal to adopt the new, lower risk procedure.

Without the addition of the disconfirming evidence that Jolene presented at the second meeting, it is likely that her proposed change in procedure would never have been implemented. The *inertia* (tendency to remain in the same state rather than to move toward change) exhibited by the Clinical Practice Committee is not unusual (Pearcey & Draper, 1996).

Provision of Psychological Safety

When a proposed change threatens the basic human needs of individuals or groups of individuals in some way, resistance can be lowered by reducing that threat, leaving people feeling more comfortable about the proposed change. Although each situation poses different kinds of threats and requires different actions to reduce these threats, the following is a list of common strategies that help increase psychological safety and reduce resistance to change:

- Point out the similarities between the old and new procedures.

- Express approval of people's concern for providing the best care possible.

- Recognize the competence and skill of the people involved.

- Provide assurance (if possible) that no one will lose his or her position because of the change.

- Suggest ways in which the change can provide new opportunities and challenges (that is, new ways to increase self-esteem and self-actualization).

- Express your valuing of each individual's and group's contributions in general and to the proposed change.

• Ensure involvement of as many people as possible in both the design of the change and the implementation.

• Provide opportunities for people to express their feelings and ask questions about the proposed change.

• Allow time for practice and learning of any new procedures, if possible, before a change is implemented.

• Provide a climate of acceptance in which some mistakes can be made without negative consequences for individuals.

When all of the preceding items are done in a climate of trust and acceptance of each other's differences, changes are far easier to implement.

Use of Command

This is an entirely different approach to change. People in authority within an organization can simply *require* people to make a change in what they are doing or can reassign people to new positions (Porter-O'Grady, 1996). This is effective in many situations but may not work well if there are ways for people to resist:

• When passive resistance can undermine the change

• When high motivational levels are necessary to make the change successful

• When people can refuse to obey the order without negative consequences.

Communicating a sense of urgency and necessity regarding the change to be made will reinforce the use of authority (Kotter, 1999).

The following is an example of an unsuccessful attempt to bring about change by command:

A new and still insecure nurse manager believed that her staff members were taking advantage of her inexperience by taking more than the two 15-minute coffee breaks allowed during an 8-hour shift. She decided that staff members would have to sign in and out for their coffee breaks as well as for their 30-minute meal break.

The staff members were outraged by this change. Most had been taking fewer than two 15-minute coffee breaks and 30 minutes for meals because of the heavy client care demands of the unit.

Staff members refused to sign the coffee break sheet. When asked why they hadn't signed it, they replied "I forgot," "I couldn't find it," or "I was called away before I had a chance." This organized passive resistance was sufficient to overcome the nurse manager's authority. The nurse manager decided that the coffee break sheet had been a mistake, removed it from the bulletin board, and never spoke of it again.

For people in authority, acting by command often seems to be the easiest way to bring about change: just tell people what to do and don't listen to any arguments about it. There is risk in this approach, however. High levels of involvement in planning the change may slow down the process of implementation (and sometimes results in a standoff and no change), but it usually produces a high level of commitment to the change once it is accepted (Conger, Spreitzer, & Lawler, 1999). Even when staff members do not resist authority-based change, overuse of commands can lead to staff members who are passive, dependent, unmotivated, and unempowered. Providing high-quality patient care requires staff members who are active, motivated, and highly committed to their work, just the opposite of the results of authority-based change.

■ Leading the Implementation of Change

Given the current climate of "change, change, and more change," even experienced leaders can find themselves overwhelmed unless they approach it in an organized fashion and keep the ultimate goal in mind (Porter-O'Grady, 2003). New graduates may find themselves given responsibility for bringing about change. Following are some examples of the kinds of changes that you might be asked to assist in implementing:

• Revising an old procedure or adding a new technical procedure.

- Devising new ways to record, store, and retrieve patient data.

- Developing new policies for staff evaluation and promotion.

- Participating in quality improvement projects.

- Preparing for accreditation visits and inspections.

Now that you understand how change can affect people and have learned some ways to lower their resistance to change, we can discuss taking a leadership role in successful implementation of change.

The entire process of bringing about change can be divided into four phases: designing the change itself, deciding how to implement the change, the actual implementation of the change, and following through to ensure that the change has been integrated into the regular operation of the facility (Fig. 5–3).

Designing the Change

This is the starting point in the change process. The leader communicates a vision and guides the process of change (Holland, 2002). The first step in bringing about change is to carefully craft the change itself. Not every change is for the better: some changes

DESIGN THE CHANGE

PLAN THE IMPLEMENTATION

IMPLEMENT THE CHANGE

INTEGRATE THE CHANGE

Figure 5–3 Four phases of planned change.

fail because they are poorly conceived in the first place.

Ask yourself:

- What is the purpose of this change? What are we trying to accomplish?

- Is the change necessary?

- Is the change technically correct?

- Will this change work?

- Is there a better way to do this?

This is a good time to use creativity and innovation (Handy, 2002). Encourage people to talk about the changes planned, to express their doubts, and to provide their input (Fullan, 2001). Those who do are usually enthusiastic supporters later on in the process.

Planning the Implementation

The next step is to prepare a careful plan to implement the change. All the information presented previously about sources of resistance and ways to overcome that resistance should be taken into consideration when deciding how to implement a change.

Ask yourself:

- Why might people resist this change?

- Would their resistance be justified?

- What can be done to prevent or overcome this resistance?

The context in which the change will take place is another factor to consider when assessing resistance to change (Lichiello & Madden, 1996). This includes the amount of change occurring at the same time, the organizational climate, and the environment surrounding the organization. For example, there may be external pressure to change because of the competitive nature of the health care market in your community. In other situations, government regulations may make it difficult to bring about a desired change.

Almost everything that you have learned about effective leadership is useful in planning the implementation of change: setting the vision (Sproat, 2001), motivating people, involving people in decisions that affect them, dealing with conflict, eliciting cooperation, providing coordination, and fostering teamwork. Remember, you do have to move people out of their comfort zone to unfreeze the situation and get them ready to change (Flower & Gillaume, 2002). Consider all of these things when formulating a plan to implement a proposed change, then act on them in the next step: implementing the change.

Implementing the Change

Now, finally, you are ready to make the change that has been carefully planned. In addition to the strategies to lower resistance, increase motivation, and help people work well together, consider the following factors related to change.

Ask yourself:

• What is the magnitude of this change? Is this a major change that affects almost everything people do, or is it a minor one with little impact on what people do every day?

• What is the complexity of this change? Is this a difficult change to make? Does it require much new knowledge or skill, or both? How long will it take for people to acquire the necessary knowledge and skill?

• What is the pace of the change? How urgent is this change? Can it be done gradually or must it be implemented all at once?

• What is the current stress level of the people involved in this change? Is this the only change that is taking place, or is it just one of many changes taking place? How stressful are these changes? How can you help people keep their stress levels within tolerable bounds?

As indicated earlier, some discomfort is likely to occur with almost any change, but it is important to keep it within tolerable limits. You need to have sufficient pressure to make people pay attention to the change process but not so much that they are overstressed by it. In other words, you want to raise the heat enough to get them moving but not so high that they boil over (Heifetz & Linsky, 2002).

Integrating the Change

Don't forget this last step. After the change has been made, it is important to make sure that everyone has moved into a new "comfort zone."

Ask yourself:

• Is the change well integrated into everyday operations?

• Are people comfortable with it now?

• Is it well accepted? If not, why not? What can be done to increase acceptance? Is there any residual resistance that could still undermine full integration of the change? If there is, how can this resistance be overcome?

As Kotter noted, change "sticks" when, instead of being the new way to do something, it has become "the way we always do things around here" (1999, p. 18).

◼ Conclusion

Change is an inevitable part of living and working. How people respond to change, the amount of stress it causes, and the amount of resistance it provokes can be influenced by your leadership. Handled well, most changes can become opportunities for professional growth and development rather than just additional stressors with which nurses and their clients have to cope.

Study Questions

1 Why is change inevitable? What would happen if no change at all occurred in health care?

2 Why do people resist change?

3 How can leaders overcome resistance to change?

4 Describe the process of implementing a change from beginning to end. Use an example from your clinical experience to illustrate this process.

Critical Thinking Exercise

A large health care corporation recently purchased a small (50-bed) rural nursing home. A new director of nursing was brought in to replace the former one, who had retired after 30 years at this facility.

The new director addressed the staff members at the reception held to welcome him. "My philosophy is that you cannot manage anything that you haven't measured. Everyone tells me that you have all been doing an excellent job here. With my measurement approach, we will be able to analyze everything you do and become more efficient than ever."

The nursing staff members soon found out what the new director meant by his measurement approach. Every bath, episode of incontinence care, feeding of a resident, or trip off the unit had to be counted, and the amount of time each activity required had to be recorded. Nurse managers were required to review these data with staff members every week, questioning any time that was not accounted for. Time spent talking with families or consulting with other staff members was considered time wasted unless the staff member could justify the "interruption" in his or her work.

No one complained openly about the change, but absenteeism rates increased rapidly. Personal day and vacation time requests soared. Staff members nearing retirement crowded the tiny personnel office, overwhelming the single staff member with their requests to "tell me how soon I can retire on full benefits." The director of nursing found that shortage of staff was becoming a serious problem and that few new applications were coming in, despite the fact that this rural area offered few good job opportunities.

1 What evidence of resistance to change can you find in this case study?

2 What kind of resistance to change did the staff members of this nursing home exhibit?

3 If you were a staff nurse at this facility, how do you think you would have reacted to this change in administration?

4 Why did staff members resist this change?

5 What could the director of nursing do to increase acceptance of this change? What could the nurse managers and staff nurses do?

REFERENCES

Araujo Group. *A Compilation of Opinions of Experts in the Field of the Management of Change.* Unpublished report.

Bilchik, G.S. (May 2002). Are you the problem? *Hospitals and Health Networks Magazine,* 38–42.

Conger, J., Spreitzer, G., & Lawler, E.E. (1999). *The Leader's Change Handbook.* San Francisco: Jossey-Bass.

Dent, H.S. (1995). *Job Shock: Four New Principles Transforming Our Work and Business.* New York: St. Martin's Press.

Farrell, K., & Broude, C. (1987). *Winning the Change Game: How to Implement Information Systems with Fewer Headaches and Bigger Paybacks.* Los Angeles: Breakthrough Enterprises.

Flower, J., & Guillaume, P. (March/April 2002). Surfing the edge of chaos. *Health Forum Journal,* 17–20.

Fullan, M. (2001). *Leading in a Culture of Change.* San Francisco: Jossey-Bass.

Handy, C. (June 2002). The elephant and the flea: Looking backward to the future. *Times Literary Supplement,* no. 5157, 30.

Hansten, R.I., & Washburn, M.J. (1999). Individual and organizational accountability for development of critical thinking. *Journal of Nursing Administration,* 29(11), 39–45.

Heifetz, R.A., & Linsky, M. (June 2002). A survival guide for leaders. *Harvard Business Review,* 65–74.

Heller, R. (1998). *Managing Change.* New York: DK Publishing.

Holland, L.E. (2002). *Change Is the Rule: Practical Actions for Change: On Target, on Time, on Budget.* Chicago: Dearborn.

Kotter, J.P. (1999). Leading change: The eight steps to transformation. In J.A. Conger, G.M. Spreitzer, & E.E. Lawler (eds.). *The Leader's Change Handbook.* San Francisco: Jossey-Bass.

Lapp, J. (May 2002). Thriving on change. *Caring Magazine,* 40–43.

Lewin, K. (1951). *Field Theory in Social Science: Selected Theoretical Papers.* New York: Harper & Row.

Lichiello, P., & Madden, C.W. (1996). Context and catalysts for change in health care markets. *Health Affairs,* 15(2), 121–129.

Mander, A., Gomes, A., & Castle, D. (2002). The management of change in a community mental health team. *Australian Health Review* 25(2), 115–121.

Maslow, A.H. (1970). *Motivation and Personality.* New York: Harper & Row.

Parker, M., & Gadbois, S. (2000). Building community in healthcare workplace. Part 3: Belonging and satisfaction at work. *Journal of Nursing Administration,* 30, 466–473.

Pearcey, P., & Draper, P. (1996). Using the diffusion of innovation model to influence practice: A case study. *Journal of Advanced Nursing,* 23, 724–726.

Porter-O'Grady, T. (1996). The seven basic rules for successful redesign. *Journal of Nursing Administration,* 26(1), 46–53.

Porter-O'Grady, T. (2003). A different age for leadership, part 1. *Journal of Nursing Administration,* 33(2), 105–110.

Sproat, S.B. (2001). Using organizational artifacts to influence change. *Journal of Nursing Administration,* 31, 524–526.

Tappen, R.M. (2001). *Nursing Leadership and Management: Concept and Practice.* Philadelphia: F.A. Davis.

Tombes, M.B., & Gallucci, B. (1993). The effects of hydrogen peroxide rinses on the normal oral mucosa. *Nursing Research,* 42, 332–337.

Trinh, H.Q., & O'Connor, S.J. (2002). Helpful or harmful? The impact of strategic change on the performance of U.S. urban hospitals. *Health Services Research,* 37(1), 145–171.

UNIT II

Working Within the Organization

6 Organizations, Power, and Empowerment

7 Delegation of Client Care

8 Managing Client Care

9 Time Management

10 Work-Related Stress and Burnout

11 The Workplace

CHAPTER 6

Organizations, Power, and Empowerment

OBJECTIVES

After reading this chapter, the student should be able to:

- Recognize differences in sponsorship, culture, goals, structure, and informal processes in various health care organizations.

- Define power and empowerment.

- Identify sources of power in a health care organization.

- Describe several ways in which nurses can be empowered.

OUTLINE

Understanding Organizations
Types of Health Care Organizations
Organizational Cultures
Goals
Structure
  The Traditional Approach
  More Innovative Approaches
Processes
Power
Definition
Sources
Empowering Nurses
Professional Organizations
Collective Bargaining
Participation in Decision Making
Shared Governance
Enhancing Expertise
Conclusion

CHAPTER 6 SELF ASSESSMENT
How Empowered Do You Feel?

Choose an organization in which you actively participate—school, job, religious organization, or large social club—and rate your sense of empowerment in that organization:

1. Do you feel that you are an important member of this organization?
   Yes _____ No _____

2. If you made a suggestion for change, would this suggestion be given serious consideration?
   Yes _____ No _____

3. Do you feel that you have a voice in deciding the direction of the organization?
   Yes _____ No _____

4. Do you have a say in the way in which you function/participate/work in this organization?
   Yes _____ No _____

5. Can you decide or at least influence your future direction/roles in the organization?
   Yes _____ No _____

The subjects of this chapter—organizations, power, and empowerment—are not as remote from a nurse's everyday experience as you may first think. Consider two scenarios, which are analyzed later in the chapter.

SCENARIO 1

In school, Hazel Rivera had always received high praise for the quality of her nursing care plans. "Thorough, comprehensive, systematic, holistic—beautiful!" was the comment she received on the last one she wrote before graduation.

Now Hazel is a staff nurse on a busy orthopedic surgery unit. Although her time to write comprehensive care plans during the day is limited, Hazel often stays after work to complete them. Her friend Carla refuses to stay late with her. "If I can't complete my work during the shift, then they have given me too much to do," she said.

At the end of their 3-month probationary period, Hazel and Carla received written evaluations of their progress and comments about their value to the organization. To Hazel's surprise, her friend Carla received a higher rating than she did. What happened?

Were the disappointments experienced by Hazel Rivera and the critical care department staff predictable? Could they have been avoided? Without a basic understanding of the organizations within which we work and of the part that power plays in the decision-making processes that occur within health care institutions, we are doomed to be continually surprised by the responses to our well-intentioned efforts. As you read this chapter, you will learn why Hazel Rivera and the critical care department staff were disappointed.

SCENARIO 2

The nursing staff of the critical care department of a large urban hospital formed a research utilization group about a year ago. They had made many changes in their practice based on reviews of the research on several different procedures and were quite pleased with the results.

"Let's look at the bigger picture next month," their nurse manager suggested at one of their meetings. "This time, let's look at the research on different models of client care. We might get some good ideas for our unit." The staff nurses agreed. It would be a nice change to look at the way they organized client care in their department.

The nurse manager found a wealth of information on different models for organizing nursing care. One research study about a model for caring for the chronically critically ill (Rudy et al., 1995) particularly interested them because they had had many clients in that category.

Several nurses volunteered to form an ad hoc committee to design a similar unit for the chronically critically ill within their critical care department. When the plan was presented, both the nurse manager and the staff thought it was excellent. The nurse manager offered to present the plan to the vice president for nursing. The staff eagerly awaited the vice president's response.

The nurse manager returned with discouraging news. The vice president did not support their concept and said that, although they were free to continue developing the idea, they should not assume that it would ever be implemented. What happened?

We begin by looking at some of the characteristics of the organizations in which nurses work and how these organizations operate. Then we zero in on the subject of power within organizations: what it is, how one obtains it, and how nurses can become empowered.

◼ Understanding Organizations

One of the attractive features of nursing as a career is the wide variety of settings in which nurses can work. From rural migrant health clinics to organ transplant units, nurses' skills are needed wherever there are concerns about people's health. Relationships with clients may extend for months or years, as they do in school health or in nursing homes, or they may be brief and never repeated, as often happens in doctors' offices, clinics, and emergency departments.

Types of Health Care Organizations

Although some nurses work as independent practitioners, as consultants, or in the corporate world, the majority are employed by health care organizations. These organizations can be classified into three types on the basis of their sponsorship and financing:

1 Private not-for-profit. Many health care organizations were founded by civic, charitable, or religious groups. Some have been in existence for generations. Many of our hospitals, long-term care facilities, home care services, and community agencies began this way.

2 Publicly supported. Government-operated service organizations range from county public health departments to complex medical centers, such as those operated by the Veterans Administration, a federal agency.

3 Private for-profit. Increasing numbers of health care organizations are operated for profit like any other business. These include large hospital and nursing home chains, health maintenance organizations (HMOs), and many freestanding centers that provide special services, such as surgical and diagnostic centers.

The differences between these categories have become blurred for many reasons:

- All compete for clients, especially for clients with health care insurance or the ability to pay their own health care bills.

- All are feeling the effect of cost constraints.

- All may provide services that are eligible for government reimbursement, particularly Medicaid and Medicare funding, if they meet government standards.

Organizational Cultures

The size and complexity of many health care organizations make them difficult to understand. One way to begin to develop an understanding is to find a colorful image or metaphor that sums up their characteristics in a few well-chosen words. Morgan (1997) suggested using animals or other familiar images to describe an organization. For example, an aggressive organization that crushes its competitors could be likened to a bull elephant, whereas a timid organization in danger of being crushed by that bull elephant could be described as a mouse. Using another metaphor, an organization adrift without a clear idea of its future could be described as a "rudderless boat on a stormy sea," whereas an organization with its sights set clearly on exterminating its competition could be described as a "guided missile."

Organizational cultures differ a great deal. Some are very traditional, preserving their customary ways of doing things even when these processes no longer work well. Others are very progressive, eternally chasing the newest management fad or buying the latest high-tech equipment. Some seem to be warm, friendly, and open to new people and new ideas. Others are cold, defensive, and indifferent or even hostile to the outside world (Tappen, 2001). These very different organizational cultures have a considerable effect on the employees and the people served by the organization. The culture shapes people's behavior, especially their responses to each other, a particularly important factor in health care.

The culture of an organization is intangible; you cannot see it or touch it but you will recognize it when you bump up against it. Also called the "soul" or "personality" of an organization, its culture is a unique constellation of roles, norms, and values (Atchison, 2002; Haslam, 2001; Stegall, 2002). To find out what the culture of an organization is when

you are applying for a new position or trying to familiarize yourself with your new workplace, you can ask several people who work there or have considerable familiarity with the organization to describe it in just a few words. Once you have grasped the totality of an organization in terms of its overall culture, you are ready to analyze it in a little more detail. This involves understanding the *roles* (place and function of different people in the organization), *norms* (expected attitudes and behaviors), and *values* (principles intended to guide the operation of the organization) (Haslam, 2001), and identifying the organization's goals, structure, and processes.

Goals

Try answering this true-or-false question:

Question: The primary goal of any health care organization is to keep people healthy, restore them to health, or assist them in dying as comfortably as possible. True or false?

Answer: False. The previous statement is only partially correct. Most health care organizations have several goals, some more immediately apparent than others.

What other goals might a health care organization have? Following are some examples:

- **Survival.** Organizations have to maintain their own existence, a goal that is threatened when, for example, reimbursements are reduced, competition increases, or the organization fails to meet the Joint Commission on Accreditation of Healthcare Organizations' (JCAHO) standards or is unable to collect money owed by its clients (Trinh & O'Connor, 2002).

- **Growth.** The chief executive officers (CEOs) of many organizations also want their organizations to grow by expanding into new territories, adding new services, and bringing in new clients.

- **Profit.** For-profit organizations are expected to return some profit to their owners. Not-for-profit organizations have to be able to pay their bills and to avoid slipping into too much debt. This is sometimes difficult for an organization.

• **Status.** The leaders or owners of many health care organizations also want to be known as the best in their field, for example, by having the best open-heart surgeon, providing "the best nursing care in the world" (Frusti, Niesen, & Campion, 2003, p 34), having top-notch nurses, or providing the most attractive patient rooms in town.

• **Dominance.** Some organizations also want to drive others out of the health care business or gobble them up, surpassing the goal of survival and moving toward dominance of a particular market by driving out the competition.

These additional goals are not discussed in public as often as the first, more lofty statement of goals in our true-or-false test. However, they still drive the organization, especially the way the organization handles its finances and treats its employees.

These goals may have profound effects on every one of the organization's employees, nurses included. For an example, let's return to the story of Hazel Rivera. Why did she receive a less favorable rating than her friend Carla?

After comparing ratings with her friend Carla, Hazel scheduled another meeting with her nurse manager to discuss her evaluation. The nurse manager explained the rating: Hazel's care plans were very well done, and she genuinely appreciated Hazel's efforts to make them so. The problem was that Hazel had to be paid overtime for this work according to the union contract, and this had reduced the amount of overtime pay the nurse manager had available when the patient care load was especially high. "The corporation is very strict about staying within the budget," she said. "In fact, my rating is higher when I don't use up all of the budgeted overtime hours."

When Hazel asked what she could do to improve her rating, the nurse manager offered to help her streamline the care plans and manage her time better so that the care plans could be done during her shift.

Structure

The Traditional Approach

Virtually all health care organizations have a hierarchical structure of some kind (Box 6–1). In a *traditional hierarchical structure,* employees are ranked from the top to the bottom, as if they were on the various steps of a ladder (Fig. 6–1; see page 81). The number of people on the bottom rungs of the ladder is almost always much greater than the number at the top. The president or CEO is usually at the top of this ladder; the maintenance crew is usually at the bottom. Nurses fall somewhere in the middle of most health care organizations, higher than the cleaning people, aides, and technicians but lower than physicians and administrators.

The people at the top of the ladder have authority to issue orders, spend the organization's money, and hire and fire people. Much of this authority is delegated to people below them, but they retain the right to reverse a decision or regain control of these activities whenever they deem it necessary.

The people at the bottom have little authority and usually play no part in deciding how money is spent or who will be hired or fired but are responsible for carrying out the directions from people above them on the ladder. The people at the bottom are not entirely without power or the ability to influence people higher up on the ladder, however. Without the people at the bottom of the ladder, the organization could not function. If there was no one at the bottom, the work of the organization would not get done. The people at the top depend on the people lower on the ladder to do most of the work.

Some degree of bureaucracy is characteristic of the formal operation of virtually every organization, even the most deliberately informal, because it promotes smooth operations within a large and complex group of people.

BOX 6–1
What Is a Bureaucracy?

Although it seems as if everyone complains about "the bureaucracy," not everyone is clear about what a bureaucracy really is. Max Weber defined a *bureaucratic organization* as having the following characteristics:

- **Division of labor.** Specific parts of the job to be done are assigned to different individuals or groups. For example, nurses, physicians, therapists, dietitians, and social workers all provide portions of the health care needed by an individual patient.
- **Hierarchy.** All employees are organized and ranked according to their degree of authority within the organization. For example, administrators and directors are at the top of most hospital hierarchies, whereas aides and maintenance workers are at the bottom.
- **Rules and regulations.** Acceptable and unacceptable behavior and the proper way to carry out various tasks are defined, often in writing. For example, procedure books, policy manuals, bylaws, statements, and memos prescribe many types of behavior, from acceptable isolation techniques to vacation policies.
- **Emphasis on technical competence.** People with certain skills and knowledge are hired to carry out specific parts of the total work of the organization. For example, a community mental health center will have psychiatrists, social workers, and nurses to provide different kinds of therapies and clerical staff to do the typing and filing.

Some degree of bureaucracy is characteristic of the formal operation of virtually every organization, even the most deliberately informal, because it promotes smooth operations within a large and complex group of people.

Source: Weber, M. (1969). Bureaucratic organization. In Etzioni, A. (ed.). *Readings on Modern Organizations.* Englewood Cliffs, N.J.: Prentice-Hall. Adapted by permission of Pearson Education, Inc., Upper Saddle River, N.J.

More Innovative Approaches

There is much interest in restructuring organizations, not only to save money but also to make the best use of a health care organization's most valuable resource, its people. This begins with hiring the right people. It also involves providing them with the resources they need to function and the kind of leadership that can inspire the staff and unleash their creativity (Rosen, 1996).

Increasingly, people recognize that organizations need to be not only efficient but also adaptable and innovative. Organizations need to be prepared for uncertainty, for rapid changes in their environment, and for quick, creative responses to these challenges. In addition, they need to provide an internal climate that not only allows but also motivates employees to work to the best of their ability. They need to stop thinking, to paraphrase Parker and Gadbois, of the managers as the brains of the organization and employees as the muscle (2000, p. 428).

Innovative organizations have adapted an increasingly *organic structure* that is more dynamic, more flexible, and less centralized than the static traditional hierarchical structure (Yourstone & Smith, 2002). In these organically structured organizations, decisions are made by the people who will implement them, not by their bosses and not by their bosses' boss.

The organic network emphasizes increased flexibility of the organizational structure, decentralized decision making, and autonomy for working groups or teams. Once rigid department or unit structures are reorganized into autonomous teams made up of professionals from different departments and disciplines, each team is given a specific task or function to perform (e.g., a hospital infection control team, a child protection team in a community agency). These teams are responsible for their own self-correction and self-control, although they may also have a designated leader. Together, team members make decisions about work assignments and how to deal with any problems that arise. In other words, the teams supervise and manage themselves.

Supervisors, administrators, and support staff have different functions in an organic network than in a hierarchical organization. Instead of spending their time observing and controlling other people's work, they become planners and resource people. They are responsible for providing the conditions re-

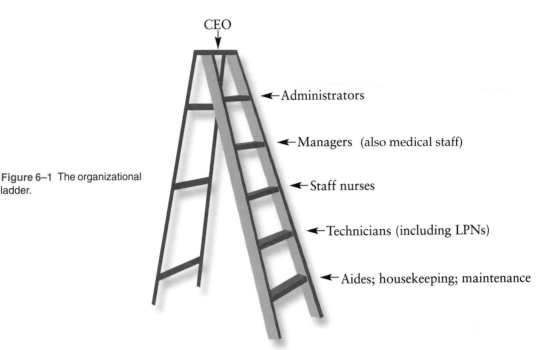

CEO

←Administrators

←Managers (also medical staff)

←Staff nurses

←Technicians (including LPNs)

←Aides; housekeeping; maintenance

Figure 6–1 The organizational ladder.

quired for the optimal functioning of the teams, and they are expected to ensure that the support, information, materials, and budgeted funds needed to do the job well are available to the teams. They also act as coordinators between the teams so that the teams are cooperating rather than blocking each other, working toward congruent goals, and not duplicating effort.

Very large organizations can also be separated into functional *divisions* that operate as though they were smaller, independent organizations. This allows each division to be better integrated internally when integration of the organization as a whole becomes almost impossible because of its great size, complexity, and diversity. However, communication among these divisions can become more difficult. This is a downside of organic structure. If not done well, there is a potential for creating chaos and confusion instead of creativity (Senge et al., 1999).

Organic networks have been compared to spider plants with their central cluster and offshoots (Morgan, 1997). Each cluster could represent a discipline (e.g., nursing, social work, occupational therapy) or a service (e.g., psychiatry, orthopedics). For example,

Figure 6–2 shows an organic network for a wellness center. Each cluster represents a separate set of services. A client might use just one or all of them to develop a personal plan for wellness. Staff members may move from one cluster to another, or the entire configuration of interconnected clusters may be reorganized as the organization shapes and is shaped by the environment.

Processes

In much the same way that organizations have some publicly announced goals as well as less publicized ones, they also have formal processes for getting things done and informal ways to get around the formal processes (Perrow, 1969). The *formal processes* are the written policies and procedures that virtually all health care organizations have. The *informal* processes are neither written nor discussed most of the time. They exist in virtually all organizations as a kind of "shadow" organization that is harder to see but equally important to recognize and understand (Purser & Cabana, 1999).

The informal process often is much simpler and faster than the formal one. Because

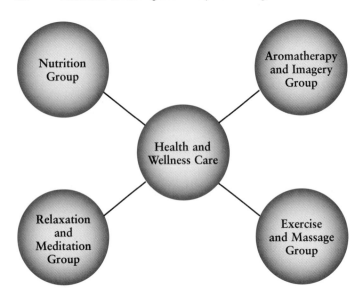

Figure 6–2 An organic organizational structure for a nontraditional wellness center. (Based on Morgan, A. (1993). *Imaginization: The Art of Creative Management.* Newbury Park, Calif.: Sage.)

the informal ways of getting things done are seldom discussed (and certainly not a part of your new employees' orientation), it may take some time for you to figure out what they are and how to use them. Once you are aware of the existence of these informal processes, they may be easier for you to identify. The following is an example:

Jocylene noticed that Harold seemed to get stat laboratory results back on his patients faster than she did. Although the results she requested came back quickly, the turnaround time for Harold's clients seemed almost instantaneous. At lunch one day, Jocylene asked Harold why that happened.

"That's easy," he said. "The people in our lab feel unappreciated. I always tell them how helpful they are. Also, if you call and let them know that the specimens are coming, they will get to them faster. They can't monitor their e-mail constantly."

Harold has just explained an informal process to Jocylene.

Sometimes, the informal processes are less obvious and people are unwilling to discuss them. However, careful observation of the most experienced, "system-wise" individuals in your organization will eventually reveal them to you. This will help you do things as efficiently as they do.

Power

Although the leadership and management techniques discussed so far will help you to achieve your goals, there are times when these attempts to influence others are overwhelmed by other forces or individuals. Where does this power come from? Who has it? Who does not?

In the earlier section on hierarchy (The Traditional Approach, which appeared under Structure), it was noted that, although people at the top of the hierarchy have most of the *authority* in the organization, they do not have all of the power. In fact, the people at the bottom of the hierarchy also have some sources of *power*. In this section, we explain how this can be true. First, we define power and then we consider the sources of power available to people on the lower rungs of the ladder.

Definition

Power is the ability to influence other people despite resistance on the part of the other person. In other words, one person or group can impose its will on another person or group (Haslam, 2001). Power may be actual or potential, intended or unintended (Lukes, 1986). It may also be used for good or for evil, for serious purposes or for selfish ones.

Sources

There are many sources of power. Many of them are readily available to nurses, but some of them are not. The following is a list derived primarily from the work of French as well as Raven and Etzioni (Barraclough & Stewart, 1992):

- **Authority.** The power granted to an individual or a group by virtue of position (within the organizational hierarchy, for example).
- **Reward.** The promise of money, goods, services, recognition, or other benefits.
- **Expertise.** The special knowledge an individual is believed to possess. As Sir Francis Bacon said long ago, "Knowledge is power" (Bacon, 1597, quoted in Fitton, 1997, p. 150).
- **Coercion.** The threat of pain or of harm, which may be physical, economic, or psychological.

Let's look at various groups of people in a health care organization in terms of the types of power that may be available to them:

- *Managers* are able to reward people with salary increases, promotions, and recognition. They can also cause economic or psychological pain for the people who work for them, particularly through their authority to evaluate and fire people.
- *Patients* at first appear to be relatively powerless in a health care organization. However, if patients refused to use the services of a particular organization, that organization would eventually cease to exist. Patients reward health care workers by praising them to their supervisors. They can also cause discomfort by complaining about them.
- *Nurses* have expertise, power, and authority over licensed practical nurses, aides, and other personnel by virtue of their position in the hierarchy. They are critical to the operation of most health care organizations and could cause considerable trouble if they refused to work, another source of power.
- *Assistants and technicians* may appear to be relatively powerless because of their low position in the hierarchy. Imagine, however, how the work of the organization (e.g., hospital, nursing home) would be impeded if all the nursing aides failed to appear one morning.

Fralic (2000) offered a good example of the power of information that nurses have:

> Florence Nightingale showed very graphically in the 1800s that wherever her nurses were, far fewer died, and wherever they were not, far more died.
>
> Think of the power of that information. Immediately people were saying, "What would you like, Miss Nightingale? Would you like more money? Would you like a school of nursing? What else can we do for you?" She had solid data, she knew how to collect it, and she knew how to interpret and distribute it in terms of things that people valued. (p. 340)

Empowering Nurses

In this last section, we look at several ways in which nurses, either individually or collectively, can maximize their power and increase their feelings of empowerment, both individually and as a group.

First, however, we should distinguish between the concepts of power and empowerment. *Power* is the actual or potential ability to "recognize one's will even against the resistance of others," according to Max Weber (quoted in Mondros & Wilson, 1994, p. 5). *Empowerment* is a psychological state, a feeling of competence, control, and entitlement. Given these definitions, it is possible to be powerful and yet not feel empowered. *Power* refers to action, and *empowerment* refers to feelings. Both are of interest to nursing leaders and managers.

Feeling empowered includes the following (Spreitzer & Quinn, 2001):

- **Self-determination.** Feeling free to decide how to do your work
- **Meaning.** Caring about your work, enjoying it, and taking it seriously
- **Competence.** Confidence in your ability to do your work well
- **Impact.** Feeling that people listen to your ideas, that you can make a difference

Nurses, like most people, want to have some power and to feel empowered. They want to be heard, to be recognized, to be valued, and to be respected. They do not want to feel unimportant or insignificant to society or to the organization in which they work.

Professional Organizations

Although we address the purpose of the American Nurses Association and other professional organizations in Chapter 16, here we look at them specifically in terms of how they can empower nurses.

Our collective voice, expressed through these organizations, can be stronger and more easily heard than is one individual's voice. By joining together in professional organizations, nurses make their viewpoint known and their value recognized. The power base of our professional organizations is derived from the number of nurses who are members and from their expertise in health matters. Why there is power in numbers may need some further explanation. Large numbers of active, informed members of an organization represent large numbers of potential voters to state and national legislators, most of whom wish to be remembered favorably in forthcoming elections. Large groups of people also have a louder voice: they can write more letters, speak to more friends and family members, make more telephone calls, and generally attract more attention than small groups can.

Professional organizations can empower nurses in a number of ways:

- Collegiality, the opportunity to work with peers on issues of importance to the profession

- Commitment to improving the health and well-being of the people served by the profession

- Representation in state legislatures and in Congress when issues of importance to nursing arise

- Representation during collective bargaining, the protection of nurses' rights and privileges as employed professionals

- Enhancement of nurses' competence through publications and continuing education

- Recognition of achievement through certification programs, awards, and the media

Collective Bargaining

Like professional organizations, collective bargaining also uses the power of numbers, in this case for the purpose of equalizing the power of employees and employer to improve working conditions, gain respect, increase job security, and have greater input into collective decisions (empowerment) and pay increases (Tappen, 2001). When people join together for a common cause, they are often more powerful than when they attempt to bring about change individually. Large numbers of people have the potential to cause more psychological or economic pain than an individual can. For example, the resignation of one nursing assistant or even one nurse may cause a temporary problem that is usually resolved rather quickly by hiring another individual. If 50 or 100 aides or nurses resign, however, the organization can be virtually paralyzed and will have much more difficulty replacing these essential workers. Collective bargaining takes advantage of this power in numbers.

An effective collective-bargaining contract can provide considerable protection to employees. However, the downside of collective bargaining (as with most uses of coercive power) is that it may encourage conflict rather than cooperation between employees and managers, an "us" against "them" environment (Haslam, 2001). Many nurses are also concerned about the effect that going out on strike might have on their clients' welfare and on their own economic security. Most administrators and managers prefer to operate within a union-free environment (Hannigan, 1998).

Participation in Decision Making

Actions can also be taken by managers and higher level administrators within an organization to increase the empowerment of the nursing staff. The amount of power available to or exercised by a given group (e.g., nurses) *within* an organization can vary considerably from one organization to the next. Three sources of power are particularly important in health care organizations:

- **Resources.** The money, materials, and human help needed to accomplish the work

- **Support.** Authority to take action without having to obtain permission

- **Information.** For example, about the organization's goals and activities of other departments

In addition, nurses also need access to *opportunities*: opportunities to be involved in decision making, to be involved in vital functions of the organization, to grow professionally, and to move up the organizational ladder (Sabiston & Laschinger, 1995). Without these, employees cannot be empowered (Bradford & Cohen, 1998). Nurses who are part-time, temporary, or contract employees are less likely to feel empowered than full-time permanent employees, who feel more secure in their positions (Kuokkanen & Katajisto, 2003).

Shared Governance

Genuine sharing of decision making is difficult to accomplish, partly because managers are reluctant to relinquish control or to trust their staff members to make wise decisions. Yet genuine empowerment of the nursing staff cannot occur without this sharing. Having some control over one's work and the ability to influence decisions are essential to empowerment (Monojlovick & Laschinger, 2002). For example, if staff members do not control the budget for their unit, they cannot implement a decision to replace aides with registered nurses without approval from higher-level management. If they want increased autonomy in decision making about the care of individual clients, they cannot do so if opposition by another group, such as

the physicians, is given greater credence by the organization's administration. In many cases, a change in the organizational culture is necessary before shared governance can work (Currie & Loftus-Hills, 2002).

Let's return to the example of the staff of the critical care department (Scenario 2). Why did the vice president for nursing tell the nurse manager that the plan would not be implemented?

Actually, the vice president for nursing thought that the plan had some merit. He believed that the proposal to implement a nurse-managed model of care for the chronically critically ill could save a little money, provide a higher quality of client care, and result in increased nursing staff satisfaction. However, the critical care department was the centerpiece of the hospital's agreement with a nearby medical school. Under this agreement, the medical school provided the services of highly skilled intensivists in return for the learning opportunities afforded their students. In its present form, the nurses' plan would not allow sufficient autonomy for the medical students, a situation that would not be acceptable to the medical school. The vice president knew that the board of trustees of the hospital believed their affiliation with the medical school brought a great deal of prestige to the organization and that they would not allow anything to interfere with this relationship.

"If shared governance were in place here, I think that we could implement this or a similar model of care," he told the nurse manager.

"How would that work?" she asked.

"If we had shared governance, the nursing practice council would review the plan and, if they approved it, forward it to a similar medical council. Then committees from both councils would work together to figure out a way for this to benefit everyone. It wouldn't necessarily be easy to do, but it could be done if we had real collegiality between the professions. I have been working toward this model but haven't convinced the rest of the administration to put it into practice as yet. Perhaps we could bring this up at the next nursing executive council meeting. I think it is time that I shared my ideas on this subject with the rest of the nursing staff."

In this case, the goals and processes existing at the time the nurses developed their proposal did not support their idea. However, they could see a way for it to be accomplished in the future. Implementation of real shared governance would make it possible for the critical care nurses to accomplish their goal. *Shared governance* is a term used to describe formal ways in which access to these sources of power and opportunity is made available to staff nurses. Under shared governance, staff nurses are included in the highest levels of decision making within the nursing department through representation on various councils that govern practice and management issues. These councils set the standard for staffing, promotion, and so forth. Under shared governance, staff nurses are also involved in decisions that affect their particular unit (Westrope, Vaughn, Bott, & Taunton, 1995).

Enhancing Expertise

Most health care professionals, including nurses, are empowered to some degree by their own professional knowledge and com-

RESEARCH EXAMPLE

Can nurse managers empower their staff? The answer is yes, according to nurse researchers who surveyed 537 staff nurses in two large hospitals. Fostering autonomy and showing confidence in the staff were especially empowering. Empowered staff worked more effectively and had lower levels of job-related tension.

Source: Laschinger, H.K.S., Wong, C., McMahon, L., & Kaufman, C. (1999). Leader behavior impact on staff nurse empowerment, job tension, and work effectiveness. *Journal of Nursing Administration*, 29(5), 28–39.

petence. First, you can take steps to enhance your own competence, thereby increasing your own sense of empowerment (Fig. 6–3)

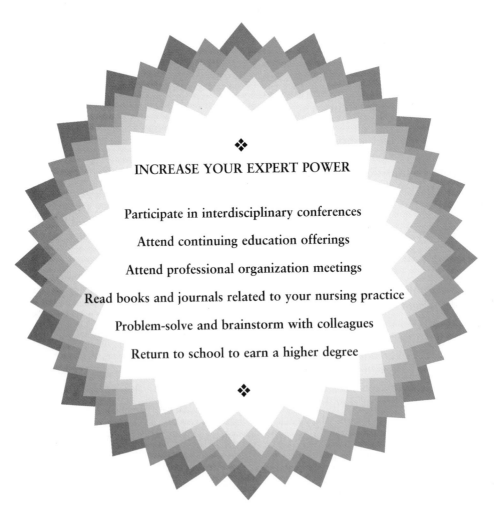

INCREASE YOUR EXPERT POWER

Participate in interdisciplinary conferences

Attend continuing education offerings

Attend professional organization meetings

Read books and journals related to your nursing practice

Problem-solve and brainstorm with colleagues

Return to school to earn a higher degree

Figure 6–3 How to increase your expert power.

• Actively participate in interdisciplinary team conferences and patient-centered conferences on your unit.

• Attend continuing education offerings selected to enhance your expertise.

• Attend local, regional, and national conferences sponsored by relevant nursing and specialty organizations.

• Read journals and books in your specialty area.

• Participate in nursing research projects related to your clinical specialty area.

• Discuss with colleagues in nursing and other disciplines how to handle a difficult clinical situation.

• Observe the practice of experienced nurses.

• Return to school to earn a bachelor's degree and higher degrees in nursing.

You can probably think of more, but this list at least gives you some ideas.

Second, you can share the knowledge and experience you have gained with other people. This means not only using your knowledge to improve your own practice but also communicating what you have learned to your colleagues in nursing and in other health care professions. It also means letting your supervisors know that you have enhanced your professional competence. You can share your knowledge with your clients, empowering them as well. You may even reach the point at which you have learned more about a particular subject than most nurses have and want to write about it for publication.

◘ Conclusion

Although most nurses are employed by health care organizations, too few have taken the time to analyze the operation of their employing organizations and the effect it has on their practice. Understanding organizations and the power relationships within them will increase the effectiveness of your leadership.

Study Questions

1 Describe the organizational characteristics of a facility in which you currently have a clinical assignment. Be sure to include the following:

   a. The type of organization it is

   b. The organizational culture

   c. How the organization is structured

   d. The formal and informal goals and processes of the organization

2 Define *power*, and describe how power affects the relationships between people of different disciplines (e.g., nursing, medicine, microbiology, administration, finance, social work) in a health care organization.

3 Discuss ways in which nurses can become more empowered. How can you use your leadership skills to do this?

Critical Thinking Exercise

Tanya Washington will finish her associate's degree nursing program in 6 weeks. Her preferred clinical area is parent-child nursing, and she hopes to become a pediatric nurse practitioner one day.

Tanya has received two job offers, both from urban hospitals with large pediatric populations. Several of her friends are already employed by these facilities, so she asked them for their impressions.

"Central Hospital is a good place to work," said one friend. "It is a dynamic, growing institution, always on the cutting edge of change. Any new idea that seems promising, Central is the first to try it. It's an exciting place to work."

"City Hospital is also a good place to work," said her other friend, "It is a strong, stable institution where traditions are valued. Any new idea must be carefully evaluated before it is adapted. It's been a pleasure to work there."

1 How would the organizational climate of each hospital affect a new graduate?

2 Which organizational climate do you think would be best for a new graduate, Central's or City's?

3 What do you need to know about Tanya before deciding which hospital would be best for her?

4 Would your answer differ if Tanya were an experienced nurse?

5 What else would you like to know about the hospitals?

REFERENCES

Atchison, T.A. (April 2002). What is corporate culture? *Trustee*, 11.

Barraclough, R.A., & Stewart, R.A. (1992). Power and control: Social science perspectives. In Richmond, V.P., & McCroskey, J.C. (eds.). *Power in the Classroom: Communication, Control and Concern*. Hillsdale, N.J.: Lawrence Erlbaum.

Bradford, D.L., & Cohen, A.R. (1998). *Power Up: Transforming Organizations Through Shared Leadership*. New York: John Wiley & Sons.

Currie, L., & Loftus-Hills, A. (2002). The nursing view of clinical governance. *Nursing Standard*, 16(27), 40–44.

Fitton, R.A. (1997). *Leadership: Quotations from the World's Greatest Motivators*. Boulder, Colo.: Westview Press.

Fralic, M.F. (2000). What is leadership? *Journal of Nursing Administration*, 30(7/8), 340–341.

Frusti, D.K., Niesen, K.M., & Campion, J.K. (2003). Creating a culturally competent organization. *Journal of Nursing Administration*, 33(1), 33–38.

Hannigan, T.A. (1998). *Managing Tomorrow's High-Performance Unions*. Westport, Conn.: Greenwood Publishing.

Haslam, S.A. (2001). *Psychology in Organizations*. Thousand Oaks, Calif.: Sage.

Kuokkanen, L., & Katajisto, J. (2003). Promoting or impeding empowerment? *Journal of Nursing Administration*, 33(4), 209–215.

Laschinger, H.K.S., Wong, C., McMahon, L., & Kaufman, C. (1999). Leader behavior impact on staff nurse empowerment, job tension, and work effectiveness. *Journal of Nursing Administration*, 29(5), 28–39.

Lukes, S. (1986). *Power*. New York: New York University Press.

Manojlovich, M., & Laschinger, H.K. (2002). The relationship of empowerment and selected personality characteristics to nursing job satisfaction. *Journal of Nursing Administration*, 32(11), 586–595.

Mondros, J.B., & Wilson, S.M. (1994). *Organizing for Power and Empowerment*. New York: Columbia University Press.

Morgan, A. (1997). *Images of Organization*. Thousand Oaks, Calif.: Sage.

Morgan, A. (1993). *Imaginization: The Art of Creative Management*. Newbury Park, Calif.: Sage.

Parker, M., & Gadbois, S. (2000). Building community in the healthcare workplace. *Journal of Nursing Administration*, 30(9), 426–431.

Perrow, C. (1969). The analysis of goals in complex organizations. In Etzioni, A. (ed). *Readings on Modern Organizations*. Englewood Cliffs, N.J.: Prentice-Hall.

Purser, R.E., & Cabana, S. (1999). *The Self-Managing Organization*. New York: Free Press (Simon & Schuster).

Rosen, R.H. (1996). *Leading People: Transforming Business from the Inside Out*. New York: Viking Penguin.

Rudy, E.B., Daly, B.J., Douglas, S., Montenegro, H.D., Song, R., & Dyer, M.A. (1995). Patient outcomes for the chronically critically ill: Special care unit versus intensive care unit. *Nursing Research,* 44, 324–331.

Sabiston, J.A., & Laschinger, H.K.S. (1995). Staff nurse work empowerment and perceived autonomy. *Journal of Nursing Administration,* 28(9), 42–49.

Senge, P., Kleiner, A., Roberts, C., Ross, R., Roth, G., & Smith, B. (1999). *The Dance of Change.* New York: Currency/Doubleday.

Spreitzer, G.M., & Quinn, R.E. (2001). *A Company of Leaders.* San Francisco: Jossey-Bass.

Stegall, M.S. (2002). Instilling a soul in your organization without losing yours to it. *Clinical Leadership and Management Review,* 16(2), 85–89.

Tappen, R.M. (2001). *Nursing Leadership and Manage-ment: Concepts and Practice,* 4th ed. Philadelphia: F.A. Davis.

Trinh, H.Q. & O'Connor, S.J. (2002). Helpful or harmful? The impact of strategic change on the performance of U.S. urban hospitals. *Health Services Research,* 37(1), 145–171.

Weber, M. (1969). Bureaucratic organization. In Etzioni, A. (ed.). *Readings on Modern Organizations.* Englewood Cliffs, N.J.: Prentice-Hall.

Westrope, R.A., Vaughn, L., Bott, M., & Taunton, R.L. (1995). Shared governance: From vision to reality. *Journal of Nursing Administration,* 25(2), 45–54.

Yourstone, S.A., & Smith, H.L. (2002). Managing system errors and failures in health care organizations: Suggestions for practice and research. *Health Care Management Review,* 27(1), 50–61.

CHAPTER 7

Delegation of Client Care

OBJECTIVES

After reading this chapter, the student should be able to:

- Define the term *delegation.*

- Define the term *unlicensed assistive personnel.*

- Understand the legal implications of making assignments to other health care personnel.

- Recognize barriers to successful delegation.

- Make appropriate assignments to team members.

OUTLINE

Introduction to Delegation

The Nursing Process and Delegation

Coordinating Assignments

The Need for Delegation

Safe Delegation

Criteria for Delegation

Task-Related Concerns

Abilities

Priorities

Efficiency

Appropriateness

Relationship-Oriented Concerns

Fairness

Learning Opportunities

Health

Compatibility

Staff Preferences

Barriers to Delegation

Experience Issues

Licensure Issues

Quality-of-Care Issues

Assigning Work to Others

Conclusion

CHAPTER 7 SELF ASSESSMENT
Delegation

1. Are you able to ask others to help you?

2. Do you need to do every task yourself?

3. If you ask someone to do something, do you check to see if the job was completed?

4. Do you take responsibility for your own behaviors?

Mary Ann is a new graduate and has just finished her orientation. She works the 7 P.M. to 7 A.M. shift on a busy monitored neuroscience unit. The client census is 48, making this a full unit. Although there is an associate nurse manager for the shift, Mary Ann is charge nurse for the shift. Her responsibilities include receiving and transcribing orders, contacting physicians with any information or requests, reviewing laboratory reports and giving them to the appropriate staff members, checking any new medication orders and placing them in the appropriate charts, relieving the monitor tech for dinner and breaks, and assigning staff to dinner and breaks.

When Mary Ann comes to work, she discovers that one registered nurse (RN) called in sick. She has two RNs and three unlicensed assistive personnel (UAPs) for staff and a full census. She panics and wants to refuse to take report. After a discussion with the charge nurse from the previous shift, she realizes that this is not an option. She sits down to evaluate the acuity of the clients and the capabilities of her staff.

◼ Introduction to Delegation

Delegation is not a new concept. In the Old Testament, Moses was instructed to identify 70 elders "so they will share with you the burden of this nation and you will no longer have to carry it by yourself" (Numbers 11: 16-17). In her *Notes on Nursing*, Florence Nightingale (1859) clearly stated:

Don't imagine that if you, who are in charge, don't look to all these things yourself, those under you will be more careful than you are . . . .

She continued by directing,

But then again to look to all these things yourself does not mean to do them yourself. If you do it, it is by so much the better certainly than if it were not done at all. But can you not insure that it is done when not done by yourself? Can you insure that it is not undone when your back is turned? This is what being in charge means. And a very important meaning it is, too. The former only implies that just what you can do with your own hands is done. The latter that what ought to be done is always done. Head in charge must see to house hygiene, not do it herself. (p. 17)

By definition, delegation is the reassigning of responsibility for the performance of a job from one person to another (ANA, 1996). Although the responsibility for the task is transferred, the accountability for the process or outcome of the task remains with the delegator, or the person delegating the activity. Nightingale referred to this delegation responsibility when she inferred that the "Head in charge" does not necessarily carry out the task but still sees that it is completed.

Delegation may be direct or indirect. *Direct delegation* is usually "verbal direction by the RN delegator regarding an activity or task in a specific nursing care situation" (ANA, 1996, p. 15). In this case, the RN decides which staff member is capable of performing the specific task or activity at this time. *Indirect delegation* is "an approved listing of activities or tasks that have been established in policies and procedures of the health care institution or facility" (ANA, 1996, p. 15).

The recent changes occurring in the health care environment continue to modify the scope of nursing practice and the activities delegated to UAPs. A main concern in almost all health care settings regarding this is that UAPs are inappropriately performing functions that belong within the legal realm of nursing (ANA, 2002).

Permitted tasks may vary from institution to institution. For example, a certified nursing assistant performs specific activities designated by the job description approved by the specific health care institution. Although the institution delineates tasks and activities in the job description, this does not mean that the RN cannot decide to assign other personnel in specific situations. Take the following example:

Mrs. Rankin was admitted to the unit from the neurological intensive care unit. She suffered a Grade II subarachnoid hemorrhage 2 weeks ago and has a left hemiparesis. She also has difficulty with swallowing. She is still receiving tube feedings through a gastrostomy tube; however, she has been advanced to a pureed diet. She needs assistance with personal care, toileting, and feeding. Although a physical therapist comes twice a day to get her up for gait training, the physician wants her in a chair as much as possible.

Assessing this situation, the RN might consider assigning a licensed practical nurse (LPN) to this client. The swallowing problems place the client at risk for aspiration, which means that feeding may present a problem. There is a potential for injury. The LPN is also capable of managing the tube feeding. While assisting with bathing, the LPN can perform range of motion exercises to all the client's extremities and assess her skin for breakdown. The LPN also knows the appropriate way to assist the client in transferring from the bed to the chair. The RN may not assign an individual to perform a task or activity not specified in his or her job description or within the scope of practice, such as allowing a nursing assistant to administer medications or perform certain types of dressing changes.

Do not confuse delegation with supervision. Supervision is more direct and requires directly overseeing the work or performance of others. Supervision includes checking with individuals throughout the day to see what activities have been completed and what may still need to be finished. For example, you have assigned a nursing assistant to take all the vital signs on the unit and give the morning baths to eight clients. Three hours into the morning, you find that she is far behind. At this point, it is important to discover why. Perhaps one of the clients required more care than expected or the nursing assistant needed to run an errand off the floor. Reevaluation of the assignment may be necessary. When working with another RN, you do not need to supervise. This is a collaborative relationship and includes consulting and giving advice when needed.

Individuals who supervise others also delegate tasks and activities. Chief nursing officers often delegate tasks to associate directors. This may include record reviews, unit reports, client acuities, and other tasks. The chief nursing officer still remains accountable for making sure that the activities are completed.

Supervision sometimes entails more direct evaluation of performance. For example, a nurse manager both supervises and delegates. Certain administrative tasks, such as staff scheduling, may be delegated to another staff member such as an associate manager. However, performance evaluations and discussions regarding individual interactions with clients and other staff members fall under supervisory duties.

Regardless of where you work, you cannot assume that only those in the higher levels of the organization delegate work to other people. You, too, will be responsible at times to delegate some of your work to other nurses, to technical personnel, or to another department. Decisions associated with this responsibility often cause some difficulty for new nurses. Knowing each person's capabilities and job description can help you decide which personnel can assist with a task.

◼ The Nursing Process and Delegation

As nurses, we understand the nursing process. The same concept can be applied to delegation (Hansten & Washburn, 1998). Before deciding who should care for a particular client, the nurse must assess each client's particular needs, set client-specific goals, and match the skills of the person assigned responsibilities with the tasks that need to be accomplished (*assessment*). After accomplishing this task, the nurse needs to mentally identify which staff member is best suited for the task or activities. Thinking this through before delegating helps prevent problems later (*plan*). Next, the nurse determines which personnel have the knowledge and skill to care for the client and assigns the tasks to the appropriate person (*implementation*). Once this is done, however, the nurse must still oversee care and determine whether client care needs have been met (*evaluation*). It is also important for the nurse to allow time for feedback during the day. This enables all personnel to see where they are and where they want to go.

Often, the nurse must first coordinate care for groups of clients before being able to delegate tasks to other personnel. By looking at the needs of each client, the nurse makes an educated decision about which staff members have the appropriate education and skill to deliver safe, quality care. The nurse also needs to consider his or her responsibilities. This includes assisting other staff members with setting priorities, clarifying instructions, and reassessing the situation.

The National Council of the State Boards of Nursing (NCSBN, 1995) published a paper addressing the issue of delegation. They developed a concept called the "Five Rights of Delegation," similar to the five rights regarding medication administration. These five "rights" are listed in Box 7–1. Before being able to delegate tasks and activities to other individuals, however, the nurse must understand the needs of each client.

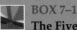

> **BOX 7–1**
> **The Five Rights of Delegation**
>
> 1 Right task
> 2 Right circumstances
> 3 Right person
> 4 Right direction/communication
> 5 Right supervision/evaluation

Coordinating Assignments

One of the most difficult tasks for new nurses to master is coordinating daily activities. Often, you not only have a group of clients for whom you are expected to provide direct care but also must supervise the work of others, such as non-nurse caregivers, LPNs, or vocational nurses. Although care plans, critical (or clinical) pathways, and computer information sheets are available to help identify client needs, these items do not provide a mechanism for coordinating the actual delivery of care. To do this, you can develop personalized worksheets that prioritize tasks for each client. Using the worksheets helps the nurse identify tasks that require the knowledge and skill of an RN and those that can be carried out by assistive personnel.

On the worksheet, tasks are prioritized on the basis of client need, not nursing convenience. For example, an order states that a client is to receive continuous tube feedings. Although it may be convenient for the nurse to fill the feeding bag with enough supplement to last 6 hours, it is not good practice and not safe for the client. Instead, the nurse should plan to check the tube feeding every 2 hours.

Remember Mary Ann in the beginning of the chapter? Here is where a worksheet helps to determine who can do what. First, Mary Ann needs to decide what particular tasks she must do. These include receiving and transcribing orders, contacting physicians with information or requests, reviewing lab reports and giving them to the appropriate staff members, and checking any new medication orders and placing them in the appropriate charts. Another RN may be able to relieve the monitor technician for dinner and breaks and a second RN may be able to assign staff to dinner and breaks. Next, Mary Ann needs to look at the needs of each client on the unit and prioritize them. Mary Ann is now ready to effectively delegate to her staff.

Some activities must be done at a certain time, and their timing may be out of your control. Examples include medication administration and clients who need special preparation for a scheduled procedure. The following are some tips for organizing your work on personalized worksheets to help you establish client priorities (Tappen, Weiss, & Whitehead, 2001):

- Plan your time around these activities.

- Do high-priority activities first.

- Determine which activities are best done in a cluster.

- Remember that you are still responsible for activities delegated to others.

- Consider your peak energy time when scheduling optional activities.

This list acts as a guideline for coordinating client care. The nurse needs to use critical thinking skills in the decision-making process. For example, activities that are usually clustered include bathing, changing linen, and parts of the physical assessment. Some clients may not be able to tolerate too much activity at one time. Take special situations into consideration when coordinating client care and deciding who should carry out some of the activities. Remember, however, even when you delegate, you remain accountable.

Figure 7–1 is an example of a personalized worksheet. (See chapter on Time Management for a complete discussion.)

▣ The Need for Delegation

The 1990s brought rapid change to the health care environment. Several forces coming together at one time contributed to these changes, including the nursing shortage, health care reform, an increased need for nursing services, and demographic trends.

These changes continue to have an impact on the delivery of nursing care, requiring institutions to hire other personnel to assist nurses with client care (Zimmerman, 1996).

Health care institutions often use UAPs to perform certain client care tasks (Habel, 2000; Huber, Blegan, & McCloskey, 1994). As the nursing shortage becomes more critical, there is a greater need for institutions to recruit the services of UAPs (ANA, 2002). A survey conducted by the American Hospital Association revealed that 97% of hospitals currently employ some form of UAP (Parkman, 1996). Because many institutions employ these personnel, many nurses feel that they know how to work with and safely delegate tasks to them. This is not the case. Therefore, many nursing organizations have developed definitions for UAPs and criteria regarding their responsibilities. The ANA defines *UAPs* as follows:

Unlicensed assistive personnel are individuals who are trained to function in an assistive role to the registered nurse in the provision of patient/client care activities as delegated by and under the supervision of the registered professional nurse. Although some of these people may be certified (e.g., certified nursing assistant [CNA]), it is important to remember that certification differs from licensure. When a task is delegated to an unlicensed person, the professional nurse remains personally responsible for the outcomes of these activities. (ANA, 1994)

As the work on the UAP issue is ongoing, the ANA has recently updated their Position Statements to define direct and indirect patient care activities that may be performed by UAPs in the health care setting. Included in these updates are specific definitions regarding UAPs and technicians and acceptable tasks.

Use of the RN to provide all the care a client needs may not be the most efficient or cost effective use of professional time. As the use of LPNs or client care extenders increases, the nurse's focus moves toward diagnosing client care needs and carrying out complex interventions (Conger, 1994). The ANA cautions against delegating nursing activities that include the foundation of the nursing process and require specialized

Nurse/Team _____ DNR 8607/Code 99

Patient Room # _____ Name _____Age _____

Allergies _____

Diagnosis _____

Diet _____ Fluids: PO _____ IV _____ Type _____

Restrictions: BR _____ BRP _____ OOB/Chair _____ Ambulate with assist _____

Activity _____

Assessment _____

Treatments

1. _____

2. _____

3. _____

4. _____

5. _____

Monitor

1. Vital signs: Temp _____ Pulse _____ AHR _____ BP _____ Parameters _____

2. Cardiac Monitor: Rhythm _____ Rate _____

3. Neurologic Status _____

4. CMS: _____ Traction: _____

Figure 7–1 Personalized patient worksheet.

knowledge, judgment, or skill (ANA, 1996, 2002). Non-nursing functions (Hayes, 1994), such as performing clerical or receptionist duties, taking trips or running errands off the unit, cleaning floors, making beds, collecting trays, and ordering supplies, however, should not be carried out by the highest paid and most educated member of the team. These tasks are easily delegated to other personnel.

Safe Delegation

In 1990, the NCSBN adopted a definition of delegation, stating that delegation is "transferring to a competent individual the authority to perform a selected nursing task in a selected situation" (p. 1). In its publication *Issues* (1995), the Council again presented this definition. Accordingly, the American Nurses Association (ANA) Code for Nurses (1985) stated, "The nurse exercises informed judgment and uses individual competence and qualifications as criteria in seeking consultation, accepting responsibilities, and delegating nursing activities to others" (p. 1). More recently, the ANA (2002) defined delegation as "The transfer of responsibility for the performance of an activity from one individual to another while retaining accountability for the outcome" (p. 1). It is important to remember that delegation still includes accountability. To delegate tasks safely, nurses must delegate appropriately and supervise adequately (Barter & Furmidge, 1994).

In 1997, the NCSBN developed a Delegation Decision-Making Grid. This grid acts as a tool to help nurses delegate appropriately. It provides a scoring instrument for seven categories that the nurse should consider when making delegation decisions. The categories for the grid are listed in Box 7–2.

Scoring the components helps the nurse evaluate the situations, the client needs, and the health care personnel available to meet the needs. A low score on the grid indicates that the activity may be safely delegated to personnel other than the RN, and a high score indicates that delegation may not be advisable. Figure 7–2 shows the Delegation Decision-Making Grid. The grid is also

> **BOX 7–2**
> **Components of the Delegation Decision-Making Grid**
>
> - Level of client acuity
> - Level of unlicensed assistive personnel capability
> - Level of licensed nurse capability
> - Possibility for injury
> - Number of times the skill has been performed by the unlicensed assistive personnel
> - Level of decision-making needed for the activity
> - Client's ability for self-care
>
> Source: Adapted from the National Council of State Boards of Nursing. *Delegation Decision-Making Grid.* National State Boards of Nursing, Inc. 1997 (http://www.ncsbn.org).

available on the NCSBN website at *http://www.ncsbn.com.*

Nurses who delegate tasks to UAPs should evaluate the activities being considered for delegation (Herrick et al., 1994). The American Association of Critical Care Nurses (AACN) (1990) recommended considering five factors affecting the decision to delegate, which are listed in Box 7–3.

It is the responsibility of the RN to be well acquainted with the state's nurse practice act and regulations issued by the state board of nursing regarding UAPs. State laws and regulations supersede any publications or opinions set forth by professional organizations. As stated earlier, the NCSBN provides criteria to assist nurses with delegation.

LPNs are trained to perform specific tasks, such as basic medication administration, dressing changes, and personal hygiene tasks. In some states, the LPN, with additional training, may start and monitor intravenous (IV) infusions and administer certain medications.

Criteria for Delegation

The purpose of delegation is not to assign tasks to others that you do not want to do yourself. When you delegate to others effectively, you should have more time to per-

Elements for Review		Client A	Client B	Client C	Client D
Activity/task	Describe activity/task:				
Level of Client Stability	Score the client's level of stability: 0. Client condition is chronic/stable/predictable 1. Client condition has minimal potential for change 2. Client condition has moderate potential for change 3. Client condition is unstable/acute/strong potential for change				
Level of UAP Competence	Score the UAP competence in completing delegated nursing care activities in the defined client population: 0. UAP - expert in activities to be delegated, in defined population 1. UAP - experienced in activities to be delegated, in defined population 2. UAP - experienced in activities but not in defined population 3. UAP - novice in performing activities and in defined population				
Level of Licensed Nurse Competence	Score the licensed nurse's competence in relation to both knowledge of providing nursing care to a defined population and competence in implementation of the delegation process: 0. Expert in the knowledge of nursing needs/activities of defined client population and expert in the delegation process 1. Either expert in knowledge of needs/activities of defined client population and competent in delegation or experienced in the needs/activities of defined client population and expert in the delegation process 2. Experienced in the knowledge of needs/activities of defined client population and competent in the delegation process 3. Either experienced in the knowledge of needs/activities of defined client population or competent in the delegation process 4. Novice in knowledge of defined population and novice in delegation				
Potential for Harm	Score the potential level of risk the nursing care activity has for the client (risk is probability of suffering harm): 0. None 1. Low 2. Medium 3. High				
Frequency	Score based on how often the UAP has performed the specific nursing care activity: 0. Performed at least daily 1. Performed at least weekly 2. Performed at least monthly 3. Performed less than monthly 4. Never performed				
Level of Decision-making	Score the decision-making needed, related to the specific nursing care activity, client (both cognitive and physical status), and client situation: 0. Does not require decision making 1. Minimal level of decision making 2. Moderate level of decision making 3. High level of decision making				
Ability for Self-Care	Score the client's level of assistance needed for self-care activities: 0. No assistance 1. Limited assistance 2. Extensive assistance 3. Total care or constant attendance				
	TOTAL SCORE				

Figure 7–2 Delegation decision-making grid.

BOX 7–3
Criteria for Determining Which Client Care Activity Can Be Delegated to Other Personnel

- Potential for harm to the patient
- Complexity of the nursing activity
- Extent of problem solving and innovation required
- Predictability of outcome
- Extent of interaction

Source: Adapted from American Association of Critical Care Nurses (AACN). (1990). *Delegation of Nursing and Non-Nursing Activities in Critical Care: A Framework for Decision-Making*. Irvine, Calif.: AACN.

form the tasks that only a professional nurse is permitted to do.

When you delegate, you must consider both the *ability* of the person to whom you are delegating and the *fairness* of the task to the individual and the team (Tappen, Weiss, & Whitehead, 2001). In other words, you need to consider both the *task aspects* of delegation (Is this a complex task? Is it a professional responsibility? Can this person do it safely?) and the *interpersonal aspects* (Does the person have time to do this? Is the work evenly distributed?).

The ANA has specified tasks that RNs may not delegate because they are specific to the discipline of professional nursing. These activities include (Boysen & Fischer, 2000):

- Initial nursing assessment and follow-up assessments if nursing judgment is indicated

- Decisions and judgments about client outcomes

- Determination and approval of a client plan of care

- Interventions that require professional nursing knowledge, decisions, or skills

- Decisions and judgments necessary for the evaluation of client care

■ Task-Related Concerns

The primary task-related concern in delegating work is whether the person assigned to do the task has the ability to complete it. Team priorities and efficiency are also important considerations.

Abilities

To make appropriate assignments, the nurse needs to know the knowledge and skill level, legal definitions, role expectations, and job description for each member of the team. It is equally important to be aware of the different skill levels of caregivers within each discipline because ability differs with each level of education. Additionally, different individuals within each level of skill possess their own particular strengths and weaknesses. Prior assessment of the strengths of each member of the team will assist in providing safe and efficient care to clients. Figure 7–3 outlines the skills of various health care personnel.

People should not be assigned a task they are not skilled in or knowledgeable to perform, regardless of their professional level. People often are reluctant to admit that they cannot do something. Instead of seeking help or saying they do not feel comfortable with the task, they may avoid doing it, delay starting it, do only part of it, or even bluff their way through it, a risky choice in health care.

Regardless of the length of time individuals have been in a position, employees need orientation when assigned a new task. Those who seek assistance and advice are showing concern for the team and the welfare of their clients. Requests for assistance or additional explanations should not be ignored, and the person should be praised, not criticized, for seeking guidance (Tappen, Weiss, & Whitehead, 2001).

Priorities

You have probably noticed that the work of a busy unit rarely ends up going as expected. Dealing with sick people, their families, physicians, and other team members all at the same time is a difficult task. Setting priorities for the day should be based on client needs, team needs, and organizational and

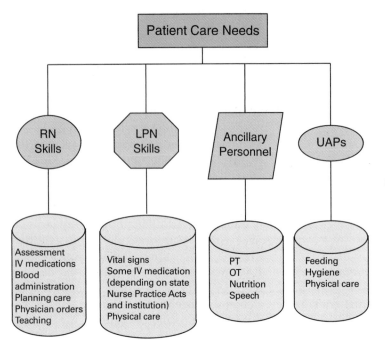

Figure 7–3 Diagram of delegation decision-making grid.

community demands. The values of each may be very different, even opposed. These differences should be discussed with team members so that decisions can be made based on team priorities.

One way to determine patient priorities is to base your decisions on Maslow's hierarchy of needs (see Fig. 5–2). Maslow's hierarchy is frequently used in nursing to provide a framework for prioritizing care to meet client needs. The basic physiologic needs come first because they are necessary for survival. Oxygen and medication administration, IV fluids, and enteral feedings are included in this group.

Identifying priorities and deciding the needs to be met first help in organizing care and in deciding which other team members can meet client needs. For example, nursing assistants can meet many hygiene needs, allowing licensed personnel to administer medications and enteral feedings in a timely manner.

Efficiency

Efficiency means that all members of the team know their jobs and responsibilities

and work together like gears in a well-built clock. They mesh together and keep perfect time.

The current health care delivery environment demands efficient, cost-effective care. Delegating appropriately can increase efficiency and save money. However, incorrect delegation can decrease efficiency and cost money in the end. When delegating tasks to individuals who cannot perform the job, the RN must often go back to perform the task. There may be legal implications if a client is injured as a result of inappropriate delegation. To date, courts have not declared nurses responsible for the negligent acts of a subordinate, provided that the nurse delegated responsibly and appropriately (Habel, 2000).

Although institutions often need to "float" staff to other units, maintaining continuity, if at all possible, is important. Keeping the same staff members on the unit all the time, for example, allows them to develop familiarity with the physical setting and routines of the unit as well as the types of clients the unit services. Time is lost when staff members are reassigned frequently to different units. Although physical layouts may be the same, client needs, unit routines, and use of space are often different, as is the availability of supplies. Time spent to orient reassigned staff members takes time away from delivery of client care. However, when staff members are reassigned, it is important for them to indicate their skill level and comfort in the new setting. It is just as important for the staff who are familiar with the setting to identify the strengths of the reassigned person and build on them.

Appropriateness

Appropriateness is another task-related concern. Nothing can be more counterproductive than floating, say, a coronary care nurse to labor and delivery. More time will be spent teaching the necessary skills than on safe mother-baby care. Assigning an educated, licensed staff member to perform non-nursing functions to protect safety is also poor use of personnel.

◙ Relationship-Oriented Concerns

Relationship-oriented concerns include fairness, learning opportunities, health concerns, compatibility, and staff preferences. Each of these is discussed next.

Fairness

Fairness means evenly distributing the workload in terms of both the physical requirements and the emotional investment in providing health care. The nurse who is caring for a dying client may have less physical work to do than another team member, but in terms of emotional care to the client and family, he or she may be doing double the work of another staff member.

Fairness also means considering equally all requests for special consideration. The quickest way to alienate members of your team is to be unfair. It is important to discuss with team members any decisions you have made that may appear unfair to others. Allow the team to participate in making decisions regarding assignments. Their participation will decrease resentment and increase cooperation. In some health care institutions, team members make such decisions as a group.

Learning Opportunities

Including assignments that stimulate motivation and learning and assisting team members to learn new tasks and take on new challenges is part of the role of the RN.

Health

Some aspects of caregiving jobs are more stressful than others. Rotating team members through the more difficult jobs may decrease stress and allow empathy to increase among the members. Special health needs, such as family emergencies or special physical problems of team members, also need to be addressed. If some team members have difficulty accepting the needs of others, the situation should be discussed with the team, bearing in mind the employee's right to privacy when discussing sensitive issues.

Compatibility

No matter how hard you may strive to get your team to work together, it just may not happen. Some people work together better than others. Helping people develop better working relationships is part of team building. Creating opportunities for people to share and learn from each other increases the overall effectiveness of the team.

As the leader, you may be forced to intervene in team member disputes. Many individuals find it difficult to work with others they do not like personally. It sometimes becomes necessary to explain that liking another person is a plus but not a necessity in the work setting and that personal problems have no place in the work environment. Take the example of Laura:

Laura had been a labor and delivery room supervisor in a large metropolitan hospital for 5 years before she moved to another city. Because a position similar to the one she left was not available, she became a staff nurse at a small local hospital. The hospital had just opened its new birthing center. The first day on the job went well. The other staff members seemed cordial enough.

As the weeks went by, however, Laura began to have problems getting other staff to help her. No one would offer to relieve her for meals or a break. She noticed that certain groups of staff members always went to lunch together, but she was never invited to join them. She attempted to speak to some of the more approachable coworkers, but she did not get much information. Disturbed by the situation, Laura went to the nurse manager.

The nurse manager listened quietly while Laura related her experiences. She then asked Laura to reflect back on some of the events of the past weeks, particularly the last staff meeting. Laura realized that she had alienated the staff during that encounter because she had monopolized the meeting and kept saying that in "her hospital" things were done in a particular way. Laura also realized that, instead of asking for help, she was in the habit of demanding it. Laura and the nurse manager discussed the difficulties of her changing positions, moving to a new place, and trying to develop both professional and social ties. Together, they came up with several solutions to Laura's problem.

Staff Preferences

Considering the preferences of individual team members is important but should not supersede the other criteria for delegating responsibly. Allowing team members to always select what they want to do may cause the less assertive members' needs to be unmet.

It is important to explain the rationale for decisions made regarding delegation so that all team members may understand the needs of the unit or organization. Box 7–4 outlines basic rights for professional health care team members. Although written originally for women, the concepts are applicable to all professional health care providers.

◙ Barriers to Delegation

Many nurses, and particularly new ones, have difficulty delegating. The reasons for this include experience issues, licensure issues, and quality-of-care issues.

Experience Issues

Many nurses received their education during the 1980s, when primary care was the

> **BOX 7–4**
> **Basic Entitlements of Individuals in the Workplace**
>
> Professionals in the workplace are entitled to:
> - Respect from others in the work setting
> - A reasonable and equitable workload
> - Wages commensurate with the job
> - Determine his or her own priorities
> - Ask for what he or she wants
> - Refuse without guilt
> - Make mistakes and be accountable for them
> - Give and receive information as a professional nurse
> - Act in the best interest of the client
> - Be human
>
> Source: Adapted from Chevernet, M. (1988). *STAT: Special Techniques in Assertiveness Training for Women in Healthcare Professions,* 2nd ed. St. Louis, Mo.: Mosby.

major delivery system. These nurses lacked the education and skill needed for delegation (Mahlmeister, 1999). Nurses educated before the 1970s worked in settings with LPNs and nursing assistants, where they routinely delegated tasks. However, client acuity was lower and the care less complex. Older nurses have considerable delegation experience and may be used as a resource for younger nurses.

The added responsibility of delegation creates some discomfort for nurses. Many believe that they are unprepared to assume this responsibility, especially when it comes to deciding the competency of another person. To decrease this discomfort, nurses need to participate in establishing the guidelines for UAPs within the institution. The ANA Position Statements on Unlicensed Assistive Personnel address this. Table 7–1 lists the direct and indirect client care activities that may be performed by UAPs.

Licensure Issues

Today's health care environment requires nurses to delegate. Many nurses voice concerns about the personal risk regarding their licensure if they delegate inappropriately. The courts have usually ruled that nurses are

TABLE 7–1
Direct and Indirect Client Care Activities

Direct Client Care Activities	Indirect Client Care Activities
Assisting with feeding and drinking	Providing a clean environment
Assisting with ambulation	Providing a safe environment
Assisting with grooming	Providing companion care
Assisting with toileting	Providing transport for non-critical clients
Assisting with dressing	Assisting with stocking nursing units
Assisting with socializing	Providing messenger and delivery services

Adapted from ANA. (2002). *Position Statement on Utilization of Unlicensed Assistive Personnel.* Washington, D.C.: ANA.

not liable for the negligence of other individuals, provided that the nurse delegated appropriately. Delegation is within the scope of nursing practice (Parkman, 1996). The art and skill of delegation are acquired with practice.

Quality-of-Care Issues

Nurses have expressed concern over the quality of client care when tasks and activities are delegated to others. Remember Nightingale's words earlier in the chapter, "Don't imagine that if you, who are in charge, don't look to all these things yourself, those under you will be more careful than you are." She added that you do not need to do everything yourself to see that it is done correctly. When you delegate, you control the delegation. You decide to whom you will delegate the task. Remember that there are levels of acceptable performance and not every task needs to be done perfectly.

Assigning Work to Others

This is difficult for several reasons:

1 Some nurses think they must do everything themselves.

2 Some nurses distrust subordinates to do things correctly.

3 Some nurses think that if they delegate all the technical tasks, they will not reinforce their learning.

4 Some nurses are more comfortable with the technical aspects of client care than with the more complex issues of client teaching and discharge planning.

Families and clients do not always see professional activities. They see direct client care. Nurses believe that when they do not participate directly in client care, they do not accomplish anything for the client. The professional aspects of nursing, such as planning care, teaching, and discharge planning, help to promote positive outcomes for clients and their families. Knowing the scope of practice of LPNs or vocational nurses helps in making delegation decisions.

◼ Conclusion

The concept of delegation is not new. The delegation role is essential to the RN-LPN and RN-UAP relationship. Personal organizational skills are a prerequisite to delegation. Before the nurse can delegate tasks to others, he or she needs to understand individual client needs. Using worksheets and Maslow's hierarchy helps the nurse understand these individual client needs, set priorities, and identify which tasks can be delegated to others. Using the Delegation Decision-Making Grid helps the nurse delegate safely and appropriately.

As the nurse, it is also important for you to be aware of the capabilities of each staff member, the tasks that may be delegated, and the tasks that the RN needs to perform. When delegating, the RN uses professional judgment in making decisions. Professional judgment is directed by the state nurse practice act and national standards of nursing.

Institutions develop their own job descriptions for UAPs and other health care professionals, but institutional policies cannot contradict the state nurse practice act. Although the nurse delegates the task or activity, he or she remains accountable for the delegation decision.

Understanding the concept of delegation helps the new nurse organize and prioritize client care. Knowing the staff and their capabilities simplifies delegation. Utilizing staff members' capabilities creates a pleasant and productive working environment for everyone involved.

Study Questions

1. What are the responsibilities of the professional nurse when delegating tasks to an LPN or a UAP?

2. What factors do you need to consider when delegating tasks?

3. If you were the nurse manager, how would you have handled Laura's situation?

4. How would you have handled the situation if you were Mary Ann?

5. Bring the client census from your assigned clinical unit to class. Using the Delegation Decision-Making Grid, decide which clients you would assign to the personnel on the unit. Give reasons for your decision.

Critical Thinking Exercise

Steven works at a large teaching hospital in a major metropolitan area. This institution services the entire geographical region, including indigent clients, and because of its renowned reputation also administers care to international clients and individuals who reside in other states. Like all health care institutions, this one has been attempting to cut costs by using more UAPs. Nurses are often floated to other units. Lately, the number of indigent and foreign clients on Steven's unit has increased. The acuity of these clients has been quite high, requiring a great deal of time from the nursing staff.

Steven arrived at work at 6:30 A.M., his usual time. He looked at the census board and discovered that the unit was filled, and bed control was calling all night to have clients discharged or transferred to make room for several clients who had been in the emergency department since the previous evening. He also discovered that the other RN assigned to his team called in sick. His team consists of himself, two UAPs, and an LPN who is shared by two teams. He has eight clients on his team: two need to be readied for surgery including preoperative and postoperative teaching, one of whom is a 35-year-old woman scheduled for a modified radical mastectomy for the treatment of breast cancer; three are second day post-ops, and two of these require extensive dressing changes, are receiving IV antibiotics, and need to be ambulated; one post-op client is required to remain on total bedrest, has a nasogastric tube to suction as well as a chest tube, is on TPN and lipids, needs a central venous catheter line dressing change, has an IV, is taking multiple IV medications, and has a Foley catheter; one client is ready for discharge and needs discharge instruction; and one client needs to be transferred to a subacute unit and report must be given to the RN of that unit. Once the latter client is transferred and the other one is discharged, the emergency department will be sending two clients to the unit for admission.

1 How should Steven organize his day? Set up an hourly schedule.

2 What type of client management approach should Steven consider in assigning staff appropriately?

3 If you were Steven, which clients and/or tasks would you assign to your staff? List all of them and explain your rationale.

4 Using the Delegation Decision-Making Grid, make staff and client assignments.

REFERENCES

American Association of Critical Care Nurses (AACN). (1990). *Delegation of Nursing and Non-Nursing Activities in Critical Care: A Framework for Decision Making.* Irvine, Calif.: AACN.

American Nurses Association (ANA). (1996). *Registered Professional Nurses and Unlicensed Assistive Personnel.* Washington, D.C.: ANA.

American Nurses Association (ANA) (2002). *Position Statements* on *Registered Nurse Utilization of Unlicensed Assistive Personnel.* Washington, D.C.: ANA.

Barter M., & Furmidge, M. (1994). Unlicensed assistive personnel. *Journal of Nursing Administration,* 24(4), 36–40.

Boysen, R., & Fischer, C. (2000). *Delegation/Practice Boundaries.* South Dakota State University College of Nursing. *http://learn.sdstate.edu/nursing/DelegationModule2.html* July 29, 2002.

Chevernet, M. (1988). *STAT: Special Techniques in Assertiveness Training for Women in Healthcare Professions,* 2nd ed. St. Louis, Mo.: Mosby.

Conger, M. (1994). The nursing assignment decision grid: Tool for delegation decision. *Journal of Continuing Education in Nursing,* 25(4), 21–27.

Habel, M. (Winter 2001). Delegating nursing care to unlicensed assistive personnel. *Continuing Education for Florida Nurses,* 39–54.

Hansten, R.I., & Washburn, M.J. (1998). *National Council of State Boards of Nursing: Concept Paper on Delegation.* Chicago: NCSBN.

Hayes, P. (1994). Non-nursing functions: Time for them to go. *Nursing Economics,* 12(3), 120–125.

Herrick, K., Hansten, R., O'Neill, L., Hayes, P., & Washburn, M. (1994). My license is on the line: The art of delegation. *Nursing Management,* 25(2), 48–50.

Huber, D., Blegan, M., & McCloskey, J. (1994). Use of nursing assistants: Staff nurse opinions. *Nursing Management,* 25(5), 64–68.

Mahlmeister, L. (1999). Professional accountability and legal liability for the team leader and charge nurse. *Journal of Obstetric, Gynecologic, and Neonatal Nursing,* 28, 300–309.

National Council of State Boards of Nursing. (1990). *Concept Paper on Delegation.* Chicago: NCSBN.

National Council of State Boards of Nursing. (1995). Delegation: Concepts and decision-making process. *Issues* (December), 1–2.

National Council of State Boards of Nursing. (1997). *Delegation Decision-Making Grid.* Chicago: National Council of State Boards of Nursing.

Nightingale, F. (1859). *Notes on Nursing: What It Is and What It Is Not.* London: Harrison and Sons. (Reprint 1992. Philadelphia: J.B. Lippincott.)

Parkman, C.A. (1996). Delegation: Are you doing it right? *American Journal of Nursing,* 96(2), 43–48.

Tappen, R., Weiss, S.A., & Whitehead, D.K. (2001). *Essentials of Leadership and Management.* Philadelphia: F.A. Davis.

Zimmerman, P.G. (1996). Delegating to assistive personnel. *Journal of Emergency Nursing,* 22, 206–212.

CHAPTER 8

Managing Client Care

OBJECTIVES

After reading this chapter, the student should be able to:

- Describe the economic climate or the health care system.

- Compare and contrast the traditional and contemporary models of client care delivery.

- Discuss the role of the nurse in continuous quality improvement and risk management.

- Discuss how continuous quality improvement methodology improves quality care.

- Explain how a critical pathway can be used to measure patient outcomes.

OUTLINE

The Economic Climate in the Health Care System
Economic Perspective
Nursing Labor Market

Models of Care Delivery
Traditional Models
  Total Care
  Functional
  Team
  Modular Nursing
  Primary Nursing
Contemporary Models
  Case Management
  Client-Focused Care
  Product Line Management
  Differentiated Practice

Monitoring and Evaluating the Quality of Care
Structured Care Methodologies
Improving Quality
Continuous Quality Improvement

Total Quality Management
Aspects of Health Care to Evaluate
  Structure
  Process
  Outcome

Quality Improvement at the Unit and Organizational Level

Risk Management

Conclusion

CHAPTER 8 SELF ASSESSMENT
Analyze Your Current Clinical Unit

1. Describe the nursing care delivery system on the unit of your current clinical site.

2. Based on your observations, how well does the model promote client and staff satisfaction?

3. What suggestions do you have for improvement?

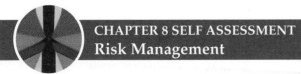

CHAPTER 8 SELF ASSESSMENT
Risk Management

Identify how you will decrease your risk in the following common areas of risk to nurses.

1. Medication errors

2. Documentation errors and/or omissions

3. Failure to correctly perform nursing care or treatments

4. Errors in patient safety that results in falls

5. Failure to communicate significant data to clients and other providers.

All the results of good nursing, as detailed in these notes, may be spoiled or utterly negated by one defect, viz.: in petty management, or in other words, by not knowing how to manage. ... How few men, or even women, understand, either in great or in little things ... . know how to carry out a "charge." To be "in charge" is certainly not only to carry out the proper measure yourself but to see that every one else does so too; to see that no one either willfully or ignorantly thwarts or prevents such measures. It is neither to do everything yourself nor to appoint a number of people to each duty, but to ensure that each does that duty to which he is appointed. (Nightingale & Barnum, 1992, pp. 20, 24)

Although Florence Nightingale wrote these words in the 1800s, they are still true today. Major changes in our health care system are occurring as administrators in all types of agencies try to find the correct balance between "lean and mean" efficiency and high-quality care (Sharp, 1994, p. 32). These efforts affect the way nursing care is delivered. The search for ways to provide safe, effective health care without spending too much money has led to the creation of new models for managing nursing care.

This chapter will help you understand and develop your role in the management of client care. The chapter begins by considering the economic context in which health care is provided. A review of the past, present, and future models for managing nursing care is presented next. This includes the traditional models of total care, primary care, functional care, and team care. The contemporary use of case management, the multidisciplinary team approach, product line management, and differentiated practice complete this section. This is followed by a discussion of the ways in which the quality of the care given is monitored and evaluated.

◼ The Economic Climate in the Health Care System

For many years, decisions about care were based primarily on providing the best quality care, whatever the cost. As the economic support for health care is challenged, however, health care providers are pressured to seek methods of care delivery that achieve quality outcomes at lower cost.

Economic Perspective

The economic perspective is rooted in three fundamental observations:

1 Resources are scarce. Due to scarce resources three choices result:

- The amount to be spent on health care services and the composition of those services

- The methods for producing those services

- The method of distribution of health care, which influences the equity of these services to various people within the population; note that health care needs are not met for more than 40 million uninsured individuals in America.

2 Resources have alternative uses. A result of the scarcity just mentioned, a choice to expend resources in one area eliminates the use of those same resources in another area. If we wish to build more nursing homes, for example, we must be willing to accept fewer hospitals, less housing, less education, or other uses of those same resources.

3 Individuals also want different things or have different preferences. Some people choose alternative treatment modalities such as acupuncture, herbal therapy, or massage therapy rather than traditional health care. The assumption exists that preferences for products and services can be influenced, which explains the extensive marketing of health care services.

During the past three decades, federal and state governments have attempted a variety of cost-containment programs to restrain the cost of health care. Some were carried out through broad federal programs, whereas others targeted specific issues or industries. Among them were:

1 Economic Stabilization Program (ESP). A broad-based federal government program, the ESP was initiated by Richard Nixon in 1971. This program froze wages and prices of all goods and services, including health care, for 90 days. Less stringent restrictions followed, and the program ended in 1974.

2 Voluntary Effort (VE). The VE program, proposed by Jimmy Carter in 1977, urged hospitals to voluntarily reduce their costs. The proposal was defeated by congress in 1979.

3 Certificate of Need (CON). The CON program aims at regulating hospital expenditures for new beds, equipment, and facility construction. The rationale is that excessive hospital growth is the root cause of hospital inflation due to empty beds and underutilized facilities that must be maintained.

4 Medicare Prospective Payment System (PPS). In 1983 the federal government changed its method of paying hospitals for treating Medicare clients. Instead of paying for actual costs, the PPS pays hospitals a fixed, pre-determined sum of money for a particular admission. If a hospital can provide the service at a cost below the fixed amount, it pockets the difference. If more resources and money are used than the predetermined amount, the hospital incurs a loss.

5 Diagnostic Related Groups (DRGs). Tied to the PPS, DRGs are the patient classification systems by which the Medicare PPS determines payment. Each of the 495 DRGs represent a particular case type.

6 Managed Care. Managed care is a system of health care that combines the financing and delivery of health services into a single entity. Currently, over 75 percent of the enrolled population in the private sector are in a managed care plan of some form. Managed care plans are seen as cost-saving alternatives to traditional fee-for-service delivery systems. Through provider networks and selective provider contracting, they attempt to control resource use and health care costs (Chang, Price, & Pfoutz, 2001).

Figure 8–1 depicts the current factors increasing and containing health care costs.

Nursing Labor Market

Registered nurses (RNs) make up 77 percent of the nurse workforce, and almost 60 percent are employed in hospitals. The nationwide unemployment rate for RNs is only 1.0

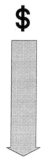

Factors Increasing Costs
• Expansion of national economy
• General inflation
• Aging population
• Growth of third-party payments
• Employer-provided health insurance
• Tax deduction for medical expenses
• Increased costs of labor and equipment
• Expansion of medical technology and products
• Malpractice insurance and litigation

Factors Containing Costs
• Federal economic stabilization program
• Voluntary effort hospital regulation program
• State-level health care payment programs
• Medicare prospective payment system (PPS) with payments of fixed amount per admission
• Diagnostic related groups (DRGs) for hospital payments
• Resource-based relative value scale (RBRVS) for physician payments
• Managed care plans

Design by S.H. Johnson

Figure 8–1 Factors affecting the cost of health care. (From Chang, C.F., Price S.A., & Pfoutz, S.K. *Economics and Nursing: Critical Professional Issues.* Philadelphia: F.A. Davis, 2001, p. 79.)

percent. Even with this low unemployment rate, vacancy rates nationwide are reported at anywhere from 13 to 20 percent and rising. A serious nursing shortage is here, and will continue at least until 2020. The demand for nurses is expected to increase even more dramatically as the baby boomers reach their sixties, seventies, and beyond. From now until 2030, the population aged 65 and older will double. What has caused the nursing shortage?

• **Enrollments declining in nursing programs.** Opportunities for young women outside of nursing have expanded. Enrollments in associate degree nursing programs have declined 11 percent in the past 2 years (Heinrich, 2001). Enrollment in bachelor of science in nursing (BSN) programs has declined 19 percent in the same period.

• **High acuity of clients in hospitals.** Medically complex clients require skilled nursing care.

• **Increased demand for nurses.** As health care moves to a variety of community settings, only the most acute clients remain in the hospital. The transfer of less acute patients to nursing homes and community settings create additional job opportunities and increased demand for nurses.

• **Aging nursing workforce.** In 2000, fewer than one in three RNs was younger than 40 years of age. The percentage of nurses age 40 to 49 is currently over 35 percent.

• **Job dissatisfaction.** Staffing levels, heavy workloads, increased use of overtime, lack of sufficient support staff, and salary discrepancies between nurses and other health care professionals have contributed to growing dissatisfaction and retention of nurses.

• **Reduction in nursing faculty.** Currently there are more than 425 unfilled faculty positions with more than 550 resignations/retirements expected in the coming 2 years (*http://www.nln.org/ slides/ speach.htm;* Heinrich, 2001).

The need to control spiraling health care costs along with the issues of supply and demand for nursing services will continue well into this century. According to the American Nurses Association (ANA), over 40 percent of nurses initially graduate from associate degree nursing programs. You, personally, not only will be affected by trends in health care delivery but also can be a major voice in decision-making (Nelson, 2002). As in the past, cost control and demand for nursing services will most likely involve changing the nurse staffing, the model of care, or professional nursing practice (Ritter-Teitel, 2002).

◪ Models of Care Delivery

Nursing care delivery systems provide the structure that allows nurses to plan and deliver nursing care to groups of clients. Even today, there is no one right way to structure and deliver nursing care. The institution size, staff availability, environment, budget, and organizational goals all affect the model of nursing care delivery. The current acute

nursing shortage continues to fuel the frenzy of work redesign in acute care hospitals across the nation. As we begin the 21st century, some of the more traditional models are reappearing. Regardless of the model, a delivery system focuses on four organizing principles (Manthey, 2001, p. 425):

1 Decision-making. Who is responsible for making what decisions?

2 Care allocation. Who gives what care to the client?

3 Communication. Who tells what to whom?

4 Management. Who is overseeing the process?

Traditional Models

Although the following models are categorized as traditional, this does not imply that the models are old or outdated. Many models are still used today, and all have historical significance in the development of the more contemporary models.

Total Care

The total care, or case, method was one of the earliest models of nursing care delivery. One nurse assumes total responsibility for the planning and delivery of care to a particular client or group of clients. This method may be used today in community health nursing, in private duty, in intensive care and isolation units, and in making assignments for students in nursing school. The client may have different nurses within a 24-hour period, but each nurse provides all of the care needed for the time period assigned. The case method is considered a precursor of primary nursing. Although the method has the advantage of being extremely client focused, it is not considered the most efficient use of staff and is not used in the majority of health care settings today.

Functional

The functional method of care delivery grew out of the 1950s' emphasis on an assembly line style of management that focused on division of labor specifics and tasks that need to be completed. The nurse manager is responsible for making work assignments. Roles such as those of the medication nurse and treatment nurse are part of the functional delivery approach. Job descriptions, procedures, policies, and lines of communication are clearly defined. The functional model is generally considered efficient, economical, and productive. The disadvantage is that this model leads to fragmentation of care because the client receives care from several different types of nursing personnel. In addition, the emotional needs of both the staff members and the client are overlooked in the interest of time management and task completion (Loveridge & Cummings, 1996).

Team

In the later 1950s and into the 1960s, the emphasis moved from a task focus to group dynamics and promotion of job satisfaction. In response to the fragmentation of the functional method and the continued scarcity of RNs after World War II, the team method was developed. Each team consists of a mix of staff members, such as an RN, a licensed practical nurse (LPN), and a nursing assistant. The team is responsible for providing care to a group of assigned clients during the shift. The team leader, usually the RN, is responsible for making assignments for the team based on the team members' abilities and the needs of the clients. Compared with the functional method, the team method emphasizes holistic care and increases client and employee satisfaction.

Modular Nursing

A more current version of team nursing is modular nursing. Modular nursing takes into account the actual structure of the unit, allowing nurses to be located nearer the clients with a wider range of responsibility delegated to them. Modular nursing is often used when primary nursing is not an option. Each RN, assisted by paraprofessional team members, delivers care to a group of clients. The geographical grouping of one 50-bed unit into three modular substations may allow staff to even further emphasize effi-

ciency in this era of RN scarcity (Huber, 2000; Loveridge & Cummings, 1996).

Primary Nursing

Primary nursing became popular in the 1960s and 1970s as nurses voiced concern over the fragmentation of care provided to their clients. In this model, an RN is assigned care of a client for 24 hours a day for the client's entire hospital stay, including discharge planning. This RN is responsible for developing the care plan and managing the associate nurses and other staff members who provide additional care for the client. Primary nursing decreases the number of persons who have contact with each client and usually increases accountability and client satisfaction. However, primary nursing severely limits the number of clients each nurse can serve and can place the client in jeopardy if the primary nurse is not capable of meeting the client's needs. As the pressures for cost containment and restructuring increased in the late 1980s and early 1990s, the primary care concept was almost totally eliminated in acute care settings (Huber, 2000; Loveridge & Cummings, 1996).

Contemporary Models

As health care administrators search for the model of care delivery that will ensure quality, promote client and staff satisfaction, and contain costs, new models emerged. Among the newer (or reemerging) models are case management, client-focused care with cross-training, product line management, and differentiated practice.

Case Management

The term *case management* is used to describe a variety of health care delivery systems in acute, long-term, and community settings. Case management is not a new concept. Public health programs have used case management to provide care since the early 1900s. As early as 1970, insurance companies began case management in an attempt to control long-term, expensive cases. When mental health services moved out of institutions into the community in the 1960s, case management programs became important to psychiatric-mental health nursing as well (Lyon, 1993). These examples of "external" case management were models for the "internal" case management that began in the 1980s within the acute care setting.

The ANA defined case management as "provision of quality care along a continuum, decreased fragmentation of care across many settings, enhancement of the quality of life, and cost containment" (Lynam, 1994, p 48). The process of case management is easily placed within the framework of the nursing process (Table 8–1).

According to Newell (1996), the primary functions of case managers include:

- **Negotiation services and/or treatments.** Obtain maximum quality services at an acceptable cost (e.g., negotiate RN hourly rates for home care services, obtain prices for equipment such as a wheelchair).

- **Communication.** Communicate with service providers, clients, families, and information systems.

- **Coordination of care.** Oversee services and resources to avoid duplication and breakdowns in quality.

- **Clinical expertise.** Possess technical knowledge of disease processes and interventions to assess, plan, and evaluate client services.

- **Holistic approach.** Be able to understand human beings' biologic, social, and behavioral needs.

- **Ethics with caring.** Maintain a focus on advocacy, honesty, and understanding in dealing with clients.

- **Coaching.** This important skill affects all of the preceding functions; be successful in working with clients, families, staff, and physicians.

Nursing care management is designed to decrease fragmentation of care, use of hospitalization, and cost through better coordination and monitoring of client care. Effective nursing case management can improve the quality of services, the quality of life for clients, and the functioning of the interdisciplinary team.

Case management systems must act like human beings who are functioning well: they are focused on the task at hand, interact without duplicity, learn and respond to new situations and information, and are honest and forthright in communicating with all parties. Well-functioning case managers and case management systems may not always do everything right, but they strive to do the right thing, thus affecting others in the system to also act with integrity (Newell, 1996).

Nursing care management is a system for delivering nursing care that is based on the philosophy of case management. The goals of nursing care management follow (Girard, 1994):

- **Outcomes based on standards of care.** Evaluation of the quality of nursing practice is based on desired measurable outcomes and accepted practices of the nursing profession.

TABLE 8–1

Comparison of Nursing Process and Nursing Case Management Process

Assessment/Diagnosis	Planning	Intervention	Evaluation
Determine physical, emotional, psychological needs	Determine resources	Link clients to services	Ensure needs are met
Reassess and begin process again	Develop care plans, critical pathways	Act as a "broker" and advocate	Monitor and document cost effectiveness and client progress

Source: Adapted from Mass, S., & Johnson, B. (November 1998). Case management and clinical guidelines. *Journal of Care Management*, 18.

• **Well-coordinated continuity of care through collaborative practice.** All providers of services work together to plan services and meet client needs. Effective collaboration requires that providers also work together to meet each other's needs.

• **Efficient use of resources to reduce wasted time, energy, and materials.** Continued monitoring of material and personnel resources can eliminate duplication of steps and services, resulting in increased efficiency and job satisfaction.

• **Timely discharge within prospective payment guidelines.** Grouping of medical conditions into categories that have allowable lengths of stay and payment schedules designated by Medicare has been in effect since the 1980s. Enabling clients to be discharged safely within the designated length of stay is an ongoing challenge for the nursing care manager.

• **Professional development and satisfaction.** Through coordination of services and collaboration with providers, family, and clients, use of the case management model can enhance clients' quality of life (Christensen & Bender, 1994).

Although many different health care personnel claim to have in-depth knowledge of client and family care needs and understanding of organizational and financial services and community resources, the RN is ideally suited to serve as care manager. "In an era of decreasing reimbursements and increasing accreditation requirements, hospital administrators view nurse case managers as one answer to balancing cost and quality" (Wayman, 1999, p. 236).

Nursing has traditionally considered the client from a total-systems perspective of person, environment, and health with a focus on the multidisciplinary efforts needed to optimize care for the individual. Nurses, accustomed to focusing on a holistic approach to nursing care, are best able to use a whole-system approach to care delivery rather than a parts-oriented approach (Newell, 1996).

The case management system of care helps clients learn to cope with the challenges of their illness. Case management services can be delivered in a variety of settings. *External case management* involves activities that are external to provider organizations. For example, case managers may work with victims of catastrophic motor vehicle accidents, workers' compensation patients, major medical insurance patients, and individual clients with complex chronic conditions. *Internal case managers* provide services within the walls of institutions or provider organizations. Internal case managers work in acute care, subacute care, rehabilitation, long-term care, home care, and managed care organizations (Newell, 1996).

The following is a case management example:

Maria is a 71-year-old Salvadoran-American woman with a history of childhood rheumatic heart disease. She has given birth to four children, the last one when Maria was 41. During that pregnancy, she spent the last trimester on bedrest. She complained of fatigue, shortness of breath, and swelling in her feet and ankles after her last child was born; 4 years after the birth of this child, she had a mitral commissurotomy to open the calcified mitral valve.

Since then, she has complained of the same symptoms, and she has been unable to walk up the flight of stairs in her two-story home. Maria and her husband depend on his small pension and social security for their living expenses. Their home is paid for, and the children are always sending "gifts," but money is limited. The couple joined a Medicare health maintenance organization (HMO) to cover the cost of drugs and to avoid having to carry a supplemental policy to augment traditional Medicare coverage.

As Maria's condition deteriorated, she experienced liver enlargement, sleep apnea, and petechiae on her face. She was very depressed regarding her continued illness. The HMO physician tried to talk Maria into a mitral valve replacement. She stated emphatically, "I will never go through what I did when I had that surgery, so don't even mention it!" The physician asked the nurse case manager to see Maria.

The nurse case manager met with Maria and her husband in their home. She observed that, although the house appeared clean, Maria complained that she is unable to keep house like she used to and feels useless as a wife and mother. The case manager helped Maria and her husband evaluate their options for treatment of Maria's illness. She made several visits to their home and, after forming a positive relationship with them, began to discuss the potential benefits of surgery and the possibility of improving Maria's quality of life. Maria finally consented to having a cardiac catheterization, which showed that both the mitral and tricuspid valves were leaking. She agreed to surgery, which was successful. The case manager continues to call Maria on a monthly basis to monitor her progress. Maria said recently, "I owe my new life to my wonderful nurse."

Client-Focused Care

In the client-focused care model, services and staff are organized around client needs, rather than the other way around. Traditionally, hospitals have been organized by departments, which the client goes to for services. In the client-focused care model, the services are brought to the client (Greenberg, 1994). Clients with similar needs are placed on the same nursing units, with ancillary and support services present on the unit. The traditional boundaries between disciplines are blurred. Although licensed members of the team retain their professional expertise and function within state and national practice acts and accrediting agency requirements, members of the team share all non-regulated tasks. Members of disciplines such as nursing, physical therapy, respiratory therapy, and pharmacy are unit-based. They receive additional training so that they can provide services across disciplinary lines. Their combined functions may range from clinical to managerial responsibilities and may be of higher, lower, or parallel levels when compared with their original functions.

In addition, new all-purpose "client care technicians" or unlicensed assistive personnel (UAP) roles are usually created. These new workers perform tasks such as meal delivery, cleaning and maintenance of rooms, and assisting clients with comfort needs. Under the supervision of licensed personnel, patient care technicians may also perform skilled tasks that are not restricted by various practice acts, such as insertion of indwelling urinary catheters or simple dressing changes (Christensen & Bender, 1994; Flarey, 1995).

Response to this new model of care delivery has been mixed. Some nursing administrators say that staff dissatisfaction and stress have increased, whereas others report favorable client experiences and staff satisfaction (Christensen & Bender, 1994). Since

its inception in 1989, the use of the client-focused care model has increased, but further research on its effectiveness is needed (Clouten & Weber, 1994). The following is a client-focused care example:

Esperanza has been the nurse manager on a 50-bed medical-surgical unit for 5 years. Since the advent of the prospective payment system, reimbursement for care has been limited. Patients come in sicker and go home more quickly. Esperanza just left a management meeting in which the chief executive officer informed them that nursing costs make up over half of the hospital's total budget. To cut costs and maximize effectiveness, the nurse managers must decrease the number of nurses on each shift, making sure that RNs do only those tasks that require an RN. A consultant will be brought in to implement a new system called *client-focused care*.

Each unit formed a committee of management personnel, staff nurses, and nursing assistants to meet with the consultant. In addition, representatives of other services, such as rehabilitation services, respiratory care, pharmacy, and housekeeping were included. The consultant made clear that the decisions made would be what worked for this organization, and not a blueprint from another organization.

The committees met weekly. Specific indirect and direct client care activities that could be delegated to non-licensed personnel in accordance with the state nurse practice act were identified. The committees decided that there would be two levels of clinical assistants. Job descriptions and work standards were developed for each level. Training workshops were developed, and a skill competency workshop was required for all new personnel. The hospital worked in conjunction with the local community college to offer certificates for the two clinical assistant levels. By the end of the program, 9.6 full-time RN positions were converted into 15.6 clinical assistant positions. The hospital predicted savings in recruitment, orientation, and training costs as well as increased job satisfaction for all participants. Esperanza felt that only time would tell if the program works for both the staff and the clients.

Product Line Management

Product line management is used in business to create a center to plan, manage, and market a specific product within the larger company. In health care delivery, use of this system results in a new organizational structure in which components of various clinical services or departments are merged to create a distinct "product line," such as drug abuse treatment, women's health care, or pediatric care. For example, the orthopedic product line would include nursing care, therapies, technician services, orthotic and prosthetic devices, and educational programs. In this type of delivery system, a product line manager directs these operations.

Unlike traditional systems in which the RN was the manager, the product line manager may be a member of a discipline other than nursing. In some instances, the manager may not even have a related health care background (Christensen & Bender, 1994, p. 68). The non-nurse manager may have a great deal of business and financial background and make purely business decisions regarding client care. Unfortunately, the non-nurse manager may have difficulty focusing on client and family needs that are incongruent with business decisions.

Differentiated Practice

Differentiated practice is the structuring of nursing roles and functions based on the individual's education, experience, and competence. Differentiated practice was the model behind development of the initial associate degree nursing programs. For example, a nurse with an associate degree would care for clients in the hospital setting under the supervision of a BSN nurse manager, whereas the nurse with a baccalaureate degree would plan the client's care in the home. The reasons for implementing a differentiated practice model focus on organizational and professional benefits (Huber, 2000):

- **Organizational benefits.** Decreasing costs while increasing efficiency, this argument describes differentiated practice as a means of better utilizing nursing resources.

- **Professional benefits.** This argument focuses on the need to decide what nursing is and what it is not. The professional benefits argument further focuses on delineating the role of the RB based on education.

The most common models of differentiated nursing practice are based on nursing education (AONE, 1994).

- *Associate degree nurse.* The associate

nurse is responsible for the shift of service, with a strong emphasis on meeting the physiological and comfort needs of the client assigned by the primary nurse. The associate nurse role is to implement nursing care plans developed by the nurse clinician and primary nurse.

- *Baccalaureate degree nurse or primary nurse.* The primary nurse's responsibility extends from admission to discharge, focusing on coordination of medical and nursing orders, client education, and a well-planned, timely discharge. The primary nurse must be able to match client needs with staff abilities using an interdisciplinary team approach.

- *Master's degree nurse.* This advanced practice role may include the advanced registered nurse practitioner (ARNP), advanced practice nurse (APN), and certified nurse midwife (CNM). The APN assumes the role of case manager and client advocate. The role of the ARNP extends beyond the acute care setting into multiple health care arenas.

Informally, differentiated practice among RNs exists in almost every setting. It occurs each time a nurse manager plans staff assignments according to the knowledge, competence, and licensure of the staff members involved, for example. Other members of the health care team and even clients develop a sixth sense about the abilities of the nurses with whom they interact (McClure, 1991).

The controversy over RN licensure has raged within the profession since 1965, when the ANA endorsed the concept of two levels of educational preparation and licensure. Forty years later, the organization is still fighting the idea that "a nurse is a nurse is a nurse." Regardless of educational preparation or background, nurses are often used interchangeably in the workplace. The result is that they are not used in a cost-effective manner, and many are not challenged to reach their full potential. As the nursing shortage continues, differentiated practice models are expanding to include LPNs, unlicensed personnel, and other specially trained nurse extenders.

The rationale for implementing differentiated nursing practice is both professional and economic. Professionally, differentiated practice for the RN may lead to increased satisfaction and improved client care. Used effectively, differentiated practice models also ensure efficient use of nursing resources (Allender, Egan, & Newman, 1995; Koerner et al., 1995; Ray & Hardin, 1995; Vena & Oldaker, 1994). Table 8–2 outlines the advantages and disadvantages of each model. Regardless of the patient care delivery system, the shortage of professional nurses will continue to increase the use of UAPs. The ANA defines UAPs as "individuals trained to function in an assistive role to the registered professional nurse in the provision of patient/client care activities as delegated by

and under the supervision of the registered professional nurse" (Kido, 2001, p. 28). State nurse practice acts define the legal scope of nursing in each state and enumerate the nursing activities that cannot be delegated to UAPs.

In March 1994, the ANA Board of Directors launched a major multiphase initiative to investigate the impact of health care restructuring on the safety and quality of patient care as well as on nursing. Through a program called Nursing's Safety and Quality Initiative, ANA highlights the strong linkages between nursing actions and patient outcomes. Through this initiative, many state nurses associations now collect data on nursing-sensitive quality indicators. These indicators are the outcomes most affected by nursing care. The current list of 10 indicators is described in Box 8–1.

TABLE 8–2
Advantages and Disadvantages of Nursing Care Delivery Systems

Delivery System	Major Concept	Advantages	Disadvantages
Total Care	One RN with total responsibility for care	Continuity of care	Costly; not efficient use of staff
Functional	Division of tasks with clearly defined roles	Efficient, economical, productive	Fragments care
Team	TN team leader supervises ancillary staff	More holistic	RN must take time to delegate appropriately
Modular Nursing	Derivative of team nursing; takes structure of unit into account	More efficient than team	Substations must be organized on unit
Primary Care	RN maintains 24 hour responsibility for client(s)	Emphasis on accountability and client satisfaction	Extremely costly; Primary nurse must be capable of meeting all client's needs
Case Management	Management and coordination of care for episode of illness	Focuses on entire episode of illness; goal is achievement of outcomes	Nurse must be knowledgeable in coordinating care throughout illness
Client-Focused Care	Services and staff organized around client needs	Interdisciplinary team approach	RN must be able to delegate and supervise; ancillary staff must trained; organization of all services must be present on unit
Product Line Management	Components of clinical services and departments organized around a distinct product	Makes distinct services available	Manager may not be a nurse or even have a health care background
Differentiated Practice	Nursing roles and functions based on education, experience, and competence	Recognizes roles and functions of RN	Hard to overcome mentality of "a nurse is a nurse is a nurse"

BOX 8–1
Nursing Sensitive Quality Indicators

1. Staffing mix of RNs, LPNs, and UAPs
2. Total nursing care hours/day
3. Maintenance of skin integrity
4. Patient injury rate
5. Nosocomial infections
6. Pain management
7. Patient satisfaction with nursing care
8. Patient satisfaction with education
9. Patient satisfaction with overall care
10. Nurse staff satisfaction with work environment

Source: Adapted from *http://www.nursingworld.org/readroom/fssafe99.htm*; Kido, 2001.

The use of UAPs need not affect patient safety or quality care. RNs must be actively involved in the training, educating, monitoring, and supervising of UAPs. Above all, the belief in the nurse-patient relationship as the foundation of professional nursing practice and the value placed on the delivery of direct patient care by the decision-maker is central to maintaining positive outcomes for both clients and nurses (Scott, J., Sochalski, J., & Aiken, L., 1999).

◼ Monitoring and Evaluating the Qualityof Care

Structured Care Methodologies

As you can see, various health care delivery models have surfaced in an attempt to streamline processes, reduce costs, and ensure quality service. Whether an institution uses a traditional model of care delivery or moves to one of the more contemporary models discussed, most agencies have implemented tools for tracking outcomes. These tools are called *structured care methodologies* (SCMs). SCMs are interdisciplinary tools used to "identify best practices, facilitate standardization of care, and provide a mechanism for variance tracking, quality enhancement, outcomes measurement, and outcomes research" (Cole & Houston, 1999, p. 53). SCMs include guidelines, critical pathways, algorithms, protocols, standards of care, and order sets.

• **Guidelines.** Guidelines first appeared in the 1980s as statements to assist health care providers and clients in making appropriate health care decisions. Guidelines are based on current research strategies and are often developed by experts in the field. The use of guidelines is seen as a way to decrease variations in practice.

• **Protocols.** Protocols are specific, formal documents that outline how a procedure or intervention should be conducted. Protocols have been used for many years in research and specialty areas but have moved into the general health care arena as a way to standardized approaches to achieve desired outcomes. An example seen in many facilities today is chest pain protocols.

• **Algorithms.** Algorithms are systematic procedures that follow a logical progression based on additional information or client responses to treatment. They were originally developed in the mathematics area and are frequently seen in emergency medical services. Advanced cardiac life support algorithms are now widely used in health care agencies.

• **Standards of care.** Standards of care are often discipline related and help to operationalize patient care processes and provide a baseline for quality care. Lawyers often refer to the discipline's standards of care in evaluating whether a client has received appropriate services.

• **Critical (or clinical) pathways.** Critical pathways were first used in manufacturing during the late 1950s and appeared in health care in the 1980s. A critical pathway is a "multidisciplinary map" that outlines the expected course of treatment for clients with similar diagnoses. The critical pathway should easily orient the nurse to the client outcomes for the day. In some institutions, nursing diagnoses with specific time frames are incorporated into the critical pathway. This standardized "map" is designed to describe the course of events that lead to successful client outcome within the diagnosis-related group (DRG)-defined time frame. For the client with an uncomplicated myocardial infarction (MI), a proposed course of events leading to successful client outcomes within the 4-day DRG-defined time frame might be as follows (Doenges, Moorhouse, & Geissler, 1997):

- Patient states that chest pain is relieved.

- ST and T wave changes resolve and pulse oximeter reading is greater than 90 percent; have clear breath sounds.

- Patient ambulates in hall without experiencing extreme fatigue or chest pain.

- Patient verbalizes feelings about having an MI and future fears; patient identifies effective coping strategies.

- Ventricular dysfunction, dysrhythmia, or crackles are resolved.

Critical pathways are clinical protocols involving all disciplines. They are designed for tracking a planned clinical course for clients based on average and expected lengths of stay. Financial outcomes can be evaluated from critical pathways by assessing any variances from the proposed length of stay. The health care agency can then focus on problems within the system that extend the length of stay or drive up costs because of overutilization or repetition of services.

Mr. J. was admitted to the telemetry unit with a diagnosis of MI. He had no previous history of heart disease and no other complicating factors such as diabetes, hypertension, or elevated cholesterol levels. His DRG prescribed length of stay was 4 days. He had an uneventful hospitalization for the first 2 days. On the third day, he complained of pain in the left calf. The calf was slightly reddened and warm to the touch. This condition was diagnosed as thrombophlebitis, which increased his length of hospitalization. A review of the events leading up to the complaints of calf pain by the case manager indicated that, although the physician ordered compression stockings for Mr. J., they never arrived and no one followed through on the order. The variances related to his proposed length of stay were discussed with the team providing care, and measures were instituted to make sure that this oversight did not occur again.

Critical pathways provide a framework for communication and documentation of care. They are also excellent teaching tools through which staff members from various disciplines can learn about the expected care of given client populations and an institution's practice patterns. Critical pathways can be used by an institution to evaluate the cost of care for different client populations (Capuano, 1995; Crummer & Carter, 1993; Flarey, 1995; Lynam, 1994).

Most institutions have adopted a chronological, diagrammatic format for presenting a critical pathway. Time frames may range from daily (day 1, day 2, day 3) to hourly, depending on client needs. Key elements of the critical pathway include discharge planning, patient education, consultations, activities, nutrition, medications, diagnostic tests, and treatment (Crummer & Carter, 1993). Table 8–3 is an example of a critical pathway. Although originally developed for use in acute care institutions, critical pathways can be developed for home care and long-term care settings as well. The client's nurse is usually responsible for monitoring and recording any deviations from the critical pathway. When deviations occur, the reasons are discussed with all members of the health care team, and the appropriate changes in care are made. The nurse must also identify general trends in client outcomes and develop plans to improve the quality of care to reduce the number of deviations in critical pathways. Through this close monitoring, the health care team can avoid last-minute surprises that may delay client discharge and can more effectively predict lengths of stay.

SCMs may be used alone or together. A client who is admitted for an MI may have care planned using a critical pathway for his acute MI, a heparin protocol, and a dysrhythmia algorithm. In addition, the nurses may refer to the standards of care in developing a traditional nursing care plan.

SCMs can improve physiologic, psychologic, and financial outcomes. Services and interventions are sequenced to provide safe and effective outcomes in a designated time and with most effective use of resources. They also give an interdisciplinary perspec-

TABLE 8–3

Sample Critical Pathway: Heart Failure, Hospital. ELOS 4 Days Cardiology or Medical Unit

ND and Categories of Care	Day 1 _____	Day 2 _____	Day 3 _____	Day 4 _____
Decreased cardiac output R/T decreased myocardial contractility, altered electrical conduction, structural changes	Goals Participate in actions to reduce cardiac workload	Display VS within acceptable limits; dysrhythmias controlled; pulse oximetry within acceptable range Meet own self-care needs with assist as necessary	→ Dysrhythmias controlled or absent → Free of signs of respiratory distress Demonstrate measurable increase in activity tolerance	→
Fluid volume Excess R/T compromised regulatory mechanism	Verbalize understanding of fluid/food restrictions	Verbalize understanding of general condition and healthcare needs Breath sounds clearing Urinary output adequate Wt loss (reflecting fluid loss)	Plan for lifestyle/ behavior changes Breath sounds clear Balanced I & O Edema resolving	Plan in place to meet post-discharge needs Wt stable (continued loss if edema present)
Referrals	Cardiology Dietitian	Cardiac rehab Occupational therapist (for ADLs) Social services Home care	Community resources	
Diagnostic studies	ECG Echo-Doppler CXR ABGs/Pulse oximetry Cardiac enzymes BUN/Cr CBC, electrolytes Mg++ PT/aPTT Liver function studies Serum glucose Albumin Uric acid Digoxin level (as indicated)	Echo-Doppler (if not done day 1) or MUGA Cardiac enzymes (if ↑) BUN/Cr Electrolytes PT/aPTT (if on anticoagulants)	CXR BUN/Cr Electrolytes PT/aPTT (as indicated) Repeat digoxin level (if indicated)	

(Continued on following page)

TABLE 8–3

Sample Critical Pathway: Heart Failure, Hospital. ELOS 4 Days
Cardiology or Medical Unit (Continued)

ND and Categories of Care	Day 1 _____	Day 2 _____	Day 3 _____	Day 4 _____
Additional assessments	UA			
	Apical pulse, heart/breath sounds q8h	→	→ bid	→
	Cardiac rhythm (telemetry) q4h	→ →	→	D/C	→
	B/P, P.R *q2h till stable, q4h*	q8h	→	→
	Temp q8h			
	I & O *q8h*	→	→	→ D/C
	Weight *qAM*	→	→	→
	Peripheral edema *q8h*	→	→ bid	→ qd
	Peripheral pulses *q8h*	→	→ bid	→ D/C
	Sensorium *q8h*	→	→ bid	→ D/C
	DX check *qd*	→	→	→
	Response to activity	→	→	→
	Response to therapeutic interventions	→	→	→
Medications / Allergies: _____ _____	IV diuretic	po	→	→
	ACE inhibitor	→	→	→
	Digoxin	→	→	→
	PO/Cutaneous nitrates	→	→	→
	Morphine sulfate	→	→ D/C	
	Daytime/HS sedation	→	→	→ D/C
	PO/low dose anticoagulant	→	→ PO or D/C	→
	IV/PO potassium	→	→ D/C	
	Stool softener/laxative	→	→	→
Patient education	Orient to unit/room Review advanced directives Discuss expected outcomes, diagnostic tests/results Fluid/nutritional restrictions/needs	Cardiac education per protocol Review medications: dose, time, route, purpose, side effects Progressive activity program Skin care	Signs/systems to report to healthcare provider Plan for home-care needs	Provide written instructions for homecare Schedule for follow-up appointments

TABLE 8–3
Sample Critical Pathway: Heart Failure, Hospital. ELOS 4 Days
Cardiology or Medical Unit (Continued)

ND and Categories of Care	Day 1 _____		Day 2 _____		Day 3 _____		Day 4 _____
Additional nursing actions	Bed/chair rest	→	BPR/Ambulate as tol, cardiac program	→	Up ad lib/graded program	→	
	Assist with physical care	→		→		→	(send home)
	Egg-crate mattress	→		→		→	
	Dysrhythmia/ angina care per protocol	→		→	D/C		
	Supplemental O₂	→		→		→	
	Cardiac diet	→		→		→	

Source: Doenges, M., E., Moorhouse, M.F., and Geissler, A.C. (2002). *Nursing Care Plans: Guidelines for Individualizing Patient Care,* ed. 6, pp. 59–60. Philadelphia: F.A. Davis, with permission. CP = critical path; ELOS = estimated length of stay; ND = nursing diagnosis.

tive that is not found in the traditional nursing care plan. Computer programs allow health care personnel to track variances (differences from the identified standard) and use these variances in planning quality improvement (QI) activities.

The use of structured care methodologies does not take the place of the expert clinical judgment of the RN. The fundamental purpose of the SCM is to assist health care providers in implementing practices identified with good clinical judgment, research-based interventions, and improved client outcomes. Data from SCMs allow comparisons of outcomes, development of research-based decisions, identification of high-risk patients, and identification of issues and problems before they escalate into pending disasters. Do not be afraid to learn and understand the different SCMs. They can be invaluable tools to your already expert nursing knowledge. Box 8–2 reviews the uses of SCMs.

Improving Quality

Quality management activities have been part of nursing care since Florence Nightin-

gale evaluated the care of soldiers during the Crimean War (Nightingale, 1992). Quality monitoring and standard setting occurs through many avenues:

1 Professional organizations

2 Federal and state governments

3 State licensure

4 Private accreditation

BOX 8–2
Structured Care Methodologies

• Link the process of care and the outcome
• Allow for measuring quality of care
• Increase the predictability of service needs
• Clarify the responsibilities of interdisciplinary team
• Facilitate communication among team members
• Decrease documentation time
• Provide a systematic approach to measurement

Source: Adapted from Mass, S., & Johnson, B. (November 1998). Case management and clinical guidelines. *Journal of Care Management,* p. 19.

Involvement in quality improvement (QI) begins at the staff nurse level. QI procedures are used to address not only whether the appropriate interventions took place and the desired outcomes occurred but also how long it took and how much it cost.

In 1951, the Joint Commission on Accreditation of Healthcare Organizations (JCAHO) was established. The focus of its evaluation at that time was on structural measures of quality, assessment of the physical plant, number of client beds per nurse, credentialing of service providers, and other standards for each department. Since that time, this system of evaluation has given way to a more process- and outcome-focused model: continuous quality improvement (CQI). Shortly after the establishment of JCAHO, the ANA and National League for Nursing (NLN) began publishing standards related to nursing. Table 8–4 identifies current standards published by the American Nurses Credentialing Center.

Today, JCAHO accredits more than 19,000 health care organizations. Evaluation of nursing services is an important part of the accreditation. JCAHO-accredited agencies are measured against national standards set by health care professionals. Hospitals, health care networks, long-term care facilities, ambulatory care centers, home health agencies, behavioral health care facilities, and clinical laboratories are among the organizations seeking JCAHO accreditation. Although the accreditation by JCAHO is voluntary, Medicare and Medicaid reimbursement cannot be sought by organizations not accredited by JCAHO.

On the subjective level, most nurses would agree that they recognize high-quality

TABLE 8–4

Certifications Available from the American Nurses Credentialing Center (AACC)

Specialty Certifications RN, BC	Specialty Certifications Associate/Diploma RN, C	Modular Certification RN, C	Advanced Practice Certification	Clinical Nurse Specialist
Cardiac and Vascular Nurse	Gerontology Nurse	Nursing Case Management	Acute Care NP	Community Health Nurse
College Health Nurse	Pediatric Nurse	Ambulatory Nursing	Adult NP	Gerontological Nurse
General Nursing Practice	Psych/Mental Heath Nurse		Family NP	Home Health Nurse
Gerontology Nurse	Medical-Surgical Nurse		Gerontological NP	Medical-Surgical Nurse
Home Health Nurse	Perinatal Nurse		Pediatric NP	Pediatric Nurse
Informatics Nurse			Psych Mental Health NP	Psych/Mental Health Nurse
			Adult	Adult
			Family	Family
Medical-Surgical Nurse				
Nursing Administration				
Nursing Professional Development				
Pediatric Nurse				
Perinatal Nurse				
Psych/Mental Health Nurse				
School Nurse				

Adapted from American Nurses Credentialing Center, http://nursingworld.org/ancc/faqs.htm#bac

care when they see it. More objectively, however, quality in nursing care has been difficult to define. Quality encompasses effectiveness, efficiency, optimality (a balance between cost and effectiveness), acceptability, legitimacy (conformance to social norms and ethical principles), and equity (Donabedian quoted in Mark, Salyer, & Geddis, 1997). Should we strive for perfection in health care? Is it good enough to provide just adequate care? Leebov (1991) asked us to consider the following before answering these questions:

- How many babies is it okay to drop?

- How many medication errors are allowable in a week or a month?

- How many rude comments to patients is too many?

- How long can a call light be ignored?

QA (quality assurance), QI (quality improvement), CQI (continuous quality improvement), and TQM (total quality management) are acronyms you will hear in almost any health care setting in the United States.

Continuous Quality Improvement

Continuous quality improvement (CQI) is a process of identifying areas of concern (indicators), collecting data on these indicators on an ongoing basis, analyzing and evaluating the data, and implementing needed changes. When the indicator no longer is a concern, another indicator is selected. Common indicators include the number of falls, medication errors, and infection rates. Indicators can be identified by the accrediting agency and/or by the facility itself. The purpose of CQI is to continuously improve the capability of everyone involved in providing care, including the organization itself, to provide the highest quality health care. CQI consists of four basic elements (Kinlaw, 1992).

1 Use of interdisciplinary team approach

2 Inclusion of patient perspective

3 Measurement of work structures, processes, and outcomes

4 Availability of resources for implementation

Employees are empowered to make decisions to improve quality. Education, training, participation at all levels, and empowerment of staff members are keys to CQI success. Improvements are accomplished through the use of QI teams. Their purpose is to identify processes that may be too costly or ineffective, in order to change them. With these supporting data, decisions can be made regarding changes needed to improve quality. These teams comprise representatives from every area involved in the process under study.

CQI relies on collecting information and analyzing it. The time frame used in a QI program can be retrospective (evaluating past performance), concurrent (evaluating current performance), or prospective (future oriented, collecting data as they come in). The procedures used to collect data will depend on the purpose of the program. Data may be obtained using a variety of methods such as observation, performance appraisals, client satisfaction surveys, statistical analyses of length-of-stay and costs, surveys, peer reviews, and chart audits (Huber, 2000).

Although you may think this is the responsibility of number crunchers not nurses, in the CQI framework, data collection becomes everyone's responsibility. You may be asked to brainstorm your ideas with other nurses or members of the interdisciplinary team, complete surveys or check sheets, or even keep a time log of your daily activities for a week or longer. Collecting comprehensive, accurate, and representative data is the first step in revisiting the process. How do you actually administer medications to a group of clients? What steps are involved? Are the medications always available at the right time and in the right dose, or do you have to wait for the pharmacy to bring them to the floor? Is the pharmacy technician delayed by emergency orders that must be processed? Looking at the entire process and actually mapping it out on paper in the form of a flowchart may be part of the CQI process for your organization (Fig. 8–2).

JCAHO does not mandate a specific model to accomplish QI. They do, however, have standards that address organizational performance in specific areas. The goal of the survey is not just to assess what the organization says it does but also to see what it actually accomplishes. The dimensions of performance that JCAHO has defined are efficacy, appropriateness, availability, timeliness, effectiveness, continuity, safety, efficiency, respect, and caring (Simms, Price, & Ervin, 2000, p. 307). Table 8–5 describes JCAHO dimensions of quality performance.

◼ Total Quality Management

When the idea of CQI becomes a management philosophy that permeates every as-

ASSIGN RESPONSIBILITIES
⬇
IDENTIFY VITAL AREAS
⬇
DEFINE SCOPE OF CARE
⬇
ANALYZE AREA IN TERMS OF:
⬇
ASPECTS
STANDARDS
INDICATORS
CRITERIA
⬇
MEASURE ACTUAL PERFORMANCE
&
MEASURE PATIENT OUTCOMES
⬇
EVALUATE PERFORMANCE AND OUTCOMES
⬇
RECOMMEND AND IMPLEMENT ACTIONS
⬇
EVALUATE DEGREE OF IMPROVEMENT

Figure 8–2 Unit level quality improvement process. (Adapted from Hunt, D.V. (1992). *Quality in America: How to Implement a Competitive Quality Program.* Homewood, Ill.: Business One Irwin; and Duquette, A.M. (1991). Approaches to monitoring practice: Getting started. In Schroeder, P. (ed.). *Monitoring and Evaluation in Nursing.* Gaithersburg, Md.: Aspen.)

pect of a health care organization, CQI becomes total quality management (TQM).

Aspects of Health Care to Evaluate

As just mentioned, three different aspects of health care can be evaluated in a QI program: the structure within which the care is given, the process of giving that care, and the outcome of that care. To be comprehensive, an evaluation program must include all three aspects of health care (Brook, Davis, & Kamberg, 1980; Donabedian, 1969, 1977, 1987). When focused on nursing care, the independent, dependent, and interdependent functions of nurses may be added to the model (Irvine, 1998). Each of these dimensions is described here and their interrelationship is illustrated in Table 8–6.

Structure

Structure refers to the setting in which the care is given and the resources (human, financial, and material) that are available. The questions related to structure are "Is the structure in place that will allow quality to exist? and Is the structure of the organization set up to allow quality of care?" (Huber, 2000, p. 618). It is the easiest of the three aspects to measure and yet is still overlooked in some evaluation procedures. The following is a list of some of the structural aspects of a health care organization that can be evaluated:

- **Facilities.** Includes comfort, convenience of layout, accessibility of support services, safety

- **Equipment.** Includes adequate supplies, state-of-the-art equipment, and staff ability to use it

- **Staff.** Includes credentials, experience, absenteeism, turnover rate, staff-client ratios

- **Finances.** Includes salaries, adequacy, sources

Although none of these structural factors alone can guarantee that good care will be

TABLE 8–5
JCAHO Dimensions of Quality Performance

Dimensions	The Questions
Appropriateness	To what degree is the intervention relevant to client needs?
Availability	To what degree are the appropriate interventions available to meet client needs?
Continuity	To what degree are the interventions coordinated between organizations, among care providers, and across time?
Effectiveness	To what degree is the intervention provided in the correct manner to achieve the intended client outcome?
Efficacy	To what degree has the intervention been shown to accomplish the intended outcome?
Efficiency	To what degree does the care have the desired effect with a minimum of effort, expense or waste?
Respect and Caring	To what degree are the clients involved in the health care decisions and treated with sensitivity and respect for their individual needs, expectations, and differences by health care providers?
Safety	To what degree are the risks of the interventions and the environment reduced for both client and health care provider?
Timeliness	To what degree are appropriate interventions available to meet client needs?

Source: Adapted from Joint Commission on Accreditation of Healthcare Organizations (JCAHO). (1997). *Accreditation Manual for Hospitals.* Chicago: JCAHO.

given, they can make good care more likely. A higher level of nurses each shift and a higher proportion of RNs in the skill mix are structural factors that are associated with shorter lengths of stay; higher proportions of RNs are also related to fewer adverse patient outcomes (Lichtig, Knauf, & Milholland, 1999).

A common pitfall in evaluating structural factors, however, has been to neglect the other two aspects, process and outcome. The following example illustrates the problems that occur when only structure is evaluated:

A hospital measured the quality of nursing care given in its eight-bed critical care unit by comparing its staffing ratio with the standard ratio of one nurse to two clients. The inadequacy of this structural measure became apparent during a period when the unit had six (out of a total of eight) clients who each required the care of one nurse. Under the standard that was set, only four nurses were on duty, which created a severe staff shortage because seven nurses were actually needed to provide adequate care.

Process

Process refers to the activities carried out by the health care providers. It includes all

TABLE 8–6
Dimensions of Quality Improvement in Nursing: Examples

	Independent Function	Dependent Function	Interdependent Function
Structure	Pressure ulcer risk assessment form available	High-speed automatic dial-up system puts nurses in touch with physicians rapidly	Nursing case management model of care adopted on rehabilitation unit
Process	Assesses risk for development of pressure ulcer and implements preventive measure	Order to increase dosage of pain medication obtained and processed within 1 hour	Communicates with therapists about need for customized wheelchair
Outcome	Skin intact at discharge	Relief from pain	Able to enter narrow doorway to bathroom unassisted

Source: Adapted from on Irvine, D. (1998). Finding value in nursing care: A framework for quality improvement and clinical evaluation. *Nursing Economics,* 16(3), 110–118.

activities carried out and decisions made from the time an individual approaches the health care system through assessment, diagnosis, treatment, and follow-up care (Irvine, 1998). Examples include the following:

- Setting an appointment

- Conducting a physical assessment

- Ordering a radiograph and magnetic resonance imaging scan

- Administering a blood transfusion

- Completing a home environment assessment

- Preparing the patient for discharge

- Telephoning the patient post discharge

Each of these processes can be evaluated in terms of timeliness, appropriateness, accuracy, and completeness (Irvine, 1998). Process variables include psychosocial interventions such as teaching and counseling, as well as physical care measures. It can include leadership activities such as interdisciplinary team conferences. When process data are collected, a set of objectives, procedures, or guidelines is needed to serve as a standard or gauge against which to compare the activities. This set of objectives can be highly specific, such as listing all the steps in a catheterization procedure, or it can be a list of objectives, such as "offer information on breast-feeding to all expectant parents" or "conduct weekly staff meetings."

The ANA Standards of Care are process standards. These standards answer the question "What should the nurse be doing and what process should he/she follow to ensure quality care?"

Outcome

An outcome is the result of the activities in which the health care providers have been involved. Outcome measures evaluate the effectiveness of these nursing activities by answering such questions as: Did the patient recover? Is the family more independent now? Has team functioning improved? Outcome standards address indicators such as physical and mental health status, social and physical function, health attitudes/knowledge/behavior, utilization of services, and customer satisfaction (Huber, 2000).

These questions are very general and reflect overall goals of health care providers and the organizations in which they work. The outcome questions asked during an actual evaluation should be far more specific and should measure observable behavior, such as the following:

Client: Wound healed; blood pressure within normal limits; infection absent
Family: Increased time between visits to the emergency department; applied for food stamps
Team: Decisions reached by consensus; attendance at meetings by all team members

You can see that some of these outcomes, such as blood pressure or time between emergency department visits, are easier to measure than are other, equally important outcomes, such as increased satisfaction or changes in attitude. Although these less tangible outcomes cannot be measured as precisely, it is still important to include them. Although these less tangible outcomes cannot be measured as precisely, it is still important to include them so that the full spectrum of biologic, psychologic, and social aspects are represented (Strickland, 1997). For this reason, considerable effort has been put into identifying the patient outcomes that are affected by the quality of nursing care. As mentioned earlier, the ANA has identified 10 quality indicators in acute care that are likely to relate to the availability and quality of professional nursing services in hospitals (see Table 8–3). Across the United States, data is now being collected from nursing units using these quality indicators.

A major problem in using and interpreting outcome measures in evaluation is that outcomes are influenced by many factors. For example:

The outcome of client teaching done by a nurse on a home visit is affected by the client's interest and ability to learn, the quality of the teaching materials, the presence or absence of family support, the information given by other caregivers (which may conflict), and the environment in which the teaching is done. If the teaching is successful, can the nurse be given full credit for the success? If it is not successful, who has failed?

It is necessary to evaluate the process as well as the outcome to determine why an intervention such as client teaching succeeds or fails. A comprehensive evaluation includes all three aspects: structure, process, and outcome.

◼ Quality Improvement at the Unit and Organizational Level

In this section, we consider how the process of QI works at the unit level, where nursing is often the central focus. For the sake of simplicity, we focus almost exclusively on the effect of nursing on client care, although it is generally recommended that QI be interdisciplinary for maximum effectiveness. As a staff member, you will be expected to participate in the QI initiatives for your unit.

Once the policies and procedures for implementing QI projects are defined at the organizational level, much of the responsibility for carrying them out may be delegated to staff members of each unit. At the unit level, the first step is to assign responsibility to various staff members. All staff members may be brought together to act as a quality circle, or a representative group may be appointed to a committee to implement QI activities in consultation with the rest of the nursing staff. It is preferable to have as high a level of staff participation as possible, including representation from all three shifts in an inpatient setting.

Once staff members understand the purpose of QI, they can begin to identify areas for study. Staff members may use their own judgment about which areas are in greatest need of evaluation, or they may conduct preliminary surveys to determine the most problem-prone areas. Some guidance from the nurse manager may be needed to select a priority area and to prevent a difficult problem or one that is hard to define from being missed.

Some broad examples of areas for study might include the highest risk clients, the most common client problems, or the source of a high number of incident reports (Elrod, 1991). Other, more selectively focused examples might be physical restraint use, dysphagia, ventilator-assisted breathing, respiratory treatments, preoperative teaching, human immunodeficiency virus (HIV)-positive clients, or urinary incontinence. Each of these defines the scope of the problem to be evaluated (Duquette, 1991).

Once the scope is defined, the problem itself is further analyzed in terms of its important aspects, the generally accepted standards of care for these aspects, indicators (evidence) that these standards have been met, and the criteria (threshold) for determining whether they were met. For example:

Let's say that one area chosen for study by an outpatient clinic staff is patient teaching with newly diagnosed hypertensive clients. Three important aspects of this area of care include teaching the client about the disease process, about lifestyle modifications, and about pharmacological treatment (Johanssen, 1993). In regard to lifestyle modification, the standard of care would state, "the client will receive information about exercise, dietary modifications, smoking cessation, alcohol moderation, and stress reduction." Indicators for the dietary modification portion would be that the client can describe the recommended modifications, modifies diet as recommended, and maintains weight within 10 percent of ideal weight. A criterion or threshold for this last indicator would be that at least 50 percent of clients would achieve this level within 6 months of the original recommendation.

A standard of nursing practice describes what nurses do for or with clients and their families. This is in contrast to a nursing standard of care, which describes the kind of care clients can expect and do receive from nurses (JCAHO, 1994). The first function and major reason for setting standards is to increase objectivity by defining as clearly as possible what is acceptable and what is not acceptable. Without these standards, judgments made in the evaluation process may be variable, subjective, and susceptible to the whims and biases of the evaluators. Consistent application of these standards of care is essential for CQI.

A second function of these standards is to communicate clearly to all stakeholders (staff, administrators, consumers, accreditors, and regulators) what level of service is expected at that organization.

An *indicator* is an objective, measurable variable of care. The listed indicators are those variables on which data will be collected in a QI project. If data are to be collected on a continuing basis, the process is usually referred to as *monitoring*. The criteria, or threshold, set a predetermined level of the indicator that will be considered an acceptable level of care (Betta, 1992). For some indicators, such as documenting patient response to a blood infusion, a 100 percent level of achievement is expected. In other cases, such as weight reduction or smoking cessation, a 75 percent level of achievement is considered excellent.

Once these variables are well defined, a plan for data collection is devised. Usually, a worksheet is designed to facilitate data collection. For example:

A form (Fig. 8–3) could be devised to list each newly diagnosed hypertensive client, the client's weight at diagnosis, ideal weight, and weight at subsequent clinic visits. A final column for noting whether the client is within 10 percent of ideal weight could be added to indicate how many met the criteria after 6 months.

After data are collected, the staff reviews the findings and evaluates the degree to which the criteria were met. For example, if only 25 percent of the newly diagnosed hypertensive clients were within 10 percent of their ideal weight in 6 months, the clinic staff might decide to offer weight reduction classes or a support group. They might also decide to invite the clinic psychologist and nutritionist to participate in the group. Figure 8–4 is an example of QI guidelines.

Establishing an organization-wide QI program is primarily an administrative responsibility. This is a circular process as described in Figure 8–5. Starting with a statement of the organization's philosophy regarding QI, the mechanisms to implement quality are then set up. From an organiza-

Patient Identification Number	Weight at 1st Visit	Ideal Weight	Difference Ideal vs. Actual Weight	Weight at 2nd Visit	Weight at 3rd Visit	Weight at 4th Visit	Weight at 5th Visit	Weight at Six Months
01723	135	130	5	136	137	135	133	130
01799	210	145	65	205	204	201	199	197
23045	175	165	10	173	175	176	178	180

Figure 8–3 Personalized patient worksheet.

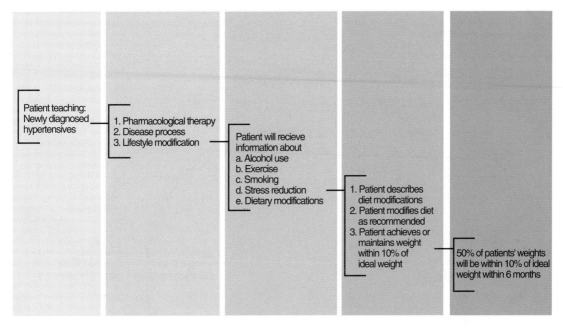

Figure 8–4 Example of quality improvement guidelines. (From Tappen, R.M. *Nursing Leadership and Management: Concepts and Practice*, 4th ed., Philadelphia: F.A. Davis, 2001, p. 403.

tion-wide quality council, subcouncils and unit teams are organized. The feedback from the grassroots involvement is sent back to the quality council or other administrative body for evaluation. Changes may then be implemented, policies revised, and the cycle begins again. The cost of QI efforts in terms of both time and commitment to the process is considerable. Over the long-term, however, QI efforts should improve patient outcomes.

■ Risk Management

An important part of QI is risk management. Defined as a process of identifying, analyzing, treating, and evaluating real and potential hazards, *risk management* addresses liability and financial loss. JCAHO recommends the integration of a quality control-risk management program in order to monitor and maintain continuous feedback and communication.

Risk events are categorized according to severity. Although all untoward events are important, not all carry the same severity of outcomes (Benson-Flynn, 2001).

1 Service occurrence. A service occurrence is an unexpected occurrence that does not result in a clinically significant interruption of services and that is without apparent patient or employee injury. Examples of a service occurrence include minor property or equipment damage, unsatisfactory provision of service at any level, or inconsequential interruption of service. Most occurrences in this category are addressed within the client complaint process.

2 Serious incident. A serious incident results in a clinically significant interruption of therapy or service, minor injury to a client or employee, or significant loss or damage of equipment or property. Minor injuries are usually defined as needing medical intervention outside of hospital admission or physical or psychological damage.

3 Sentinel events. A sentinel event is an unexpected occurrence involving death or serious/permanent physical or psychological injury, or the risk thereof. The phrase, "or the risk thereof" includes any process variation for which a recurrence would carry a significant chance of a serious adverse outcome.

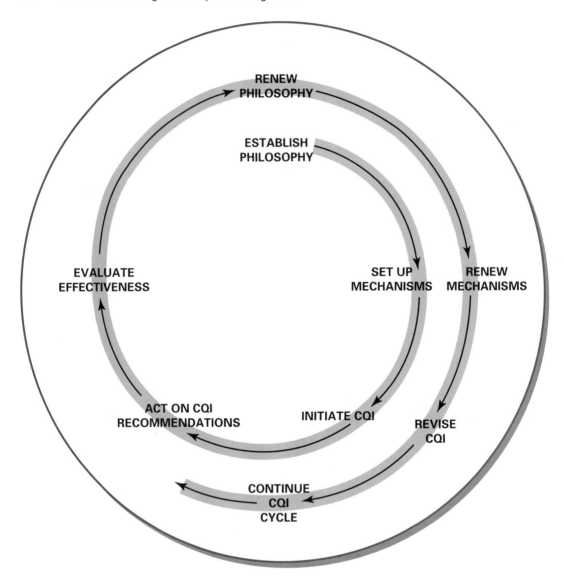

Figure 8–5 Continuous quality improvement (CQI) cycle. (From Tappen, R.M. *Nursing Leadership and Management: Concepts and Practice,* 4th ed., Philadelphia: F.A. Davis, 2001, p. 406.

Such events are called sentinel because they signal the need for immediate investigation and response. When a sentinel event occurs in a health care organization, it is necessary that appropriate individuals within the organization be made aware of the event, they investigate and understand the causes that underlie the event, and they make changes in the organization's systems and processes to reduce the probability of such an event in the future (*http://www. jcaho.org/ptsafety_frm.html*).

The subset of sentinel events that is sub-

ject to review by JCAHO includes any occurrence that meets any of the following criteria:

- The event has resulted in an unanticipated death or major permanent loss of function, not related to the natural course of the patient's illness or underlying condition.

- The event is one of the following (even if the outcome was not death or major permanent loss of function):

  - Suicide of a patient in a setting where the patient receives around-the-clock

CURRENT RESEARCH

Long, C., Anderson, C., Greenberg, E., & Woomer, N. (2002). Defining and monitoring indwelling catheter-related urinary track infections. *Home Healthcare Nurse, 20,* 255–262.

Defining and monitoring infection rates in home care is of major importance with the implementation of Adverse Event Outcome Reports. This study identified the collective effort of home care quality improvement nurses in defining standard indicators for urinary tract infections (UTIs) and the ways to monitor these infections within and across home care agencies for evaluation and benchmarking. The first step was to establish a case definition of UTI and develop appropriate data collection instruments. The subsequent steps were to establish agency participation rules and methods for data aggregation, analysis, and benchmarking.

This study produced several qualitative and quantitative findings. Overall, home care agency quality managers were able to develop a consensus definition for catheter-related UTIs in the home, providing criteria in which to measure and report findings. In addition, the method for reporting the results, or the UTI rate, was verified and executed uniformly throughout the duration of the UTI Benchmarking Project.

Home care and infection control practitioners are progressing tremendously in the uncharted territory of home care–acquired infections. Achieving consensus on infection definitions from empirical findings, epidemiological fundamentals, and current standards of process continues to be a need. As the field of infection control in the home matures, whereby protocols for measurement are established and definitions for home care–acquired infections are refined, quality managers and agency administrators are challenged to develop strategies for measurement within and comparison among other home care agencies.

care (e.g., hospital, residential treatment center, crisis stabilization center)

• Infant abduction or discharge to the wrong family

• Rape

• Hemolytic transfusion reaction involving administration of blood or blood products having major blood group incompatibilities

• Surgery on the wrong patient or wrong body part (*http://www.jcaho.org/ptsafety_frm.html*)

Adhering to nursing standards of care as well as the policies and procedures of the institution greatly decrease the nurse's risk. Common areas of risk for nursing include:

• Medication errors

• Documentation errors and/or omissions

• Failure to correctly perform nursing care or treatments

• Errors in patient safety that result in falls

• Failure to communicate significant data to clients and other providers (Swansburg & Swansburg, 2002).

Risk management programs also include attention to areas of employee wellness and prevention of injury. Latex allergies, repetitive stress injuries and carpal tunnel syndrome, barrier protection for tuberculosis, back injuries, and the rise of antibiotic-resistant organisms all fall under the attention of risk management (Huber, 2000).

Adhering to standards of care and exercising the degree of care that a reasonable nurse would demonstrate under the same or similar circumstances can protect the nurse from negligent litigation. Understanding what actions to take when something goes wrong is imperative. The main goal is client safety. Reporting and remediation must occur quickly (Huber, 2000).

Once an incident has occurred, an incident report must be completed. The incident report is used to collect and analyze data for future determination of risk. The incident report should be completed in a timely manner. It should be accurate, objective, complete, and factual. If there is future litigation, the plaintiff's attorney can subpoena the report. The incident report should be prepared in only a single copy and never placed in the medical record (Swansburg & Swansburg, 2002). It is kept with internal hospital correspondence.

You have a responsibility to remain education and informed and to become an active participant in understanding and identifying potential risks both to your clients and to yourself. Ignorance of the law is no excuse. Maintaining a knowledgeable, professional, and caring nurse-patient relationship is the first step in decreasing your own risk.

◘ Conclusion

Pressure from JCAHO, health care consumers, health care payers, and health care providers has caused the focus in the health care system to shift from patient care to issues of cost and quality. Experts tell us that quality promotes decreased costs and increased satisfaction. View this as an opportunity for nurses to become more professional and for nurses to become empowered to organize and manage client care so that it is safe, efficient, and of the highest quality.

Regardless of the care model used or the indicators selected, in patient care delivery, focus attention on the following (Hansten, R. & Washburn, M., 2001, p 24D):

1 Think critically. Use your creative, intuitive, logical, and analytical processes continually in working with clients.

2 Plan and report outcomes. Emphasizing results is a necessary part of managing resources in today's cost-conscious environment. Focusing on the outcomes moves the nurse out of the mindset of just focusing on tasks.

3 Make introductory rounds. Begin each shift with the health care team members introducing themselves, describing their roles, and providing clients updates.

4 Plan in partnership with the client. In conjunction with the introductory rounds, spend a few minutes early in the shift with each client discussing shift objectives and long-term goals. This event becomes the center of the nursing process for the shift and ensures that the client and nurse are working toward the same outcomes.

5 Communicate the plan. Avoid confusion among members of the team by communicating the intended outcomes and the important role that each member plays in the plan.

6 Evaluate progress. Schedule time during the shift to quickly evaluate outcomes and the progress of the plan and to make revisions as necessary.

Study Questions

1 What problems have you identified during your clinical experiences that could be considered issues to be addressed using CQI?

2 How would you begin discussion of these problems with the nurse manager?

3 What structured care methodologies have you seen implemented in practice? Which ones might you use to assist you in planning of care?

4 How would you develop your career goals based on the concepts of differentiated practice discussed in this chapter?

5 What issues may arise when the care delivery system is changed? What does the RN need to consider when implementing these changes?

6 How would you utilize the six points discussed in the conclusion in working as part of a team?

7 Review the unit on risk management. in what areas of risk do you feel you are the most vulnerable? How will you work on correcting your risk?

Critical Thinking Exercise

The director of QI has called a meeting of all the staff members on your floor. Based on last quarter's statistics, the length of stay of clients with uncontrolled diabetes is 2.6 days longer than that of clients for the first half of the year. She has requested that the staff identify members who wish to participate in looking at this problem. You have volunteered to be a member of the QI team. The team will consist of the diabetes educator, a client-focused care assistant, a pharmacist, and you, the staff nurse.

1 Why were these people selected for the team?

2 What data need to be collected to evaluate this situation?

3 What are the potential outcomes for clients with uncontrolled diabetes?

4. Develop a flowchart of a typical hospital stay for a client with uncontrolled diabetes.

WEBSITES

http://www.afip.org/Departments/legalmed/jnrm.html Legal Medicine: The Journal of Nursing Risk Management

http://www.jcaho.org/ Joint Commission on Accreditation of Healthcare Organizations

http://www.ahcpr.gov/ Agency for Healthcare Research and Quality

http://www.nursingworld.org American Nurses Association

http://nursingworld.org/ancc/faqs.htm#bac American Nurses Association Credentialing Center

REFERENCES

Allender, C., Egan, E., & Newman, M. (1995). An instrument for measuring differentiated nursing practice. *Nursing Management,* 26(4), 42–45.

American Organization of Nurse Executives (AONE). (1994). Differentiated competencies for nursing practice. *Nursing Management,* 25(9), 34.

Benson-Flynn, J. (2001). Incident reporting: Clarifying occurrences, incidents, and sentinel events. *Home Healthcare Nurse,* 19, 701–706.

Betta, P.A. (1992). Developing a successful ambulatory QA program. *Nursing Management,* 23(4), 31–33, 47–54.

Brook, R.H., Davis, A.R., & Kamberg, C. (1980). Selected reflections on quality of medical care evaluations in the 1980s. *Nursing Research,* 29(2), 127.

Capuano, T.A. (1995). Clinical pathways. *Nursing Management,* 26(1), 34–37.

Chang, C., Price, S., Pfoutz, S. (2001). *Economics and Nursing.* Philadelphia: FA Davis.

Christensen, P., & Bender, L. (1994). Models of nursing care in a changing environment: Current challenges and future directions. *Orthopaedic Nursing,* 13(2), 64–70.

Clouten, K., & Weber, R. (1994). Patient-focused care . . . playing to win. *Nursing Management,* 25(2), 34–36.

Cole, L., & Houston, S. (1999). Structured care methodologies: Evolution and use in patient care delivery. *Outcomes Management for Nursing Practice,* 3(2), 53–60.

Crummer, M.B., & Carter, V (1993). Critical pathways: The pivotal tool. *Cardiovascular Nursing,* 7(4), 30–37.

Doenges, M.E., Moorhouse, M.F., & Geissler, A.C. (1997). *Nursing Care Plans: Guidelines for Individualizing Patient Care,* 4th ed. Philadelphia: F.A. Davis.

Donabedian, A. (1969). A guide to medical care administration. In *Medical Care Appraisal: Quality and Utilization* (Vol. II). New York: American Public Health Association.

Donabedian, A. (1977). Evaluating the quality of medical care. *Milbank Memorial Fund Quarterly,* 44 (part 2), 166.

Donabedian, A. (1987). Some basic issues in evaluating

the quality of health care. In Rinke, L.T. (ed.). *Outcome Measures in Home Care.* New York: National League of Nursing.

Duquette, A.M. (1991). Approaches to monitoring practice: Getting started. In Schroeder, P. (ed.). *Monitoring and Evaluation in Nursing.* Gaithersburg, Md.: Aspen.

Elrod, M.E.B. (1991). Quality assurance: Challenges and dilemmas in acute care medical-surgical environments. In Schroeder, P. (ed.). *Monitoring and Evaluation in Nursing. Gaithersburg,* Md.: Aspen.

Flarey, D.L. (1995). *Redesigning Nursing Care Delivery.* Philadelphia: J.B. Lippincott.

Girard, N. (1994). The case management model of patient care delivery. *AORN Journal,* 60, 403–415.

Greenberg, L. (1994). Work redesign: An overview. *Journal of Emergency Nursing,* 20(3), 28A–32A.

Hansten, R., & Washburn, M. (2001). Outcomes-based care delivery. *American Journal of Nursing,* 101(2), 24A–D.

Heinrich, J. (2001). *Nursing Workforce: Emerging Nurse Shortages Due to Multiple Factors.* Report to the Chairman, Subcommittee on Health, Committee on Ways and Means, House of Representatives. July 2001. ERIC Document ED 455 385.

Huber, D. (2000). *Leadership and Nursing Care Management.* 2nd ed. Philadelphia: W.B. Saunders.

Hunt, D.V. (1992). *Quality in America: How to Implement a Competitive Quality Program.* Homewood, Ill.: Business One Irwin.

Irvine, D. (1998). Finding value in nursing care: A framework for quality improvement and clinical evaluation. *Nursing Economics,* 16(3), 110–118.

Johanssen, J.M. (1993). Update: Guidelines for treating hypertension. *American Nursing,* 93(3), 42–49.

Joint Commission on Accreditation of Healthcare Organizations (JCAHO). (1994). *Framework for Improving Performance: A Guide for Nurses.* Chicago: JCAHO.

Kido, V. (2001). The UAP dilemma. *Nursing Management,* 32(11), 27–29.

Kinlaw, D.C. (1992). *Continuous Improvement and Measurement for Total Quality.* Homewood, Ill.: Business One Irvine.

Koerner, J., Bunkers, L., Gibson, S., Jones, R., Nelson, B., & Santema, K. (1995). Differentiated practice: The evaluation of a professional practice model for integrated client care services. In Flarey, D.L. (ed.). *Redesigning Nursing Care Delivery.* Philadelphia: J.B. Lippincott.

Leebov, W. (1991). *The Quality Quest: A Briefing for Health Care Professionals.* Chicago: American Hospital Publishing.

Lichtig, L.K., Knauf, R.A., & Milholland, D.K. (1999). Some impacts of nursing on acute care hospital outcomes. *Journal of Nursing Administration,* 29(2), 25–33.

Long, C., Anderson, C., Greenberg, E., & Woomer, N. (2002). Defining and monitoring indwelling catheter-related urinary tract infections. *Home Healthcare Nurse,* 20, 255–262.

Loveridge, C., & Cummings, S. (1996). *Nursing Management in the New Paradigm.* Gaithersburg, Md.: Aspen.

Lynam, L. (1994). Case management and critical pathways: Friend or foe. *Neonatal Network,* 13(8), 48–51.

Lyon, J.C. (1993). Models of nursing care delivery and case management: Clarification of terms. *Nursing Economics,* 11(3), 163–169.

Manthey, M. (2001). A core incremental staffing plan. *Journal of Nursing Administration,* 31, 424–425.

Mark, B. A., Salyer, J., & Geddis, N. (1997). Outcomes research: Clues to quality and organizational effectiveness? *Nursing Clinics of North America,* 32, 589-601.

Mass, S., & Johnson, B. (November 1998). Case management and clinical guidelines. *Journal of Care Management,* 18–26.

McClure, M. (1991). Models of practice. In American Academy of Nursing. *Differentiating Nursing Practice.* Kansas City, Mo.: AAN.

Nelson, M. (2002). Educating for professional nursing practice: Looking backward into the future. *Online Journal of Issues in Nursing,* May 31, 2002, *http://www.nursingworld.org/ojin/topic18/tpc18_3.htm* accessed 5/27/02.

Newell, M. (1996). *Using Nursing Case Management to Improve Health Outcomes.* Gaithersburg, Md.: Aspen.

Nightingale, F., & Barnum, B.S. (1992). *Notes on Nursing: What It Is, and What It Is Not,* Commemorative Edition. Philadelphia: Lippincott-Raven.

Ray, G., & Hardin, S. (1995). Advanced practice nursing. *Nursing Management,* 26(2), 45–47.

Ritter-Teitel, J. (2002). The impact of restructuring on professional nursing practice. *Journal of Nursing Administration,* 32(1), 31–41.

Scott, J., Sochalski, J., & Aiken, L. (1999). Review of magnet hospital research: Findings and implications for professional nursing practice. *Journal of Nursing Administration,* 29(1), 9–19.

Sharp, M. (1994). Every citizen deserves care and every patient deserves a nurse. *Nursing Management,* 25(9), 32–33.

Simms, Price, & Ervin, 2000, p. 307.

Strickland, O. (1997). Challenges in measuring patient outcomes. *Nursing Clinics of North America,* 32, 495–512.

Swansburg, R., & Swansburg, R. (2002). *Introduction to Management and Leadership for Nurse Managers,* 3rd ed. Boston: Jones and Bartlett.

Tappen, R.M. *Nursing Leadership and Management: Concepts and Practice,* 4th ed., Philadelphia: F.A. Davis, 2001

Vena, C., & Oldaker, S. (1994). Differentiated practice: The new paradigm using a theoretical approach. *Nursing Administration Quarterly,* 19(1), 66–73.

Wayman, C. (1999). Hospital-based nursing case management: Role clarification. *Nursing Case Management,* 4, 236–241.

CHAPTER 9

Time Management

OBJECTIVES

After reading this chapter, the student should be able to:

- Describe his or her perception of time.

- Set short- and long-term personal career goals.

- Analyze activities at work using a time log.

- Organize work to make more effective use of available time.

- Set limits on the demands made on one's time.

- Create a personal calendar using a computerized calendar system

OUTLINE

The Tyranny of Time

How Do Nurses Spend Their Time?

Organizing Your Work
Setting Your Own Goals
Lists
Long-Term Planning Systems
Schedules and Blocks of Time
Filing Systems

Setting Limits
Saying No
Eliminating Unnecessary Work

Streamlining Your Work
Keeping a Time Log
Reducing Interruptions
Categorizing Activities
Finding the Fastest Way
Automating Repetitive Tasks
The Rhythm Model for Time Management

Conclusion

Coming onto the unit, Celia, the evening charge nurse, already knew that a hectic day was in progress. Scattered throughout the unit were clues from the past 12 hours. Two clients on emergency department stretchers were parked outside observation rooms already occupied by clients who had been admitted the previous day in critical condition. Stationed in the middle of the hall was the code cart, with its drawers opened and electrocardiograph paper cascading down the sides. Approaching the nurses' station, Celia found Guillermo buried deep in paperwork. He glanced at her with a face that had exhaustion written all over it. His first words were, "Three of your RNs called in sick. I called staffing for additional help, but only one is available. Good luck!"

Celia surveyed the unit, looked at the number of staff members available, and reviewed the client acuity level of the unit. She decided not to let the situation upset her. She would take charge of her own time and reallocate the time of her staff. She began to mentally reorganize her staff and alter the responsibilities of each member. Having taken steps to handle the problem, Celia felt ready to begin the shift.

Business executives, managers, students, and nurses know that time continues to be a valuable resource. Time cannot be saved and used later, so it must be used wisely. As a new nurse, you may at times find yourself sinking in the "quicksand" of a time trap, knowing what needs to be done but just not having the necessary time to do it (Ferrett, 1996). In today's fast-paced health care environment, time management skills are critical to a nurse's success. Learning to take charge of your time is the key to time management (Gonzalez, 1996). Many nurses feel as though they never have enough time to accomplish the tasks that need to be completed. Like the White Rabbit in *Alice in Wonderland,* they are constantly in a rush against time. Time management is simply organizing and monitoring time so that client care tasks can be scheduled and implemented in a timely and organized fashion (Bos & Vaughn, 1998).

◘ The Tyranny of Time

Newton stated that time was absolute and that it occurred whether the universe was there or not. Many years later, Einstein theorized that time has no independent existence apart from the order of events by which we measure it (Smith, 1994). It really does not

matter which theory is correct because as nurses our professional and personal lives are guided by time.

How often do you look at your watch during the day? Do you divide your day into blocks of time? Do you steal a quick glance at the clock when you come home after putting in a full day's work? Do you mentally calculate the amount of time left to complete the day's tasks of grocery shopping, driving in a car pool, making dinner, and leaving again to take a class or attend a meeting? In our society, calendars, clocks, watches, newspapers, television, and radio all remind us of our position in time. Our perception of time is important because it affects our use of time and our response to time (Box 9–1).

Computers complete operations in a fraction of a second, and we can measure speeds to the nanosecond. Time clocks that record the minute we enter and leave work are commonplace, and few excuses for being late are really considered acceptable. Timesheets and schedules are part of most health care givers' lives. We are expected to follow precisely set schedules and meet deadlines for virtually everything we do, from distributing medications to doing reports on time. Many agencies produce vast quantities of computer-generated data that can be analyzed to determine the amount of time spent on various activities. It is no wonder some of us seem obsessed with time.

Individual personality, culture, and environment all interact to influence our perceptions of time (Matejka & Dunsing, 1988). Each of us has an internal tempo (Chappel, 1970). Some internal tempos are quicker than others. Environment also affects the way we respond to time. A fast-paced environment influences most of us to work at a faster pace, despite our internal tempo. For individuals with a slower tempo, this pace can cause discomfort. If you are a high-achievement–oriented person, you are likely to have already set some career goals for yourself and to have a mental schedule of deadlines for reaching these goals ("go on to complete my bachelor of science in nursing [BSN] in 4 years; a master of science in nursing [MSN] in 6 years").

BOX 9–1
Time Perception

Webber (1980) collected a number of interesting tests of people's perception of time. You may want to try several of these:

- Do you think of time more as a galloping horseman or a vast motionless ocean?
- Which of these words best describes time to you: sharp, active, empty, soothing, tense, cold, deep, clear, young, or sad?
- Is your watch fast or slow? (You can check it with the radio.)
- Ask a friend to help you with this test. Go into a quiet room without any work, reading material, radio, food, or other distractions. Have your friend call you after 10 to 20 minutes have elapsed. Try to guess how long you were in that room.

Webber test results interpreted. A person who has a circular concept of time would compare it to a vast ocean. A galloping horseman would be characteristic of a linear conception of time, emphasizing speed and motion forward. A fast-tempo, achievement-oriented person would describe time as clear, young, sharp, active, or tense rather than empty, soothing, sad, cold, or deep. These same fast-tempo people are likely to have fast watches and to overestimate the amount of time that they sat in a quiet room.

Source: Adapted from Webber, R.A. (1980). *Time Is Money! Tested Tactics That Conserve Time for Top Executives.* New York: Free Press

Many health care professionals are linear, fast-tempo, achievement-oriented people. Simply working at a fast pace, however, is not necessarily equivalent to achieving a great deal. Much energy can be wasted in rushing around and stirring things up but actually accomplishing very little. The rest of this chapter looks at ways in which you can use your time and energy wisely to accomplish your goals.

■ How Do Nurses Spend Their Time?

Nurses are the largest group of health care professionals. Because of the number of nurses needed and the shift variations, attention concerning the efficiency and effectiveness of their time management is needed. The effect of rotating shifts has long been a concern in nursing. Nurses who rotate shifts are twice as likely to report medication errors as those who do not rotate. Night-shift staff members and rotating-shift staff members also report getting less sleep, getting a poorer quality of sleep, using more sleep medication, and having problems with nodding off at work or while driving home after work ("Sleeping on the job," 1993).

Today's labor market for skilled health

care professionals remains tight. Institutions face new challenges of not "trimming the fat, but compensate for loss of muscle" (Baldwin, 2002, p.1). Current shortages of nurses, radiology technicians, pharmacists, and other health care specialists show all the signs of a long-term problem. Health care institutions now need to change their thinking on how to manage work. Most are looking toward technology to help cope with staffing shortages (Baldwin, 2002).

A new graduate worked the 7 A.M. to 3 P.M. shift and rotated every third week to the 11 P.M. to 7 A.M. shift in a medical intensive care unit, working 7 days straight before getting 2 days off. It was not difficult to remain awake during the entire shift the first night on duty, but each night thereafter staying awake became increasingly more difficult. After the 2 A.M. vital signs were taken and recorded, the new graduate inevitably fell asleep at the nurses' station. He was so tired that he had to check and re-check client medications and other procedures for fear of making a fatal error. He became so anxious over the possibility of injuring someone that sleep during the day became impossible. Because of his obsession with re-checking his work, he had difficulty completing tasks and was always behind at the end of the shift (of course, napping didn't help his time management).

A number of studies have examined how nurses use their time, especially nurses in acute-care settings. For example, a study by

Arthur Andersen found that only 35 percent of nursing time is spent in direct client care (including care planning, assessment teaching, and technical activities). Documentation accounts for another 20 percent of nursing time. The remainder of time is spent on transporting clients, processing transactions, performing administrative responsibilities, and undertaking hotel services (Brider, 1992) (Fig. 9–1). Categories may change from study to study, but the amount of time spent on direct client care is usually less than half the workday. As hospitals continue to re-evaluate the way they deliver health care, nurses are finding themselves more involved with tasks that are not directly client-related, such as determining quality improvement, developing critical pathways, and so forth. These are added to their already existing client care functions. The critical nursing shortage has compounded these issues. The result is that in some cases, nurses are able to meet only the highest priority client needs, particularly in certain clinical settings such as short-stay units or ambulatory care centers (Curry, 2002).

Any change in the distribution of time spent on various activities can have a considerable impact on client care and on the organization's bottom line. Prescott (1991) offered the following example: If more unit management responsibilities could be shifted from nurses to non-nursing personnel, about 48 minutes per nurse shift could be redirected to client care. In a large hospital with 600 full-time nurses, the result would be an additional 307 hours of direct client care *a day.* Calculating the results of this timesaving strategy in another way shows an even greater impact: the changes would contri-

Daily Time Log

	Activities	Comments
6:30		
7:00		
7:30		
8:00		
8:30		
9:00		
9:30		
10:00		
10:30		
11:00		
11:30		
12:00		
12:30		
1:00		
1:30		
2:00		
2:30		
3:00		
3:30		
4:00		
4:30		
5:00		

Figure 9–1 Time Log. (Adapted from Robichaud, A.M. (1986). Time documentation of clinical nurse specialist activities. *Journal of Nursing Administration*, 16(1), 31–36.)

bute the equivalent of the work of 48 additional full-time nurses to direct client care.

Many health care institutions are considering integrating units with similar patient populations and having them managed by a non-nurse manager, someone with business and management expertise and not necessarily nursing skills. However, as a group, nurses respect managers who have nursing expertise and who are able to perform as nurses. They feel that a nurse-manager has a greater understanding of both client and professional staff needs. To address these service concerns, many educational institutions have developed dual graduate degrees combining nursing and management.

◼ Organizing Your Work

Setting Your Own Goals

It is difficult to decide how to spend your time because there are so many things that need time. A good first step is to take a look at the situation and get an overview. Then ask yourself, "What are my goals?" Goals help clarify what you want and give you energy, direction, and focus. Once you know where you want to go, set priorities. This is not an easy task. Remember Alice's conversation with the Cheshire Cat in Lewis Carroll's *Alice in Wonderland?*

"Would you tell me please, which way I ought to go from here?" asked Alice.

"That depends a good deal on where you want to go to," said the Cat.

"I don't care where," said Alice.

"Then it doesn't matter which way you go," said the Cat.

How can you get somewhere if you do not know where you want to go? It is important to explore your personal and career goals. This can help you make decisions about the future. This concept can be applied to day-to-day activities as well as help in career decisions. Ask yourself questions about what you want to accomplish over a particular time period. Personal development skills include discipline, goal setting, management and organizational skills, self-monitoring,

and a positive attitude toward the job (Bos & Vaughn, 1998). Many of the personal management and organizational skills related to the workplace focus on time management and scheduling. Most new nurses have the skills required to perform the job but lack the personal management skills necessary to get the job done, specifically when it comes to time management.

To help organize your time, you need to set both short- and long-term goals. Short-term goals are those that you wish to accomplish within the near future. Setting up your day in an organized fashion is a short-term goal, as is scheduling a required "Medical Errors" or "Domestic Violence" course.

Long-term goals are those you wish to complete over a long period of time. Advanced education and career goals are examples. A good question to ask yourself is, "What do I see myself doing 5 years from now?" Every choice you make requires a different allocation of time (Moshovitz, 1993).

Eleanor, a licensed practical nurse returning to school to obtain her associate's degree in nursing, was faced with a multitude of responsibilities. A wife, a mother of two toddlers, and a full-time staff member at a local hospital, Eleanor suddenly found herself in a situation in which there just were not enough hours in a day. She became convinced that becoming a registered nurse was an unobtainable goal. When asked where she wanted to be in 5 years, she answered, "At this moment, I think, on an island in Tahiti!"

Several instructors helped Eleanor develop a time plan. First, she was asked to list what she did each day and how much time each task required. This list included basic childcare, driving children to and from daycare, shopping, cooking meals, cleaning, hours spent in the classroom, study hours, work hours, and time devoted to leisure. Once this was established, she was asked which tasks could be allocated to someone else (e.g., her husband), which tasks could be clustered (e.g., cooking for several days at a time), and which tasks could be shared.

Eleanor's husband was willing to assist with car pools, grocery shopping, and cleaning. Eleanor previously had never asked him for help. Cooking meals was clustered: Eleanor made all the meals in 1 day and then froze and labeled them to be used later. This left time for other activities.

Eleanor graduated at the top of her class and has subsequently completed her BSN and become a clinical preceptor for other associate degree students on a pediatric unit in a county hospital. She never did get to Tahiti, though.

Employers pay nurses for their time. Does that mean that nurses "sell" their time? If so, then nurses "own" their time. Looking at time from this perspective changes the point of view about time, as nurses then manage their own time to accomplish client care tasks.

Time management means we need to handle time with a measure of proficiency. Therefore, time management means skillfully meeting client care needs during a nursing shift (Navuluri, 2001). Organizing your work can eliminate extra steps or serious delays in completing your work. It can also reduce the amount of time spent doing things that are neither productive nor satisfying.

Working on the most difficult tasks when you have the most energy decreases frustration later in the day when you may be more tired and less efficient. To begin managing your time, you need to develop a clearer understanding of how you use your time. Creating a personal time inventory helps you estimate how much time you spend on typical activities. Keeping the inventory for a week gives a fairly accurate estimate of how you spend your time. The inventory also helps identify "time wasters" (Gahar, 2000). To avoid time wasters, take control. It is important to prevent endless activities and other people controlling you. Every day, set priorities to help you meet your goals.

Lists

One of the most useful organizers is the "to do" list. You can make this list either at the end of every day or at the beginning of each day before you do anything else. Some people say they do it at the end of the day because something always interferes at the beginning of the next day. Do not include routine tasks because they will make the list too long and you will do them without the extra reminder. If you are a team leader, place the unique tasks of the day on the list: team conference, telephone calls to families, discussion of a new project, or in-service demonstration on a new piece of equipment. You may also want to arrange these things to

do in order of their priority, starting with those that must be done on that day. Ask yourself the following questions regarding the tasks on the list (Moshovitz, 1993):

- What is the relative importance of each of these tasks?
- How much time will each task require?
- When must each task be completed?
- How much time and energy has to be devoted to these tasks?

If you find yourself postponing an item for several days, decide whether to give it top priority the next day or drop it from the list as an unnecessary task.

The list itself should be in a user-friendly form: on your electronic organizer, in your pocket, or on a clipboard. Checking the list several times a day quickly becomes a good habit. Computerized calendar-creator programs help in setting priorities and guiding daily activities. These programs can be set to appear on the desktop when you turn on your computer and give an overview of the day, week, or month. This calendar acts as an automated to do list. Your daily to do list may become your most important time manager. Box 9–2 summarizes ways to determine how to distribute your time.

Long-Term Planning Systems

At the beginning of the semester, students are told the examination dates and when papers will be due. Many students find it helpful to enter the dates on a semester-long calendar so that they can be seen at a glance. Then the students can see when clusters of assignments are due at the same time. This

BOX 9–2
Determining How to Speed Your Time

- Set goals.
- Make a schedule.
- Write a "to do" list.
- Revise and modify the "to do" list; do not throw it out.

allows for advance planning or perhaps requests to change dates or get extensions.

Many individuals prefer computerized planning systems. A variety of calendar-creator programs have been developed for this purpose. Many of these are found on the Internet or intranet of an institution.

Personal digital assistants (PDAs), or handheld organizers, have become quite popular. These devices allow both short-term and long-term scheduling. PDAs permit storing of personal notes and reminders, contact data, Internet access, and other program files. Handheld devices permit synchronization with personal computers and Internet-based calendars.

Schedules and Blocks of Time

Without some type of schedule, you are more likely to drift through a day or bounce from one activity to another in a disorganized fashion. Assignment sheets, worksheets, flow sheets, and critical pathways are all designed to help you plan client care and schedule your time effectively. The critical pathway is a guide to recommended treatments and optimal client outcomes (see Chapter 7). *Assignment sheets* indicate the clients for whom each staff member is responsible. *Worksheets* are then created to organize the daily care that must be given to the assigned clients (see Chapters 2 and 7 for examples of worksheets). *Flow sheets* are lists of items that must be recorded for each client.

Effective worksheets and flow sheets schedule and organize the day by providing reminders of various tasks and when they need to be done. The danger in using them, however, is that the more they divide the day into discrete segments, the more they fragment the work and discourage a holistic approach. If a worksheet becomes the focus of attention, the perspective of the whole and of the individuals who are our clients may be lost. Some activities must be done at a certain time. These activities structure the day or week to a great extent, and their timing may be out of your control. However, in every job there are tasks that can be done whenever

you want to do them, as long as they are done on time.

In certain nursing jobs, reports and presentations are often required. For these activities, you may need to set aside blocks of time during which you can concentrate on the task. Trying to create and complete a report in 5- or 10-minute blocks of time is unrealistic. By the time you reorient yourself to the project, the time allotted is over and nothing has been accomplished. Setting aside large blocks of time to do complex tasks is much more efficient.

Consider energy levels when beginning a big task. Start when levels are high and not at, say, 4:00 in the afternoon if that is when you find yourself winding down (Baldwin, 2002). For example, if you are a morning person, plan your demanding work in the morning. If you get energy spurts later in the morning or early afternoon, plan to work on larger or heavier tasks at that time. Nursing shifts may be designed in 8-, 10-, or 12-hour blocks. Many nurses working the night shifts (11 P.M. to 7 A.M., or 7 P.M. to 7 A.M.) find they have more energy a little later into their shift rather than at the beginning, whereas nurses working the day shifts (7 A.M. to 3 P.M.; 7 A.M. to 7 P.M.) find they have the most energy at the beginning of their shift. Also, learn to delegate tasks that do not require professional nursing skills.

Some people go to work early to have a block of uninterrupted time. Others take work home with them for the same reason. This extends the workday and cuts into leisure time. The higher your stress level, the less effective you will be on the job—don't bring your work home with you. You need some time off to recharge your batteries (Turkington, 1996).

Filing Systems

Filing systems are helpful to keep track of important papers. Every professional needs to maintain copies of licenses, certifications, and continuing education credits as well as current information about their specialty area. Keeping these organized in an easily retrievable system saves time and energy when you need to refer to them. Using color-coded folders is often helpful. Each color holds documents that are related to one another. For example, all continuing education credits might be placed in a blue folder, anything pertaining to licensure in a yellow folder, and so on.

◼ Setting Limits

To set limits, it is necessary first to identify your objectives and arrange the actions needed to meet them in order of their priority (Haynes, 1991; Navuluri, 2001). The focus of time management exists on two levels: temporal and spatial. Nurses to need focus on client care needs during the shift (temporal) or within the boundaries of the working environment (spatial). This viewpoint automatically sets limits to our time. Therefore, it is important to stick to our objectives and keep our focus on our time both temporally and spatially.

Saying No

Saying no to low-priority demands on your time is an important but difficult part of setting limits. Assertiveness and determination are necessary for effective time management. Learn to tactfully say no at least once a day (Hammerschmidt & Meador, 1993). Client care is a team effort. Effective time management requires you to look at other members of the time who may be able to take on the task.

The wisdom of time management is that we may have to let others help us manage our time, however, only to the extent that we never give up the ownership of our time. In other words, although our supervisors and managers may tell us what we need to do, how we accomplish this remains up to us (Navuluri, 2001). Is it possible to say no to your supervisor or manager? It may not seem so at first, but actually many requests are negotiable. Requests sometimes are in conflict with career goals. Rather than sit on a committee in which you have no interest, respectfully decline and volunteer for one that holds promise for you as well as meets the needs of your unit.

Can you refuse an assignment? Your manager may ask you to work overtime or to come in on your scheduled day off, but you can refuse. You may not refuse to care for a group of clients or to take a report because you think the assignment is too difficult or unsafe. You may, however, discuss the situation with your supervisor and together work out alternatives. You can also confront the issue of understaffing by filing an unsafe staffing complaint. Failure to accept an assignment may result in accusations of abandonment.

Some people have difficulty saying no. Ambition keeps some people from declining any opportunity, no matter how overloaded they are. Many individuals are afraid of displeasing others and therefore feel obligated to continuously take on all forms of additional assignments. Still others have such a great need to be needed that they continually give of themselves, not only to clients but also to their coworkers and supervisors. They fail to stop and replenish themselves and then they become exhausted. Remember, no one can be all things to all people at all times without creating serious guilt, anger, bitterness, and disillusionment. "Anyone who says it's possible has never tried it" (Turkington, 1996, p. 9).

Eliminating Unnecessary Work

Some work has become so deeply embedded in our routines that it appears essential, although it is really unnecessary. Some nursing routines fall into this category. Taking vital signs, giving baths, changing linens, changing dressings, performing irrigations, and doing similar basic tasks are more often done according to schedule rather than according to client need, which may be much more or much less often than the routine specifies. Some of these tasks may be appropriately delegated to others:

- If clients are ambulatory, bed linens may not need to be changed daily. Incontinent and diaphoretic clients need to have fresh linens more frequently. Not all clients need a complete bed bath every day. Elderly clients have dry, fragile skin;

giving them good mouth, facial, and perineal care may be all that is required on certain days. This should be included in the client's care plan.

• Much paperwork is duplicative, and some is altogether unnecessary. For example, is it necessary to chart nursing interventions in two or three places on the client record? Charting by exception, flow sheets, and computerized records are attempts to eliminate some of these problems.

• Socialization in the workplace is an important aspect in maintaining interpersonal relationships. When there is a social component to interactions in a group, the result is usually positive. However, too much socialization can reduce productivity in the workplace; use judgment in deciding when socializing is interfering with work.

You may create additional work for yourself without realizing it. How often do you walk back down the hall to obtain equipment when it all could have been gathered at one time? How many times do you walk to a client's room instead of using the intercom, only to find that you need to go back to where you were to get what the client needs? Is the staff providing personal care to clients who are well enough to meet some of these needs themselves?

◼ Streamlining Your Work

Many tasks cannot be eliminated or delegated, but they can be done more efficiently. There are many sayings in time management that reflect the principle of streamlining work. "Work smarter, not harder" is a favorite one that should appeal to nurses facing increasing demands on time. "Never handle a piece of paper more than once" is a more specific one, reflecting the need to avoid procrastination in your work. "A stitch in time saves nine" reflects the degree to which preventive action saves time in the long run.

Several methods of working smarter and not harder are:

• Gather materials, such as bed linens, for all of your clients at one time. As you go to each room, leave the linen so that it will be there when you need it.

• While giving a bed bath or providing other personal care, perform some of the aspects of the physical assessment, such as taking vital signs, skin assessment, and parts of the neurological and musculoskeletal assessment. Prevention is always a good idea.

• If a client does not "look right," do not ignore your instincts. The client is probably having a problem.

• If you are not sure about a treatment or medication, ask before you proceed. It is usually less time-consuming to prevent a problem than it is to resolve one.

• When you set aside time to do a specific task that has a high priority, stick to your schedule and complete it.

• Do not allow interruptions while you are completing paperwork, such as transcribing orders.

What else can you do to streamline your work? A few general suggestions follow, but the first one, a time log, can assist you in developing others unique to your particular job. If you complete the log correctly, a few surprises about how you really spend your time are almost guaranteed.

Keeping a Time Log

Our perception of time is elastic. People do not accurately estimate the time they spend on any particular task; we cannot rely on our memories for accurate information about how we spend our time. The time log is an objective source of information. Most people spend a much smaller amount of their time on productive activities than they estimate. Once you see how large amounts of your time are spent, you will be able to eliminate or reduce the time spent on nonproductive or minimally productive activities (Drucker, 1967; Robichaud, 1986). For example, many nurses spend a great deal of time searching for or waiting for missing medications, equipment, or supplies. Before beginning client care, assemble all the equipment and supplies you will need, and check the client's medication drawer against the medication administration record so that you can order anything that is missing before you begin.

Figure 9–1 is an example of a time log in which you enter your activities every half hour. This means that you will have to pay careful attention to what you are doing so that you can record it accurately. Do not postpone the recording; do it every 30 minutes. A 3-day sample may be enough for you to see a pattern emerging. It is suggested that you repeat the process again in 6 months, both because work situations change and to see if you have made any long-lasting changes in your use of time.

Reducing Interruptions

Everyone experiences interruptions. Some of these are welcome and necessary, but too many interfere with your work. A phone call from the lab with a critical value is a necessary interruption. Hobbs (1987) stated that necessary interruptions are not time wasters. Middle level managers are interrupted every 8 minutes while senior managers suffer interruptions every 5 minutes. Client care managers, the nurses, seemed to be interrupted every minute. Interruptions need to be kept to a minimum or eliminated, if possible. Closing the door to a client's room may reduce interruptions. You may have to ask visitors to wait a few minutes before you can answer their questions, although you must remain sensitive to their needs and return to them as soon as possible.

There is nothing wrong with asking a colleague who wants your assistance to wait a few minutes if you are engaged in another activity. Interruptions that occur when you are trying to pour medications or make calculations can cause errors. Physicians and other professionals often request nursing attention when nurses are involved with client care tasks. Find out if an unlicensed person may be of assistance. If not, ask the physician to wait, stating that you will be more than glad to help as soon as you complete what you are doing. Be courteous, but be firm; you are busy also.

Categorizing Activities

Clustering certain activities helps eliminate the feeling of bouncing from one unrelated task to another. It also makes your caregiving more holistic. You may, for example, find that documentation takes less time if you do it while you are still with the client or immediately after seeing a client. The information is still fresh in your mind, and you do not have to rely on notes or recall. Many health care institutions have switched to computerized charting, with the computers placed at the bedside. This set-up assists in documenting care and interventions while the nurse is still with the client. Also, try to follow a task through to completion before beginning another.

Finding the Fastest Way

Many time-consuming tasks can be made more efficient through the use of automation. Narcotic delivery systems that deliver the correct dose and electronically record the dose, the name of the client, and the name of the health care personnel removing the medication are being used in many institutions. This system saves staff time in documentation and in performing a narcotic count at the end of each shift. Bar coding is another method used by health care institutions. Bar coding allows for scanning certain types of client data, decreasing the number of paper chart entries (Baldwin, 2002; Meyer, 1992).

Efficient systems do not have to be complex. Using a preprinted color-coded sticker system helps to identify clients who must be without food or fluids (NPO) for tests or surgery, those who require 24-hour urine collections, or those who are having special cultures done. The information need not be written or entered repeatedly if stickers are used.

Everyone discusses the amount of time physicians, nurses, and other clinicians waste looking for things such as client charts, equipment, and even clients. Erica Drazen, vice president of First Consulting Group in Lexington, Massachusetts, suggested using more sophisticated wireless technology, similar to the car tracking systems used by law enforcement. Tiny transmitters can be activated from a central point to locate the items or individuals. Using electronic medical record systems (EMR) decreases the amount of time spent looking for client records. By using the approved access codes, health care personnel can obtain information from anywhere within the institution. This also minimizes time spent on paper charting.

Automating Repetitive Tasks

Developing techniques for repetitive tasks is similar to finding the fastest method, but it focuses on specific tasks that are repeated again and again, such as client teaching.

Many clients come to the hospital or ambulatory center for surgery or invasive diagnostic tests for same-day treatment. This does not give nurses much teaching time. Using videotapes and pamphlets as teaching aids can reduce the time needed to share the information, allowing the nurse to be available to answer individual questions and create individual adaptations. Many facilities are using these techniques for cardiac rehabilitation, preoperative teaching, and infant care instruction. Computer-generated teaching and instruction guides permit clients to take the information home with them. This can decrease the number of phone calls requiring repetition of information.

The Rhythm Model for Time Management

Navuluri (2001) looked at time management in terms of a Rhythm Model—a PQRST pattern: prioritize, question, re-check, self-reliance, treat. By prioritizing we are able to accomplish the most important tasks first. Questioning permits us to look at events and tasks in terms of effectiveness, efficiency, and efficacy. Re-checking unfinished tasks quickly helps us to efficiently manage our time. Self-reliance allows us to know the difference between events that are within our control and those that are not, as well as realizing our limitations. No one knows better what we are capable of doing than ourselves. Treats are part of life. It is okay to take a break or time for ourselves. It is important because it permits us to refresh. Table 9–1 summarizes the Rhythm Model for Time Management.

TABLE 9–1
The Rhythm Model for Time Management

Prioritize	List tasks in order of importance.
	Remember that some tasks must occur at specific times whereas others can occur at any time.
	Emergencies take precedence.
	Identify events controlled by you and events controlled by others.
	Use critical thinking skills to assign priorities.
Question	
Effectiveness	Did the task produce the desired outcome?
Efficiency	How can I accomplish the plan with the least expenditure of time?
	Is there a way to break this down into simpler tasks?
Efficacy	Do I have the skill and ability to obtain the desired effect?
Re-check	Mentally and physically re-check an unfinished or delegated task.
Self-reliance	Identify those tasks that are within your control and those that are not.
	Use critical thinking skills and adaptability to revise priorities.
	"Go with the flow."
Treat	Treat yourself to a break when you can.
	Treat yourself to time off.
	Treat yourself to an educational experience: Commit yourself to excellence.
	Treat others courteously and with respect.

■ Conclusion

Time can be our best friend or our worst enemy, depending on our perspective and how we manage it. It is important to identify how you feel about time and to assess your own time management skills. Nursing requires that we perform numerous activities within what often seems to be a very short period of time. Knowing this can create stress. Learn to delegate. Learn to say, "I would really like to help you; can it wait until I finish this?" Learn to say no. Most of all, learn how to make the most of your day. Finally, remember that 8 hours should be designated as sleep time and several more as personal or leisure ("time off") time.

Study Questions

1 Develop a personal time inventory. Identify your time wasters. How do you think you can eliminate these activities?

2 Create your own client care worksheet. How does this worksheet help you organize your clinical day?

3 Keep a log of your clinical day. Which activities took the most time and why? Which activities took the least time? What situations interfered with your work? What could you do to reduce the interference?

4 Identify a task that is done repeatedly in your clinical area. Think of a new, more efficient way to do that task. How could you implement this new routine? How could you evaluate its efficiency?

Critical Thinking Exercise

Antonio was recently hired as a team leader for a busy cardiac step-down unit. Nursing responsibilities of the team leader, in addition to client care, include meeting daily with team members, reviewing all admissions and discharges for acuity and length of stay, and documenting all clients who exceed length of stay and the reasons. At the end of each month, the team leaders are required to meet with unit managers to review the client care load and team member performance. This is the last week of the month, and Antonio has a meeting with the unit manager at the end of the week. He is 2 weeks behind on staff evaluations and documentation of clients who exceeded length of stay. He is becoming very stressed over his team leader responsibilities.

1 Why do you think Antonio is feeling stressed?

2 Make a "to do" list for Antonio.

3 Develop a time log for Antonio to use to analyze his activities.

4 How can Antonio organize and streamline his work?

Self-Assessment

1 Create a weekly schedule using a computerized calendar found on the Internet.

2 If you have a PDA, show your classmates how you use this to keep dates, notes, and personal information.

3 Draw the Rhythm Model for Time Management (see Table 9-1). Using the information from your clinical experience, fill in the table.

REFERENCES

Bos, C.S., & Vaughn, S. (1998). *Strategies for Teaching Students with Learning and Behavioral Problems,* ed. 4. Boston: Allyn & Bacon.

Baldwin, F.D. (2002). Making do with less. *Healthcare Informatics,* pp.1–7. Online, March 2002.

Brider, P. (1992). The move to patient-focused care. *American Journal of Nursing,* 92(9), 27–33.

Chappel, E.D. (1970). *Culture and Biological Man: Exploration in Behavioral Anthropology.* New York: Holt, Rinehart, & Winston. (Reprinted as *The Biological Foundations of Individuality and Culture.* Huntingdon, N.Y.: Robert Krieger, 1979.)

Curry, P. (March 25, 2002). Pressure cooker: Hospital's emphasis on productivity increases stress for nurses and patients. *Nurseweek News, http://www. nurseweek.com*

Drucker, P.E. (1967). *The Effective Executive.* New York: Harper & Row.

Gahar, A. (2000). *Programming for College Students with Learning Disabilities.* (Grant No.: 84-078C) *http:// www.csbsju.edu.* February, 16, 2000.

Gonzalez, S.I. (1996). Time management. *The Nursing Spectrum in Florida,* 6(17), 5.

Ferrett, S.K. (1996). *Connections: Study Skills for College and Career Success.* Chicago: Irwin Mirror Press.

Hammerschmidt, R., & Meador, C.K. (1993). *A Little Book of Nurses' Rules.* Philadelphia: Hanley & Belfus.

Haynes, M.E. (1991). *Practical Time Management.* Los Altos, Calif.: Crisp Publications.

Hobbs, S. (1987). Getting to grips with business plans, audit, and applications. *Nursing Standard.*

Matejka, J.K., & Dunsing, R.J. (1988). Time management: Changing some traditions. *Management World,* 17(2), 6–7.

Meyer, C. (1992). Equipment nurses like. *American Journal of Nursing,* 92(8), 32–38.

Moshovitz, R. (1993). *How to Organize Your Work and Your Life.* New York: Doubleday.

Navuluri, R.B. (March 2001). Our time management in patient care. *Research for Nursing Practice,* pp 1–8.

Prescott, P.A. (1991). Changing how nurses spend their time. *Image,* 23(1), 23–28.

Robichaud, A.M. (1986). Time documentation of clinical nurse specialist activities. *Journal of Nursing Administration,* 16(1), 31–36.

Sleeping on the job. (1993). *American Journal of Nursing,* 93(2), 10.

Smith, H.W. (1994). *The ten natural laws of successful time and life management: Proven strategies for increased productivity and inner peace.* New York: Warner Books.

Turkington, C.A. (1996). *Reflections for Working Women: Common Sense, Sage Advice, and Unconventional Wisdom.* New York: McGraw-Hill.

Webber, R.A. (1980). *Time Is Money! Tested Tactics That Conserve Time for Top Executives.* New York: Free Press.

CHAPTER 10

Work-Related Stress and Burnout

OBJECTIVES

After reading this chapter, the student should be able to:

- Identify signs and symptoms of stress, reality shock, and burnout.

- Describe the impact of stress, reality shock, and burnout on the individual and the health care team.

- Evaluate his or her own and colleagues' stress levels.

- Develop strategies to manage personal and professional stresses.

OUTLINE

Consider the Statistics

Stress
Effects of Stress
Responses to Stress

The Real World
Initial Concerns
Differences in Expectations
Additional Pressures on the New Graduate
Resolving the Problem

Burnout
Definition
Aspects
Stressors Leading to Burnout
    Personal Factors
    Job-Related Conditions
    Human Service Occupations
    Conflicting Demands
    Technology
    Lack of Balance in Life
Consequences
A Buffer Against Burnout

Stress Management
ABCs of Stress Management
    Awareness
    Belief
    Commitment
Physical Health Management
    Deep Breathing
    Good Posture
    Rest
    Relaxation and Time-Outs
    Proper Nutrition
    Exercise
Mental Health Management
    Realistic Expectations
    Reframing
    Humor
    Social Support

Conclusion

◼ Consider the Statistics

Fifty years ago, the term *personal anxiety* was never used to describe stress. In the decades since that time, stress has become the most common psychological complaint and a widespread health problem. Consider these current statistics (Lenson, 2001):

- 75 to 90 percent of all doctor office visits in the United States are for stress-related illnesses.

- 43 percent of all U.S. adults suffer some kind of adverse health effects related to stress.

- American businesses pay more than $300 billion each year for stress related absenteeism, reduced productivity, and health benefits.

- A month after the World Trade Center attack in September 2001, 60 to 80 percent of Americans reported suffering from some degree of posttraumatic stress disorder.

◼ Stress

Effects of Stress

Hans Selye first explored the concept of stress in the 1930s. Selye (1956) defined *stress* as the nonspecific response of the body to any demands made on it. His description of the general adaptation syndrome (GAS) has had an enormous influence on our present-day notions about stress and its effect on human beings. The GAS consists of three stages:

1 Alarm. The body awakens to the stressor and there is a slight change below the normal level of resistance.

2 Resistance. The body adjusts to the stressor and tries to restore balance.

3 Exhaustion. As the stressor continues, the body energy falls below the normal level of resistance and illness may occur.

Most people think of stress as work pressure, rush-hour traffic, or sick children. These are triggers to the stress response, the actual body reaction to the daily factors mentioned. As identified by Selye, *stress* is the fight-or-flight response in the body, caused by adrenaline and other stress hormones, causing the physiologic changes we learned in nursing school, such as increased heart rate and blood pressure, faster breathing, dilated pupils, increased blood sugar, and dry mouth.

Currently, stress is assessed on four levels: environmental, social, physiological, and psychological. *Environmental stressors* include weather, pollens, noise, traffic, and pollution. *Social stressors* include elements such as deadlines, finances, work responsibilities and interactions, and multiple demands for your time and attention. *Physiologically,* illness, aging, injuries, lack of exercise, poor nutrition, and inadequate sleep all cause stress on our bodies. The fourth cause of stress, *psychological,* are the thoughts we do to ourselves. How our brain interprets changes in the environment and body determines when our body turns on the fight-or-flight response (Davis, Eshelman, & McKay, 2000).

Epidemiological research has shown that long-term stress contributes to cardiovascular disease, hypertension, ulcers, substance abuse, immune system disorders, emotional disturbances, and job-related injuries (Crawford, 1993; Lusk, 1993). Table 10–1 lists the most common physical and psychological signs of stress (Goliszek, 1992; Martin, 1993).

"Whether the stress you experience is the result of major life changes or the cumulative effect of minor everyday hassles, it is how you respond to these experiences that determines the impact stress will have on your life" (Davis, Eshelman, & McKay, 2000).

Responses to Stress

Some people manage potentially stressful events more effectively than others (Crawford, 1993; Teague, 1992). Perceptions of events and the subsequent stress responses vary considerably from one person to another. A patient crisis that you consider stressful, for example, may not seem stressful at all to a coworker. The following is an example:

A new graduate was employed on a busy telemetry floor. Often, when clients were admitted, they were in acute distress with shortness of breath, diaphoresis, and chest pain. Family members were distraught and anxious. Each time the new graduate had to admit a client, she experienced a "sick-to-her-stomach" feeling, tightness in the chest and throat, and difficulty concentrating. She was afraid that she would miss something important and that the client would die during the admission. The more experienced nurses seemed to handle each admission with ease, even when the client's physical condition was severely compromised.

Selye also differentiated between "good" stress and "bad" stress. In 1974, Selye stated: "Stress is the spice of life. Since stress is associated with all types of activity, we could not avoid most of it only by never doing anything" (Lenson, 2001, p. 5). Good stress can push us to perform better and accomplish more. What makes an event "good stress" or "bad stress"? Lenson (2001) identified seven factors that differentiate good and bad stress:

1 We exert a high level of control over the outcomes of good stresses. With bad stresses, we enjoy little or no control.

2 We experience positive feelings when we process good stress. With bad stress, negative or ambivalent feelings occur.

3 Good stress helps us achieve positive goals. No desirable outcomes occur with bad stress.

4 We feel eager when anticipating the work we need to do to process our good stressors.

5 Bad stress leaves us with feelings of exhaustion and avoidance.

6 Good stress helps us grow; bad stress boxes us in. Good stress improves our interpersonal relationships; bad stress makes these relationships worse.

7 Processing all stress takes action on our part.

◙ The Real World

Today's health care system has adopted the corporate mindset. Both the new graduate and the seasoned professional will continue to experience redesigning, changing staffing

TABLE 10–1
Signs and Symptoms of Stress

Physical Signs and Symptoms

Rapid heart rate and respirations
Dry mouth and throat
Increased body temperature
Weakness, dizziness
Trembling hands, fingers, body
Nervous tics
Menstrual problems
Loss of appetite
Frequent urination
Diarrhea
Reduced immunity
Fatigue, low energy
Acid stomach, heartburn
Back and neck pain
Headache

Psychological/Behavioral Signs and Symptoms

Absenteeism
Alcoholism
Apathy
Irritability/Anger
Boredom
Callousness
Conflicts with workers
Cynicism
Defensiveness
Depersonalization
Depression
Feelings of helplessness and hopelessness
Decreased interest in sexual activity
Depression
Drug dependence
Nightmares
Inability to concentrate
Impaired judgment
Isolation
Withdrawal
Procrastination
Excessive worry, anxiety
Forgetfulness
Disorganized thinking
Pessimism
Unable to complete tasks

Source: Adapted from Martin, K. (May 1993). To cope with stress. *Nursing 93*, 39-41, with permission; and Goliszek, A. (1992). *Sixty-Six Second Stress Management: The Quickest Way to Relax and Ease Anxiety.* Far Hills, N.J.: New Horizon.

models, complex documentation requirements, continued nursing shortages, and the expectation that work does not end when the employee goes home (Trossman, 1999). Most agencies expect new graduates to come to the work setting able to organize their work, set priorities, and provide leadership to ancillary personnel. New graduates often say, "I had no idea that nursing would be this demanding." Even though your program of study is designed to help you prepare for the demands of the work setting, you will still need to continue to learn on the job. In fact, experienced nurses will tell you that what you learned in school is only the beginning; it provides you with the fundamental knowledge and skills needed to continue to grow and develop as you practice nursing in various capacities and work settings. Graduation signals not the end of learning but the beginning of your journey toward becoming an expert nurse (Benner, 1984).

Right now you are probably thinking, "Nothing can be more stressful than going to school. I can't wait to go to work and not have to study for tests, go to the clinical agency for my assignment, do client care plans," and so forth. In most associate degree programs, students are assigned to care for one to three clients a day, working up to six or seven clients under a preceptor's supervision by the end of their program. Compare this with your "next clinical rotation," your first real job as a nurse. You may work 7 to 10 days in a row on 8- to 12-hour shifts, caring for 10 or more clients. You may also have to supervise several technicians or licensed practical nurses. These drastic changes from school to employment cause many to experience what is called *reality shock* (Kraeger & Walker, 1993; Kramer, 1981).

Initial Concerns

The first few weeks on a new job are the "honeymoon" phase. The new employee is excited and enthusiastic about the new position. Coworkers usually go out of their way to make the new person feel welcome and overlook any problems that arise. Everything seems rosy. Unfortunately, honeymoons do not last forever. The new graduate is soon expected to behave just like everyone else and discovers that expectations for a professional employed in an organization

are quite different from expectations for a student in school. Those behaviors that brought rewards in school are not necessarily valued by the organization. In fact, some of them are criticized. The new graduate who is not prepared for this change feels confused, shocked, angry, and disillusioned. The tension of the situation can become almost unbearable if it is not resolved. Table 10–2 provides a list of ongoing and newer workplace stresses.

Graduate nurses in the first 3 months of employment identified concerns related to skills, personal and professional roles, patient care management, the shocks of bad experiences, the affirmations of good experiences, constructive evaluation, knowledge of the unit routine, and school versus work priorities (Godinez, Schweiger, Gruver, & Ryan, P., 1999; Heslop, 2001).

Well-supervised orientation programs are very helpful for newly licensed nurses. In this era of the nursing shortage, the orientation program may be cut short and the new nurse required to function on his or her own very quickly. One way to minimize initial work stress is to ask questions about the orientation program: How long will it be? Who will I be working with? When will I be on my

TABLE 10–2

Stress in the Workplace

Ongoing Sources of Stress in the Workplace	Newer Sources of Stress in the Workplace
Work overload	Changes in technology
Role conflict	Downsizing
Ineffective, hostile, incompetent supervisors	Constant changes in nursing care delivery
Lack of personal job fit, recognition, or clear job description	Work-home conflicts
Fear and uncertainly related to career progress	Elder and child care issues
Age, gender, race, religious discrimination	Workplace violence
	Lawsuits related to job stress

Source: Adapted from DeFrank, R. & Ivancevich, J. (1998). Stress on the job: An executive update. *Academy of Management Executive,* 12(3), 55.

own? What happens if at the end of the orientation I still need more assistance?

Differences in Expectations

The enthusiasm and eagerness of the first new job quickly disappear as reality sets in. Regardless of the career one chooses, there is no perfect job. The problem begins when reality and expectations collide. After 2 to 3 months, the new nurse begins to experience a formal separation from being a student and grabs hold of the professional reality of the nursing role. To cope with reality, we must recognize several facts of work life (Goliszek, 1992, pp. 36, 46):

1 Expectations are usually distortions of reality. Unless we accept this and react positively, we will go through life experiencing disappointment. As a student you had only two or three patients to care for, and you are very surprised to hear your first full day off orientation that you have five patients. Although you did hear the nurses talking about their caseload while you were a student, you expected to continue to have two or three patients for at least the next 4 months.

2 To some extent, you need to fit yourself into your work, not fit the work to suit your needs or demands. Having a positive attitude helps to maintain flexibility and a sense of humor. Your first position is at a physician's office. He is about ready to retire, and his patient load is dwindling. You wanted to apply for a position in acute care, but you have a very active social life and did not want to work weekends.

3 Regardless of the job, the way you perceive events on the job will influence how you feel about your work. Your attitude will affect whether work is a pleasant or unpleasant experience. Health care is not easy. Sick people can be cranky and demanding. Health care agencies continue to want to do more with less. How you perceive your contribution to the health care system will definitely influence your reality.

4 Feelings of helplessness and powerlessness at work cause frustration and unre-

lieved job stress. If you go to work every day feeling that you do not make a difference, it is time to reevaluate your position and your goals.

What are these differences in expectations? Kramer (1981), who studied reality shock for many years, found a number of them, which are listed in Table 10–3.

Ideally, health care should be comprehensive. It should not only meet all of a client's needs but also be delivered in a way that considers the client as a whole person, a member of a particular family that has certain unique characteristics and needs, and a member of a particular community. Most health care professionals, however, are not employed to provide comprehensive, holistic care. Instead, they are asked to give medications, provide counseling, make home visits, or prepare someone for surgery, but rarely to do all these things. These tasks are divided among different people, each a specialist, for the sake of efficiency rather than continuity or effectiveness.

When efficiency is the goal, the speed and amount of work done are rewarded rather than the quality of the work. This also creates a conflict for the new graduate, who was allowed to take as much time as needed to provide good care while in school.

Expectations are also communicated in different ways. In school, an effort is made to provide explicit directions so that students know what they are expected to accomplish. In many work settings, however, instructions on the job are brief, and many expectations are left unspoken. New graduates who

TABLE 10–3

Professional Ideals and Work Realities

Professional Ideals	Work Realities
Comprehensive, holistic care	Mechanistic, fragmented care
Emphasis on quality of care	Emphasis on efficiency
Explicit expectations	Implicit (unstated) expectations
Balanced, frequent feedback	Intermittent, often negative feedback

are not aware of these expectations may find that they have unknowingly left tasks undone or are considered inept by coworkers. The following is an example:

Brenda, a new graduate, was assigned to give medications to all the clients cared for by the team. Because this was a fairly light assignment, the graduate spent some time looking up the medications and explaining their actions to the clients receiving them. Brenda also straightened up the medicine room and filled out the order forms, which she thought would please the task-oriented team leader.

At the end of the day, Brenda reported these activities with some satisfaction to the team leader. She expected the team leader to be pleased with the way the time had been used. Instead, the team leader looked annoyed and told her that whoever passes out medications always does the blood pressures too and that the other nurse on the team, who had a heavier assignment, had to do them. Also, because supplies were always ordered on Fridays for the weekend, it would have to be done again tomorrow, so Brenda had in fact wasted her time.

Additional Pressures on the New Graduate

The first job a person takes after finishing school is often thought of as a proving ground where newly gained knowledge and skills are tested. Many set up mental tests for themselves that they feel must be passed before they can be confident of their ability to function. Passing these self-tests also confirms achievement of identity as a practitioner rather than a student.

At the same time, new graduates are undergoing testing by their coworkers, who are also interested in finding out whether the new graduate can handle the job. The new graduate is entering a new group, and the group will decide whether to accept this new member. This testing is somewhat like hazing of freshmen entering high school or college. It is usually reasonable, but sometimes new graduates are given tasks that they are not ready to handle. If this happens, Kramer (1981) recommended that new graduates refuse to take the test rather than fail it. Another opportunity for proving themselves will soon come along.

Additional problems, such as dealing with resistant staff members, cultural differ-

ences, and age differences, may also occur. Above all, the experience of loss is frequently described by new graduates. Losses are described by some of all of the following (Boychuk, 2001):

- The ideal world of caring and curing they had come to know through their education

- Their innocence

- The familiarity of academia

- The protection of clinical supervision by nursing instructors

- Externally set boundaries of care and safety

- A sense of collegiality and trusted relationships with peers

- Grounded feedback

Resolving the Problem

Before considering ways to resolve these problems, we look at some less successful ways of coping with these problems.

- **Abandon professional goals.** When faced with reality shock, some new graduates abandon their professional goals and adopt the organization's operative goals as their own. This eliminates their conflict but leaves them less effective caregivers. It also puts the needs of the organization before their needs or the needs of the client and reinforces operative goals that might better be challenged and changed.

- **Give up professional ideals.** Others give up their professional ideals but do not adopt the organization's goals or any others to replace them. This has a deadening effect; they become automatons, believing in nothing related to their work except doing what is necessary to earn a day's pay.

- **Leave the profession.** Those who do not give up their professional ideals try to find an organization that will support them. Unfortunately, a significant proportion of those who do not want to give up their professional ideals escape these conflicts by leaving their jobs and abandoning their profession. Kramer and Schmalenberg (1993) stated that there would be fewer shortages of nurses if more health care organizations met these ideals.

Instead of focusing on the bad stress you can meet the transition to professional nursing by adapting to good stress:

- **Develop a professional identity.** Opportunities to challenge one's competence and develop an identity as a professional can begin in school. Success in meeting these challenges can immunize the new graduate against the loss of confidence that accompanies reality shock.

- **Learn about the organization.** The new graduate who understands how organizations operate will not be as shocked as the naive individual. When you begin a new job, it is important to learn as much as you can about the organization and how it really operates. This not only saves you some nasty surprises but also gives you some ideas about how to work within the system and how to make the system work for you.

- **Use your energy wisely.** Keep in mind that much energy goes into learning a new job. You may see many things that you think need to be changed, but you need to recognize that to implement change also takes time and energy on your part. It is a good idea to make a list of these things so that you do not forget them later when you have become socialized into the system and have some time and energy to invest in change.

- **Communicate effectively.** Deal with the problems that can arise with coworkers. The same interpersonal skills you use in communicating with patients can be effective in dealing with your coworkers.

- **Seek feedback often and persistently.** Seeking feedback not only provides you with needed information but also pushes the people you work with to be more specific about their expectations of you.

- **Develop a support network.** Identifying colleagues who have also held onto their professional ideals and sharing not only your problems but also the work of improving the organization with them are helpful ways to cushion against reality shock. Their recognition of your work can keep you going when rewards from the organization are meager. A support network is a source of strength when resisting pressure to give up professional ideals and a source of power when attempting to bring about change. Developing your skills can help to prevent the problems of reality shock. Begin early in your career to protect yourself against reality shock.

- **Find a mentor.** A mentor is someone more experienced within or outside the organization who provides career development support, such as coaching, sponsoring advancement, providing challenging assignments, protecting protégés from adversity, and promoting positive visibility. Mentors provide guidance to the new graduate as he or she changes from student to professional nurse. Mentors can also fulfill psychosocial roles, such as personal support, friendship, acceptance, role modeling, and counseling. Many organizations have preceptors for the new employee. In many instances, the preceptor will become your mentor. However, the mentor role is much more encompassing than the preceptor role. The mentor relationship is a voluntary one and is built on mutual respect and development of the mentee. Table 10–4 identifies responsibilities of the mentor and mentee in this relationship (Scheetz, 2000; Simonetti & Ariss, 1999).

You have made it through the first 6 months of employment, and you are finally starting to feel like a "real" nurse. You are beginning to realize that a stress-free work environment is probably impossible to achieve. Shift work, overtime, distraught families, staff shortages, and pressure to do more with less continue to contribute to the stresses

TABLE 10–4
Mentor and Mentee Responsibilities

Mentor Responsibilities	Mentee Responsibilities
Has excellent communication and listening skills	Demonstrates eagerness to learn
Shows sensitivity to needs of nurses, patients, and workplace	Participates actively in the relationship by keeping all appointments and commitments
Able to encourage excellence in others	Seeks feedback and uses it to modify behaviors
Able to share an provide counsel	Demonstrates flexibility and an ability to change
Exhibits good decision-making skills	Is open in the relationship with mentor
Shows an understanding of power and politics	Demonstrates an ability to move toward independence
Demonstrates trustworthiness	Able to evaluate choices and outcomes

placed on nurses. An inability to deal with this continued stress will eventually lead to burnout.

◼ Burnout

Definition

The ultimate result of unmediated job stress is burnout. The term *burnout* became a favorite buzzword of the 1980s and continues to be part of today's vocabulary. Herbert Freudenberger formally identified it as a leadership concern in 1974. The literature on job stress and burnout continues to grow as new books, articles, workshops, and videotapes appear regularly. A useful definition of *burnout* is the "progressive deterioration in work and other performance resulting from increasing difficulties in coping with high and continuing levels of job-related stress and professional frustration" (Paine, 1984, p. 1).

Much of the burnout experienced by nurses has been attributed to the frustration that arises because care cannot be delivered in the ideal manner they learned in school. For those whose greatest satisfaction comes from caring for clients, anything that interferes with providing the highest quality care causes work stress. The often unrealistic and sometimes sexist image of nurses in the media, to which we all are exposed, adds to this frustration. Neither the school ideal nor the media image is realistic, but either may make nurses feel dissatisfied with themselves and their jobs, keeping stress levels high (Corley, Farley, Geddes, Goodloe, & Green, 1994; Fielding & Weaver, 1994; Grant, 1993; Kovner, Hendrickson, Knickman, & Finkler, 1994; Malkin, 1993; Nakata & Saylor, 1994; Skubak, Earls, & Botos, 1994).

Sharon had wanted to be a nurse for as long as she could remember. She married early, had three children, and put her dreams of being a nurse on hold. Now her children are grown, and she finally realized her dream by graduating last year from the local community college with a nursing degree. However, she has been feeling overwhelmed at work, critical of coworkers and patients, and argumentative with supervisors. She is having difficulty adapting to the restructuring changes at her hospital and goes home angry and frustrated every day. She cannot stop working for financial reasons but is seriously thinking of quitting nursing and taking some computer classes. "I'm tired of dealing with people. Maybe machines will be more friendly and predictable." Sharon is experiencing burnout.

Aspects

Goliszek (1992) identified four stages of the burnout syndrome:

1 High expectations and idealism. At the first stage, the individual is enthusiastic, dedicated, and committed to the job and exhibits a high energy level and positive attitude.

2 Pessimism and early job dissatisfaction. In the second stage, frustration, disillusionment, or boredom with the job develops, and the individual begins to exhibit the physical and psychological symptoms of stress.

3 Withdrawal and isolation. As the individual moves into the third stage, anger, hostility, and negativism are exhibited. The physical and psychological stress symptoms worsen. Through stage three, simple changes in job goals, attitudes, and behaviors may reverse the burnout process.

4 Irreversible detachment and loss of

interest. As the physical and emotional stress symptoms become severe, the individual exhibits low self-esteem, chronic absenteeism, cynicism, and total negativism. Once the individual has moved into this stage and remained there for any length of time, burnout is inevitable. Regardless of the cause, experiencing burnout leaves an individual emotionally and physically exhausted.

Stressors Leading to Burnout

Personal Factors

Some of the personal factors influencing job stress and burnout are age, gender, number of children, education, experience, and favored coping style. For example, the fact that many nurses are single parents raising families alone adds to the demands of already difficult days at work. Married nurses may have the additional stress of dual-career homes, causing even more stress in coordinating work and vacation schedules as well as daycare problems. Baby boomers are finding they need to care for elderly parents along with their children (DeFrank & Ivancevich, 1998). Competitive, impatient, and hostile personality traits have also been associated with emotional exhaustion and subsequent burnout (Borman, 1993).

Job-Related Conditions

Job-related stress is broadly defined by the National Institute for Occupational Safety and Health (NIOSH) as the "harmful physical and emotional responses that occur when the requirements of the job do not match the capabilities, resources, or needs of the worker" (*http://www.cdc.gov/niosh/ homepage.html*). Box 10–1 describes some of the circumstances that contribute to job-related stress. These are discussed further in Chapter 11.

Human Service Occupations

People who work in human service organizations consistently report lower levels of job satisfaction than do people working in other types of organizations. Much of the stress ex-

> **BOX 10–1**
> **Five Sources of Job Stress That Can Lead to Burnout**
>
> 1. **Intrinsic factors.** Characteristics of the job itself, such as the multiple aspects of complex client care that many nurses provide
> 2. **Organizational structure.** Characteristics of the organization in which you work, such as limited financial resources
> 3. **Reward system.** The way in which employees are rewarded or punished, particularly if these are obviously unfair
> 4. **Human resources system.** In particular, the number and availability of opportunities for staff development
> 5. **Leadership.** The way in which managers relate to their staff, particularly if they are unrealistic, uncaring, or unfair
>
> Source: Adapted from Carr, K., & Kazanowski, M. (1994). Factors affecting job satisfaction of nurses who work in long-term care. *Journal of Advanced Nursing, 19*, 878–883.; Crawford, S. (1993). Job stress and occupational health nursing. *American Association of Occupational Health Nurses Journal, 41*, 522–529; and Duquette, A., Sandhu, B., & Beaudet, L. (1994). Factors related to nursing burnout: A review of empirical knowledge. *Issues in Mental Health Nursing, 15*, 337–358.

perienced by nurses is related to the nature of their work: continued intensive, intimate contact with people who often have serious and sometimes fatal physical, mental, emotional, or social problems. Efforts to save clients or help them achieve a peaceful ending to their lives are not always successful. Despite our best efforts, many of our clients get worse, not better. Some return to their destructive behaviors; others do not recover but die. The continued loss of clients alone can lead to burnout. Even exposure to medicinal and antiseptic substances, unpleasant sights, and high noise levels can cause stress for some people. Health care providers experiencing burnout may become cynical and even hostile toward their coworkers and colleagues (Carr & Kazanowski, 1994; Dionne-Proulx & Pepin, 1993; Goodell & Van Ess Coeling, 1994; Stechmiller & Yarandi, 1993; Tumulty, Jernigan, & Kohut, 1994).

In some instances, human service professionals also experience lower pay, longer hours, and more extensive regulation than do professionals in other fields. Inadequate advancement opportunities for women and minorities in lower-status, lower-paid positions are apparent in many health care areas.

Conflicting Demands

Meeting work-related responsibilities and maintaining a family and personal life can increase stress when there is insufficient time or energy for all of these. As mentioned in the section on personal factors, both the single parent and the married one are at risk because of the conflicting demands of their personal and work lives. The perception of balance in one's life is a personal one.

There appear to be some differences in the way that men and women find a comfortable balance. Men often define themselves in terms of their separateness and their career progress; women are more likely to define themselves through attachment and connections with other people. Women who try to focus on occupational achievement and pursue personal attachments at the same time are likely to experience conflict in both their work and personal lives. In addition, society evaluates the behaviors of working adult men and women differently. "When a man disrupts work for his family, he is considered a good family man, while a woman disrupting work for family risks having her professional commitment questioned" (Borman, 1993, p. 1).

Technology

Decisions related to changes in technology are often made without input from employees. These same employees are then required to adapt and cope with the changes. How many of the following changes have you had to adapt to in the not-so-distant past: e-mail, voice mail, fax machines, computerized charting, desktop computers, cellular phones? Often, employees feel that their role has become secondary to technology (De-Frank & Ivancevich, 1998).

Lack of Balance in Life

When personal interests and satisfactions are limited to work, a person is more susceptible to burnout; trouble at work becomes trouble with that individual's whole life. A job can become the center of someone's world, and that world can become very small. Two ways out of this are to set limits on the commitment to work and to expand the number of satisfying activities and relationships outside of work.

Many people in the helping professions have difficulty setting limits on their commitment. This is fine if they enjoy working extra hours and taking calls at night and on weekends, but if it exhausts them, then they need to stop doing it or risk serious burnout. For example, when you are asked to work another double shift or the third weekend in a row, you can say no. At the same time as you are setting limits at work, you can expand your outside activities so that you live in a large world in which a blow to one part can be cushioned by support from other parts. If you are the team leader or nurse manager, you also need to recognize and accept staff members' need to do this as well. Ask yourself the following questions:

- Do I exercise at least three times weekly?

- Do I have several close friends that I see regularly?

- Do I have a plan for my life and career that I have told someone about?

- Do I have strong spiritual values that I carry out in practice regularly?

- Do I have some strong personal interests that I regularly enjoy?

Studies have shown that the two best indicators of customer satisfaction were related to employee satisfaction and employee work-life balance. Well-rounded employees have a different perspective on life and are perceived by employers as more trustworthy and more grounded in reality. Ultimately, you do not have to give up your personal life to excel in your professional life (Farren, 1999).

Consequences

You can see that certain combinations of personal and organizational factors can increase the likelihood of burnout. Finding the right fit between your own preferences and the characteristics of the organization you work for can be keys to preventing burnout. Health care demands adaptable, innovative, competent employees who care about their clients, desire to continue learning, and try to remain productive despite constant challenges. Unfortunately, these are the same individuals who are prone to burnout if preventive action is not taken (Lickman, Simms, & Greene, 1993; McGee-Cooper, 1993).

Burnout has financial, physical, emotional, and social implications for the professional, the clients, and the organization. Burnout can happen to anyone, not just to people with a history of emotional problems. In fact, it is not considered an emotional disturbance in the sense that depression is but, instead, a reaction to sustained organizational stressors (Duquette, Sandhu, & Beaudet, 1994).

A Buffer Against Burnout

The idea that personal hardiness provides a buffer against burnout has been explored in recent years. *Hardiness* includes the following:

- A sense of personal control rather than powerlessness

- Commitment to work and life's activities, rather than alienation

- Seeing both life's demands and change as challenges, rather than as threats

The hardiness that comes from having this perspective leads to the use of adaptive coping responses, such as optimism, effective use of support systems, and healthy lifestyle habits (Duquette, Sandhu, & Beaudet, 1994; Nowak & Pentkowski, 1994). In addition, letting go of guilt, fear of change,

and the self-blaming, wallowing in the problem syndrome will do a lot to help you buffer against burnout (Lenson, 2001).

▣ Stress Management

Although we cannot always control the demands placed on us, we can learn to manage our reactions to them and to make healthy lifestyle choices that better prepare us to meet demands.

ABCs of Stress Management

Frances Johnston (1994) suggested using the ABCs of stress management (awareness, belief, and commitment) to have as constructive a response to stress as possible (Box 10–2). Let's look at these ABCs in a little more detail.

Awareness

How do you know that you are under stress and may be beginning to burn out? The key is being honest with yourself. Asking yourself the questions in Box 10–3 and answering them honestly are one way to assess your personal risk. To further analyze your responses to stress, you may also want to answer the questions in Box 10–4. The answers to these questions require some thought. You do not have to share your answers with others unless you want to, but you do need to be completely honest with yourself when you answer them or the exercise will not be worth the time spent on it. Try to

 BOX 10–2
ABCs of Stress Management

- Acquire awareness of your own responses to stress and the consequences of too much stress.
- Believe that you can change your perspective and your behavior.
- Commit yourself to taking action to prevent conflicts that cause stress, to learning techniques that help you cope in situations over which you have no control, and to understanding that you can choose how to react in stressful situations.

BOX 10–3
Assessing Your Risk for Burnout

- Are you feeling more fatigued than energetic?
- Are you working harder but accomplishing less?
- Are you feeling cynical or disenchanted most of the time?
- Do you often feel sad or cry for no apparent reason?
- Are you feeling hostile, negative, or angry at work?
- Are you short-tempered? Withdrawing from friends or coworkers?
- Are you forgetting appointments or deadlines? Frequently misplacing personal items?
- Are you becoming insensitive, irritable, and short-tempered?
- Are you experiencing more physical symptoms, such as headaches or stomachaches?
- Do you feel like avoiding people?
- Are you laughing less? Feeling joy less?
- Are you interested in sex?
- Do you crave junk food more often?
- Are you skipping meals?
- Have your sleep patterns changed?
- Are you taking more medication than usual? Using alcohol or other substances to alter your mood?
- Do you feel guilty when your work isn't perfect?
- Are you questioning whether the job is right for you?
- Do you feel as though no one cares what kind of work you do?
- Are you constantly pushing yourself to do better, yet feel frustrated that there isn't time to do what you want to do?
- Do you feel as if you are on a treadmill all day?
- Are you using holidays, weekends, or vacation time to catch up?
- Do you feel as if you are "burning the candle at both ends"?

Source: Adapted from Golin, M., Buchlin, M., & Diamond, D. (1991). *Secrets of Executive Success*. Emmaus, Pa.: Rodale Press; and Goliszek, A. (1992). *Sixty-Six Second Stress Management: The Quickest Way to Relax and Ease Anxiety*. Far Hills, N.J.: New Horizon.

determine the sources of your stress (Goliszek, 1992):

- Is it the *time of day* when you are doing the activity?

- Is it the *reason* that you are doing the activity?

- Is it the *way* in which you are doing the activity?

- Is it the *amount of time* you need to do the activity?

Belief

Now that you have done the "A" part of stress management, you are ready to move on to "B," which is belief in yourself. Your relationship with your inner self may be the most important relationship of all. Building

your self-image and self-esteem will enable you to block out negativism (Davidhizar, 1994). You must also believe that your destiny is not inevitable but that change is possible. Be honest with yourself. Truly value your life. Ask yourself, "If I could live 1 more month, what would I do?"—and start doing it (Johnston, 1994).

Commitment

As you move forward to step "C," you will need to make a commitment to continuing to work on stress recognition and reduction. Once you have recognized the warning signs of stress and impending burnout and have gained some insight into your personal needs and reactions to stress, it is time to find the stress management techniques that are right for you.

BOX 10–4
Questions for Self-Assessment

- What does the term *health* mean to me?
- What prevents me from living this definition of health?
- Is health important to me?
- Where do I find support?
- Which coping methods work best for me?
- What tasks cause me to feel pressured?
- Can I reorganize, reduce, or eliminate these tasks?
- Can I delegate or rearrange any of my family responsibilities?
- Can I say no to less important demands?
- What are my hopes for the future in terms of:
  Career?
  Finances?
  Spiritual life and physical needs?
  Family relationships?
  Social relationships?
- What do I think others expect of me?
- How do I feel about these expectations?
- What is really important to me?
- Can I prioritize in order to have balance in my life?

The stress management techniques in the next section are divided into physical and mental health management for ease in reading and remembering them. However, bear in mind that this is really an artificial division and that mind and body interact continuously. Stress affects both mind and body, and we need to care for both if we are to be successful in managing stress and preventing burnout.

Physical Health Management

Nurses spend much of their time teaching their clients the basics of keeping themselves healthy. However, many fail to apply these principles in their own lives. We review some of the most important aspects of health promotion and stress reduction in this section: deep breathing, good posture, rest, relaxation, proper nutrition, and exercise (Davidhizar, 1994; Posen, 2000; Wolinski, 1993).

Deep Breathing

Most of the time people use only 45% of their lung capacity when they breathe. Remember all the times when you have instructed your clients to "take a few deep breaths"? Practice taking a few slow, deep, "belly" breaths. When faced with a stressful situation, people often hold their breath for a few seconds. This reduces the amount of oxygen delivered to the brain and causes them to feel more anxious. Anxiety can lead to faulty reasoning and a feeling of losing control. Often you can calm yourself by taking a few deep breaths. Try it right now. Don't you feel better already?

Good Posture

A common response to pressure is to slump down into your chair, tensing your upper torso and abdominal muscles. Again, this restricts blood flow and the amount of oxygen reaching your brain. Instead of slumping, imagine a hook on top of your head pulling up your spine, relax your abdomen, and look up. Now, shrug your shoulders a few times to loosen the muscles and picture a sunny day at the beach or a walk in the woods. Do you feel more relaxed?

Rest

Sleep needs are different for each of us. Find out how much sleep you need and work on arranging your activities so that you get enough sleep. If it is impossible to get enough sleep on a given day, perhaps a short nap or just closing your eyes for a few minutes will help. Irregular sleep cycles over the long term can be unhealthy and increase stress. Power naps of 5 to 20 minutes can be rejuvenating.

Relaxation and Time-Outs

Many people have found that relaxation with guided imagery or other forms of meditation decreases both the physiological and psychological impact of chronic stress. Guided imagery has been used in competitions for many years, in golf, ice skating, baseball, and other sports. Research studies have shown that creation of a mental image of the desired results enhances our ability to reach the goal. Positive behavior or goal attainment is enhanced even more if you imagine the details of the process of achieving your desired outcome (Vines, 1994). Box 10–5 lists useful relaxation techniques.

Imagine taking the National Council License Examination (NCLEX). You sit down at the computer, take a few deep breaths, and begin. Visualize yourself reading the questions, smiling as you identify the correct answer, and hitting the Enter key after recording your answer, and complete the examination, feeling confident that you were successful. A week later, you go to your mailbox and find a letter waiting for you: "Congratulations, you have passed the test and are now a licensed registered nurse." You imagine telling your family and friends. What an exciting moment!

Taking breaks and time-outs during the day for a short walk or a refreshment (not caffeine) break or just to daydream can help de-stress you during the day. Just as we have circadian rhythms during the night, we have circadian rhythms during the day. These cycles are peaks of energy with troughs of low energy. Watching for these low energy cycles and taking breaks at that time will help to keeping stress from building up.

Proper Nutrition

New research results endorsing the benefits of healthful eating habits seem to appear almost daily. Although the various authorities may prescribe somewhat different regimens, ultimately it appears that too little or too much of any nutrient can be harmful. Many people do not realize that simply decreasing or discontinuing caffeine can help decrease a stress reaction in the body. Some general guidelines for good nutrition are included in Box 10–6.

BOX 10–6
Guidelines for Good Nutrition

- Eat smaller, more frequent meals for energy. Six small meals are more beneficial than three large ones.
- Eat foods that are high in complex carbohydrates, contain adequate protein, and are low in fat content. Beware of fad diets!
- Eat at least five servings of fruits and vegetables daily.
- Avoid highly processed foods.
- Avoid caffeine.
- Use salt and sugar sparingly.
- Drink plenty of water.
- Make sure you take enough vitamins, including C, B, E, beta carotene, and calcium; and minerals, including copper, manganese, zinc, magnesium, and potassium.

Source: Adapted from Bowers, R. (1993). Stress and your health. *National Women's Health Report*, 15(3), 6.

Exercise

Regular aerobic exercise for 20 minutes three times a week is recommended for most people. The exercise may be walking, swimming, jogging, bicycling, stair-stepping, or low-impact aerobics. Whichever you choose, work at a pace that is comfortable for you and increase it gradually as you become conditioned. Don't overdo it. The experience should leave you feeling invigorated, not exhausted.

The physiological benefits of exercise are well-known. Exercise may not eliminate the stressors in our lives, but it is an important element in a healthy lifestyle. Exercise has been shown to improve people's mood and to induce a state of relaxation through the reduction of physiological tension. Regular exercise decreases the energy from the fight-or-flight response discussed in the beginning of this chapter.

Exercise can also be a useful distraction, allowing time to regroup before entering a stressful situation again (Long & Flood, 1993). It is important to choose an exercise that you enjoy doing and that fits into your lifestyle. Perhaps you could walk to work every day or pedal an exercise bicycle during

BOX 10–5
Useful Relaxation Techniques

- Guided imagery
- Yoga
- Transcendental meditation
- Relaxation tapes or music
- Favorite sports or hobbies
- Quiet corners or favorite places

your favorite television program. It is not necessary to join an expensive club or to buy elaborate equipment or clothing to begin an exercise program. It is necessary to get up and get moving, however.

Some people recommend an organized exercise program to obtain the most benefit. For some, however, the cost or time required may actually contribute to their stress. For others, the organized program is an excellent motivator. Find out what works for you.

Keep your exercise plan reasonable. Plan for the long haul, not just until you get past your next performance evaluation or lose that extra 5 pounds.

Mental Health Management

Mental health management begins with *taking responsibility for your own thoughts and attitudes.* Do not allow self-defeating thoughts to dominate your thinking. You may have to remind yourself to stop thinking that you have to be perfect all the time. You may also have to adjust your expectations and become more realistic. Do you always have to be in control? Does everything have to be perfect? Do you have a difficult time delegating? Are you constantly frustrated because of the way you perceive situations? If you are answering yes to many of these questions, you may be setting yourself up for failure, resentment, low self-esteem, and burnout. Give yourself positive strokes, even if no one else does (Davidhizar, 1994; Posen, 2000; Wolinski, 1993).

Realistic Expectations

One of the most common stressors in life is having unrealistic expectations. Expecting family members, coworkers, and your employer to be perfect and meet your every demand on your time schedule is setting yourself up for undue stress.

Reframing

Reframing is looking at a situation from many different ways. When we reframe stressful situations, they often become less stressful or at least more understandable. If we have an extremely heavy workday and

we think it is because the nurse manager has it in for us, the day becomes much more stressful than if we realize that, unfortunately, today we are short-staffed but staffing is usually okay most of the time.

Humor

Laughter relieves tension. Humor is a wonderful way to reduce stress both for yourself and your patients. Remember, however, that humor is very individual, and what may be funny to you may be hurtful to your patient or coworker.

Social Support

Much research has been done to show that the presence of social support and the *quality of relationships* can significantly influence how quickly we become ill and how quickly we recover. A sense of belonging and community, an environment in which we can share our feelings without fear of condemnation or ridicule, helps us maintain our well-being. Having friends with whom to share hopes, dreams, fears, and concerns and with whom to laugh and cry is paramount to our mental health and stress management. In the work environment, coworkers who are trusted and respected become part of our social support systems (Wolinski, 1993). Box 10–7 lists some additional tips for coping with work stress.

Nurses are professional caregivers. Many years ago, Carl Rogers (1977) said that you cannot care for others until you have taken care of yourself. The word *selfish* may bring to mind someone who is greedy, self-centered, and egotistical, but to take care of yourself, you have to be *creatively selfish.* Learn to nurture yourself so that you will be better able to nurture others.

Stress reduction, relaxation techniques, exercise, and good nutrition are all helpful in keeping energy levels high. However, although they can prepare people to cope with the stresses of a job, they are not solutions to the conflicts that lead to reality shock and burnout. It is more effective to resolve the problem than to treat the symptoms (Lee & Ashforth, 1993). Box 10–8 lists keys to physical and mental health management.

> **BOX 10–7**
> **Coping with Daily Work Stress**
>
> - Spend time on outside interests.
> - Increase professional knowledge.
> - Identify problem-solving resources.
> - Identify realistic expectations for your position.
> - Assess the rewards your work can realistically deliver.
> - Develop good communication skills.
> - Join rap sessions with coworkers.
> - Do not exceed your limits—you do not always have to say yes!
> - Deal with other people's anger by asking yourself, "Whose problem is this?"
> - Recognize that you can teach other people how to treat you.

> **BOX 10–8**
> **Keys to Physical and Mental Health Management**
>
> - Deep breathing
> - Posture
> - Rest
> - Relaxation
> - Nutrition
> - Exercise
> - Realistic expectations
> - Reframing
> - Humor
> - Social support

Conclusion

You already know that the work of nursing is not easy and may sometimes be very stressful. Yet nursing is also a profession filled with a great deal of personal and professional satisfaction. Periodically ask yourself the questions designed to help you assess your stress level and risk for burnout and review the stress management techniques described in this chapter.

There is no one right way to manage stress and avoid burnout. Rather, by managing small segments of each day, you will learn to identify and manage your stress. This chapter contains many reminders to help you de-stress during the day (Box 10–9). You can also help your colleagues do the same. If you find yourself in danger of job burnout during your career, you will have learned how to bring yourself back to a healthy, balanced position.

Ultimately, you are in control. Every day you are faced with choices. By gaining power over your choices and the stress they cause, you empower yourself. Instead of being preoccupied with the past or the future, acknowledge the present moment and say to yourself (Davidson, 1999):

- I choose to relish my days.

- I choose to enjoy this moment.

- I choose to be fully present to others.

- I choose to fully engage in the activity at hand.

- I choose to proceed at a measured, effective pace.

- I choose to acknowledge all I have achieved so far.

- I choose to focus on where I am and what I am doing.

- I choose to acknowledge that this is the only moment in which I can take action.

We can't live in a problem-free world, but we can learn how to handle stress. Using the suggestions in this chapter, you will be able to adopt a healthier personal and professional lifestyle. The self-assessment worksheet, Coping with Stress, can help you currently manage stress and help you understand your responses better. The worksheet, Values Clarification will help you identify how to begin to change taking into account what is most important to you.

BOX 10–9
Ten Daily De-Stress Reminders

- Express yourself! Communicate your feelings and emotions to friends and colleagues to avoid isolation and share perspectives. Sometimes another opinion helps you see the situation in a different light.
- Take time off. Taking breaks, or doing something unrelated to work, will help you feel refreshed as you begin work again.
- Understand your individual energy patterns. Are you a morning or an afternoon person? Schedule stressful duties during times when you are most energetic.
- Do one stressful activity at a time. Although this may take advanced planning, avoiding more than one stressful situation at a time will make you feel more in control and satisfied with your accomplishments.
- Exercise! Physical exercise builds physical and emotional resilience. Don't put physical activities on the back burner as you become busy.
- Tackle big projects one piece at a time. Having control of one part of a project at a time will help you to avoid feeling overwhelmed and out of control.
- Delegate if possible. If you can delegate and share in problem solving, do it! Not only will your load be lighter, but others will be able to participate in decision-making.
- It's okay to say no. Don't take on every extra assignment or special project.
- Be work-smart. Improve your work skills with new technologies and ideas. Take advantage of additional job training.
- Relax. Find time each day to consciously relax and reflect on the positive energies you need to cope with stressful situations more readily.

Source: Adapted from Bowers, R. (1993). Stress and your health. *National Women's Health Report*, 15(3), 6.

CURRENT RESEARCH

Bernsier, D. (1998). A study of coping: Successful recovery from severe burnout and other reactions to severe work-related stress. *Work & Stress*, 12(1), 50–65.

In this qualitative study, data were gathered from first-person accounts of professionals who successfully recovered from burnout. In this study, *successful recovery* was defined as being in a job situation considered satisfactory by the subject and with the subject having no desire to change jobs. Subjects had to have taken 1 month or more sick leave because of work stress or burnout, had to have solved the related problems within the past 4 years, had to be human service workers, and had to be available for interviews.

Twenty subjects were recruited and interviewed from the Province of Quebec in Canada. Grounded theory was selected as the framework. The unstructured interviews were conducted by the same person and lasted an average of 90 minutes each. Aspects of the recovery stages were:

1. A sequence of stages: (a) admitting the problem, (b) distancing from work, (c) restoring health, (d) questioning values, (e) exploring work possibilities, (f) making a break, making a change
2. Coping strategies: (a) seeking reassurance, (b) understanding causes, (c) finding support.

This study provides an interesting framework for the general stages and specific coping strategies associated with burnout. Based on what you have learned in this chapter, what recommendations would you make to these participants to deal with burnout before it occurs again

Additional examples can be found in:

Boey, K.W. (1999). Distressed and stress resistant nurses. *Issues in Mental Health Nursing*, 20(1), 33–54.

Kalliath, T., O'Driscoll, T., & Gillespie, D. (1998). The relationship between burnout and organizational commitment in two samples of health professionals. *Work and Stress*, 12(2), 179–185.

Coping with Stress

Before you begin to change how you deal with stress, consider how you currently manage stress. Below are some of the more common ways of coping with stressful events. Identify those that you use.

	Never/ Seldom	Sometimes	Frequently
1. I ignore my own needs and just work harder.			
2. I seek out family/friends for support.			
3. I eat more than usual.			
4. I do some sort of exercise.			
5. I get irritable and take it out on others.			
6. I take time to relax, breathe, and unwind.			
7. I smoke cigarettes or drink caffeinated beverages.			
8. I confront my stress and work to change it.			
9. I withdraw emotionally and just go through the motions of the day.			
10. I change my outlook on the problem and try and put it in a better perspective.			

	Never/ Seldom	Sometimes	Frequently
11. I sleep too much.			
12. I take time off.			
13. I go shopping.			
14. I use humor to take the edge off.			
15. I increase my alcohol intake.			
16. I get involved in a hobby.			
17. I take prescription drugs to help me relax or sleep.			
18. I maintain a healthy diet.			
19. I ignore the problem.			
20. I pray, meditate, or enhance my spiritual life.			
21. I worry and become anxious.			
22. I try to focus on the things I can control and accept the things I can't.			

The even numbered items tend to be more constructive tactics than the odd numbered items.

Source: Adapted from Davis, M., Eshelman, E., & McCay, M. (2000). *The Relaxation & Stress Reduction Workbook*, 5th ed. San Jose, Calif.: New Harbinger Publications.

Values Clarification

The first step in managing your time is to decide what is most worthwhile or desirable for you. Some of the values that are important to people are career, health, home, family, spirituality, finances, leisure, learning, creativity, happiness, peace of mind, communication. You may identify others. In this exercise, list the values that are most important to you. List all of them, not in any particular order.

_____   _____

_____   _____

_____   _____

_____   _____

_____   _____

Next, think carefully about how important each value is to you and rank order them. You will find that this list comes in handy when you have difficulty choosing between two or more alternatives. If family and leisure rank very high, you many not want to consider a position where you have unscheduled hours or many on-call responsibilities.

1	6
2	7
3	8
4	9
5	10

Source: Adapted from Davis, M., Eshelman, E., & McCay, M. (2000). *The Relaxation and Stress Reduction Workbook*, 5th ed. San Jose, Calif.: New Harbinger Publications.

Study Questions

1 Discuss the characteristics of health care organizations that may lead to burnout among nurses. Which of these have you observed in your clinical rotations? How could they be eliminated?

2 How can a new graduate adequately prepare for reality shock? Whose responsibility is it to prevent reality shock?

3 What qualities would you look for in a mentor? What qualities would you demonstrate as a mentee? Can you identify someone you know who might become a mentor to you?

4 What are the signs of stress, reality shock, and burnout? How are they related?

5 How can you help colleagues deal with their stress?

6 Identify the physical and psychological signs and symptoms you exhibit during stress. What sources of stress are most likely to affect you? How do you deal with these signs and symptoms?

7 Develop a plan to manage stress on a long-term basis.

Critical Thinking Exercise

Shawna, the "new kid on the block," has been working from 7 A.M. to 3 P.M. on an infectious disease floor since obtaining her RN license 4 months ago. Most of the staff she works with have been there since the unit opened 5 years ago. On a typical day, the staffing consists of a nurse manager, two RNs, an LPN, and one technician for approximately 40 clients. The majority of the clients are HIV-positive with multisystem failure. Many are severely debilitated and need help with their activities of daily living. Although the staff members encourage family members and loved ones to help, most of them are unavailable because they work during the day. Several days a week, the nursing students from Shawna's community college program are assigned to the floor.

Tina, the nurse manager, does not participate in any direct client care, saying that she is "too busy at the desk." Laverne, the other RN, says the unit depresses her and that she has requested a transfer to pediatrics. Lynn, the LPN, wants to "give meds" because she is "sick of the clients' constant whining," and Sheila, the technician, is "just plain exhausted." Lately, Shawna has noticed that the other staff members seem to avoid the nursing students and reply to their questions with terse, short answers. Shawna is feeling alone and overwhelmed and goes home at night worrying about the clients, who need more care and attention. She is afraid to ask Tina for more help because she doesn't want to be seen as incompetent or a complainer. When she confided in Lynn about her concerns, Lynn replied, "Get real—no one here cares about the clients or us. All they care about is the bottom line! Why did a smart girl like you choose nursing in the first place?"

1 What is happening on this unit in leadership terms?

2 Identify the major problems and the factors that contributed to these problems.

3 What factors might have contributed to the behaviors exhibited by Tina, Lynn, and Sheila?

4 How would you feel if you were Shawna?

5 Is there anything Shawna can do for herself, for the clients, and for the staff members?

6 What do you think Tina (the nurse manager) should do?

7 How is the nurse manager reacting to the changes in her staff members?

8 What is the responsibility of administration?

9 How are the clients affected by the behaviors exhibited by all staff members?

REFERENCES

Benner, P. (1984). *From Novice to Expert.* Menlo Park, Calif.: Addison-Wesley.

Borman, J. (1993). Chief nurse executives balance their work and personal lives. *Nursing Administration Quarterly,* 18(1), 30–39.

Bowers, R. (1993). Stress and your health. *National Women's Health Report,* 15(3), 6.

Boychuk, J. (2001). Out in the real world: Newly graduated nurses in acute-care speak out. *Journal of Nursing Administration,* 31, 426–439.

Carr, K., & Kazanowski, M. (1994). Factors affecting job satisfaction of nurses who work in long-term care. *Journal of Advanced Nursing,* 19, 878–883.

Corley, M., Farley, B., Geddes, N., Goodloe, L., & Green, P. (1994). The clinical ladder: Impact on nurse satisfaction and turnover. *Journal of Nursing Administration,* 24(2), 42–48.

Crawford, S. (1993). Job stress and occupational health nursing. *American Association of Occupational Health Nurses Journal,* 41, 522–529.

Davidhizar, R. (1994). Stress can make you or break you. *Advance Practice Nurse,* 10(1), 17.

Davidson, J. (1999). *Managing Stress,* 2nd ed. New York: Pearson Education Macmillan Company.

Davis, M., Eshelman, E., & McCay, M. (2000). *The Relaxation and Stress Reduction Workbook,* 5th ed. California: New Harbinger Publications.

DeFrank, R., & Ivancevich, J. (1998). Stress on the job: An executive update. *Academy of Management Executives,* 12(3), 55.

Dionne-Proulx, J., & Pepin, R. (1993). Stress management in the nursing profession. *Journal of Nursing Management,* 1, 75–81.

Duquette, A., Sandhu, B., & Beaudet, L. (1994). Factors related to nursing burnout: A review of empirical knowledge. *Issues in Mental Health Nursing,* 15, 337–358.

Farren, C. (1999). Stress and productivity: What tips the scale? *Strategy and Leadership,* 27(1), 36.

Fielding, J., & Weaver, S. (1994). A comparison of hospital and community-based mental health nurses: Perceptions of their work environment and psychological health. *Journal of Advanced Nursing,* 19, 1196-1204.

Freudenberger, H.J. (1974). Staff burn-out. *Journal of Social Issues,* 30(1), 159.

Golin, M., Buchlin, M., & Diamond, D. (1991). *Secrets of Executive Success.* Emmaus, Pa.: Rodale Press.

Goliszek, A. (1992). *Sixty-Six Second Stress Management. The Quickest Way to Relax and Ease Anxiety.* Far Hills, N.J.: New Horizon.

Godinez, G., Schweiger, J., Gruver, J., & Ryan, P. (1999). Role transition from graduate to staff nurse: A qualitative analysis. *Journal for Nurses in Staff Development,* 15(3), 97–110.

Goodell, T., & Van Ess Coeling, H. (1994). Outcomes of nurses' job satisfaction. *Journal of Nursing Administration,* 24(11), 36–41.

Grant, P. (1993). Manage nurse stress and increase potential at the bedside. *Nursing Administration Quarterly,* 18(1), 16–22.

Heslop, L. (2001). Undergraduate student nurses: Expectations and their self-reported preparedness for the graduate year role. *Journal of Advanced Nursing,* 36, 626–634.

Johnston, F. (May-June 1994). Stress can kill. *Today's OR Nurse,* 5–6.

Kovner, C., Hendrickson, G., Knickman, J., & Finkler, S. (1994). Nurse care delivery models and nurse satisfaction. *Nursing Administration Quarterly,* 19(1), 74–85.

Kraeger, M., & Walker, K. (1993). Attrition, burnout, job dissatisfaction and occupational therapy manager. *Occupational Therapy in Health Care,* 8(4), 47–61.

Kramer, M. (January 27–28, 1981). Coping with reality shock. Workshop presented at Jackson Memorial Hospital, Miami, Fla.

Kramer, M., & Schmalenberg, C. (1993). Learning from success: Autonomy and empowerment. *Nursing Management,* 24(5), 58–64.

Lee, R.T., & Ashforth, B.E. (1993). A further examination of managerial burnout: Toward an integrated model. *Journal of Organizational Behavior,* 14(1), 3–20.

Lenson, B. (2001). *Good Stress—Bad Stress.* New York: Marlowe and Company.

Lickman, P., Simms, L., & Greene, C. (1993). Learning environment: The catalyst for work excitement. *Journal of Continuing Education in Nursing,* 24, 211–216.

Long, B., & Flood, K. (1993). Coping with work stress: Psychological benefits of exercise. *Work and Stress,* 7(2), 109–119.

Lusk, S. (1993). Job stress. *American Association of Occupational Health Nurses Journal,* 41, 601–606.

Malkin, K.F. (1993). Primary nursing: Job satisfaction and staff retention. *Journal of Nursing Management,* 1, 119–124.

Martin, K. (May 1993). To cope with stress. *Nursing 93,*39–41.

McGee-Cooper, A. (September-October 1993). Shifting from high stress to high energy. *Imprint,* 93(5), 61–69.

Nakata, J., & Saylor, C. (1994). Management style and staff nurse satisfaction in a changing environment. *Nursing Administration Quarterly,* 18(3), 51–57.

National Institute for Occupational Safety and Health (NIOSH) *http://www.cdc.gov/niosh/homepage.html* accessed 7/27/02.

Nowak, K., & Pentkowski, A. (1994). Lifestyle habits, substance use, and predictors of job burnout in professional women. *Work and Stress,* 8(1), 19–35.

Paine, W.S. (1984). Professional burnout: Some major costs. *Family and Community Health,* 6(4), 1–11.

Posen, D. (2000). Stress management for patient and physician. (Online). Available: *http://www.mentalhealth.com/mag1/p51-str.html*

Rogers, C. (1977). *Carl Rogers on Personal Power.* New York: Dell.

Scheetz, L.J. (2000). *Nursing Faculty Secrets.* Philadelphia: Hanley & Belfus.

Selye, H. (1956). *The Stress of Life.* New York: McGraw-Hill.

Simonetti, J., & Ariss, S. (1999), *Business Horizons,* 42(6), 56–73.

Skubak, K., Earls, N., & Botos, M. (1994). Shared governance: Getting it started. *Nursing Management,* 25(5), 80I–J, 80N, 80P.

Stechmiller, J., & Yarandi, H. (1993). Predictors of burnout in critical care nurses. *Heart Lung,* 22, 534–540.

Tappen (1995).

Teague, J.B. (1992). The relationship between various coping styles and burnout among nurses. *Dissertation Abstracts International,* 1994,198402.

Trossman, S. (July/August 1999). Stress! It's everywhere! And it can be managed! *American Nurse,* 1.

Tumulty, G., Jernigan, E., & Kohut, G. (1994). The impact of perceived work environment on job satisfaction of hospital staff nurses. *Applied Nursing Research,* 7(2), 84–90.

Vines, S. (1994). Relaxation with guided imagery. *American Association of Occupational Health Nurses Journal,* 42, 206–213.

Wolinski, K. (1993). Self-awareness, self-renewal, self management. *AORN Journal,* 58, 721–730.

CHAPTER 11

The Workplace

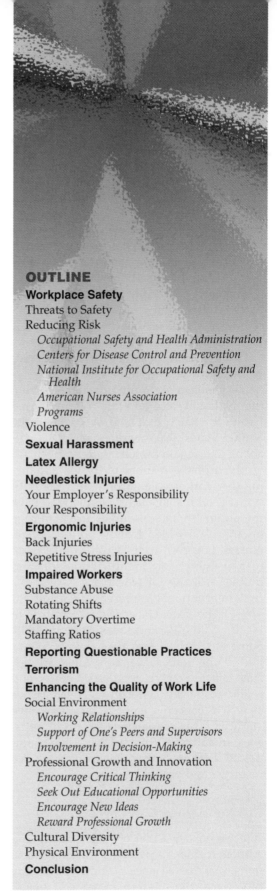

OBJECTIVES

After reading this chapter, the student should be able to:

- Recognize threats to safety in the workplace.

- Identify agencies responsible for overseeing workplace safety.

- Describe methods of dealing with violence in the workplace.

- Identify the role of the nurse in dealing with terrorism attacks.

- Recognize situations that may reflect sexual harassment.

- Make suggestions for improving the physical and social environment.

OUTLINE

Workplace Safety
Threats to Safety
Reducing Risk
   Occupational Safety and Health Administration
   Centers for Disease Control and Prevention
   National Institute for Occupational Safety and Health
   American Nurses Association
   Programs
Violence

Sexual Harassment

Latex Allergy

Needlestick Injuries
Your Employer's Responsibility
Your Responsibility

Ergonomic Injuries
Back Injuries
Repetitive Stress Injuries

Impaired Workers
Substance Abuse
Rotating Shifts
Mandatory Overtime
Staffing Ratios

Reporting Questionable Practices

Terrorism

Enhancing the Quality of Work Life
Social Environment
   Working Relationships
   Support of One's Peers and Supervisors
   Involvement in Decision-Making
Professional Growth and Innovation
   Encourage Critical Thinking
   Seek Out Educational Opportunities
   Encourage New Ideas
   Reward Professional Growth
Cultural Diversity
Physical Environment

Conclusion

Almost half our waking hours are spent in the workplace. For this reason alone, the quality of the workplace environment is a major concern. Yet it is neglected to a surprising extent in many health care organizations. It is neglected by administrators, who would never allow peeling paint or poorly maintained equipment but leave their staff, their most costly and valuable resource, unmaintained and unrefreshed. The "do more with less" thinking that has predominated in many organizations places considerable pressure on staff and management alike (Chisholm, 1992). Improvement of the workplace environment is more difficult to accomplish under these circumstances, but it is more important than ever.

Occupational hazards for health care workers are an enormous health and economic problem. According to statistics from the National Institute for Occupational Health and Safety (NIOSH), every day in the United States, 9000 workers sustain a disabling injuring on the job (Slattery, 1998).

Much of the responsibility for enhancing the workplace environment rests with upper-level management, people who have the authority and resources to encourage organization-wide growth and change. Nurses, however, have begun to take more responsibility for identification of and problem-solving for workplace issues. The first international conference, Caring for Those Who Care: Occupational Hazards to Health Care Workers, was held in 1998. Some of the most prevalent threats identified at the conference were latex allergy, back injury, violence, needlestick injury, and pollution. In the 21st century, these issues as well as concerns about bioterrorism have surfaced. This chapter focuses on these issues, in addition to sexual harassment, impaired workers, enhancement of work life quality, and diversity.

◘ Workplace Safety

Safety is not a new concept in the workplace. Although guidelines for safe working conditions have existed since the time of the early Egyptians, the modern movement began during the Industrial Revolution. In 1913, the National Council for Industrial Safety (now the National Safety Council) was formed. Through the National Safety Council, national standards for occupational safety issues are developed and statistics on accident and injury rates are collected. The National Safety Council believes that safety in the workplace is the responsibility of both the employer and the employee. The employer must ensure a safe, healthful work environment, and employees are accountable for knowing and following safety guidelines and standards (National Safety Council, 1992).

Threats to Safety

Threats to safety in the workplace can range from exposure to a potentially lethal chemical or infectious or radioactive agents to violence from clients or other staff members.

In 1993, 300 of Brigham Young Hospital's 1000 staff nurses reported the following symptoms: hives; rashes; headache; dizziness; nausea; eye, nose, and throat irritation; menstrual irregularities; urticaria; cardiac and respiratory distress; hair loss; joint pain; and memory loss. The mysterious illness began with the operating room staff and soon spread to all areas of the hospital. The hospital, undergoing reconstruction, was soon given a diagnosis of "sick building syndrome." Several nurses became so sensitized to the chemicals floating in the hospital air that they have been on permanent leave since 1994 and may never be able to return to nursing (Himali, 1995).

In spring 2001, a Florida nurse with 20 years' psychiatric nursing experience died of head and face trauma. Her assailant, a former wrestler, had been admitted involuntarily in the early morning to the private mental health care facility. An investigation reviewed that the facility did not have a policy on workplace violence and no method of summoning help in an emergency (Arbury, 2002).

Six to eight hundred thousand needlestick injuries occur annually to U.S. health care workers. Percutaneous exposure is the principal route for human immunodeficiency virus and hepatitis B virus (HIV/HBV) transmission, and most of these injuries are sustained by nurses. In fact, over 80 percent of HIV exposures in the health care field occur through this method, most of the exposures occurring with recapping of needles (OSHA: *http://www.osha.gov/SLTC/needlestick/index.html 8/3/02*).

Threats to safety in the workplace vary from one setting to another and from one individual to another. A pregnant staff member may be more vulnerable to risks from radiation; staff members working in the emergency room of a large urban public hospital are at more risk for HIV and tuberculosis than the staff members working in the newborn nursery. All staff members have the right to be made aware of potential risks. No worker should feel intimidated or uncomfortable in the workplace.

Reducing Risk

Occupational Safety and Health Administration

The Occupational Safety and Health Act of 1970 and the Mine Safety and Health Act of 1977 were the first federal guidelines and standards related to safe and healthful working conditions. Through these acts, the NIOSH and the Occupational Safety and Health Administration (OSHA) were formed. OSHA regulations apply to most U.S. employers that have one or more employee and that engage in businesses affecting commerce. Under OSHA regulations, the employer must comply with standards for providing a safe, healthful work environment. Employers are also required to keep records of all occupational (job-related) illnesses and accidents. Examples of occupational accidents and injuries include burns, chemical exposures, lacerations, hearing loss, respiratory exposure, musculoskeletal injuries, and exposure to infectious diseases.

OSHA regulations provide for workplace inspections that may be conducted with or without prior notification to the employer. However, catastrophic or fatal accidents and employee complaints may also trigger an OSHA inspection. OSHA encourages employers and employees to work together to identify and remove any workplace hazards before contacting the nearest OSHA area office. If the employee has not been able to resolve the safety or health issue, the employee may file a formal complaint, and an inspection will be ordered by the area OSHA director (U.S. Department of Labor, 1995). Any violations found are posted where all employees can view them. The employer has the right to contest the OSHA decision. The law also states that the employer cannot punish or discriminate against employees for exercising their rights related to job safety and health hazards or participating in OSHA inspections (U.S. Department of Labor, 1995).

OSHA inspections focus especially on blood-borne pathogens, lifting and ergonomic (proper body alignment) guidelines, confined-space regulations, respiratory guidelines, and workplace violence. *(http://www.osha.gov)*. Table 11–1 depicts the major categories of potential hazards found in hospitals as identified by OSHA. The U.S. Department of Labor publishes fact sheets related to various OSHA guidelines and activities. They can be obtained from your employer, at the local public library, or via the Internet at *http://www.osha.gov*.

Centers for Disease Control and Prevention

The Centers for Disease Control and Prevention (CDC) is the lead federal agency for protecting the health and safety of citizens both at home and abroad. The CDC partners with other agencies throughout the nation to investigate health problems, conduct research, implement prevention strategies, and promote safe and healthy environments. The CDC publishes continuous updates of recommendations for prevention of HIV transmission in the workplace and universal precautions related to blood-borne pathogens, as well as the most recent information on other infectious diseases in the workplace, such as tuberculosis and hepatitis. Currently, the CDC is targeting public health emergency preparedness and response related to biological and chemical agents and threats *(http://www.cdc.gov/)*. Information can be obtained by consulting the *Mortality and Morbidity Weekly Report (MMWR)*

TABLE 11–1
Potential Hospital Hazards

Hazard	Definition	Examples
Biological	Infectious/biological agents such as bacteria, viruses, fungi, parasites	Human immunodeficiency virus (HIV), vancomycin-resistant enterococcus (VRE), methicillin-resistant *Staphylococcus aureus* (MRSA), hepatitis B virus, tuberculosis
Chemical	Medications, solutions, and gases that are potentially toxic or irritating to the body system	Ethylene oxide, formaldehyde, glutaraldehyde, waste anesthetic gases, cytotoxic agents, pentamidine ribavirin
Psychological	Factors and situations encountered or associated with the work environment that create or potentiate stress, emotional strain, and/or interpersonal problems	Stress, workplace violence, shiftwork, inadequate staffing, heavy workload, increased patient acuity.
Physical	Agents that cause tissue trauma	Radiation, lasers, noise, electricity, extreme temperatures, workplace violence
Environmental, mechanical, biomedical	Factors within work environment that cause or potentiate accidents, injuries, strain, or discomfort	Tripping hazards, unsafe or unguarded equipment, air quality, slippery floors, confined spaces, obstructed work areas or passageways, awkward postures, localized contact stresses, temperature extremes, repetitive motions, lifting and moving patients

Source: Adapted from http://www.osha.gov/SLTC/healthcarefacilities/hazards.html

in the library, via the Internet *(http://www.cdc.gov/health/diseases.htm)*, or through the toll-free phone number (800-311-3435). Interested health care workers can also be placed on the CDC's mailing list to receive any free publications.

National Institute for Occupational Safety and Health

The NIOSH is part of the CDC, and is the federal agency responsible for conducting research and making recommendations for the prevention of work-related disease and injury. According the current NIOSH research, each day, an average of 9000 U.S. workers sustain disabling injuries on the job, 16 die from a work-related injuries, and 137 die from work-related diseases. Table 11–2 compares the costs of occupational injuries and diseases to several other prevalent diseases *(http://www.cdc.gov/niosh/about.html)*

Box 11–1 lists the most important federal laws enacted to protect individuals in the workplace.

American Nurses Association

When looking at agencies that are instrumental in dealing with workplace safety, the American Nurses Association (ANA) must be included. The ANA is discussed more completely in Chapter 16. For the purpose of this discussion, we need to understand that the ANA's history embodies advocacy for the nurse. Workplace advocacy is part of this total commitment. In 1999 the Commission on Workplace Advocacy was established as part of the ANA. The Commission is comprised of nine members, appointed by the ANA Board of Directors and representing constituent member associations. Additionally, state member associations often offer their own workplace advocacy information. Issues such as collective bargaining, work-

TABLE 11–2
National Institute for Occupational Health and Safety: Annual Cost of Diseases 2001

Occupational injuries and diseases	$171 billion
Cancer	$170.7 billion
Cardiac disease	$164.3 billion
Alzheimer's disease	$ 67.3 billion
AIDS	$ 33 billion

Source: Adapted from *http://www.cdc.gov/niosh/about.html*

BOX 11–1
Federal Laws Enacted to Protect the Worker in the Workplace

- Equal Pay Act of 1963: Employers must provide equal pay for equal work regardless of sex.
- Title VII of Civil Rights Act of 1964: Employees may not be discriminated against in employment on the basis of race, color, religion, sex, or national origin.
- Age Discrimination in Employment Act of 1967: Private and public employers may not discriminate against persons 40 years of age or older except when a certain age group is a bona fide occupational qualification.
- Pregnancy Discrimination Act of 1968: Pregnant women cannot be discriminated against in employment benefits if they are able to discharge job responsibilities.
- Fair Credit Reporting Act of 1970: Job applicants and employees have the right to know of the existence and content of any credit files maintained on them.
- Vocational Rehabilitation Act of 1973: An employer receiving financial assistance from the federal government may not discriminate against individuals with disabilities and must develop affirmative action plans to hire and promote individuals with disabilities.
- Family Education Rights and Privacy Act—the Buckley amendment of 1974: Educational institutions may not supply information about students without their consent.
- Immigration Reform and Control Act of 1986: Employers must screen employees for the right to work in the United States without discriminating on the basis of national origin.
- Americans with Disabilities Act of 1990: Persons with physical or mental disabilities and who are chronically ill cannot be discriminated against in the workplace. Employers must make "reasonable accommodations" to meet the needs of the disabled employee. These include such things as installing foot or hand controls; readjusting light switches, telephones, desks, table and computer equipment; providing access ramps and elevators; offering flexible work hours; and providing readers for blind employees.
- Family Medical Leave Act of 1993: Requires employers with 50 or more employees to provide up to 13 weeks of unpaid leave for family medical emergencies, childbirth, or adoption.
- Needlestick Safety and Prevention Act of 2001: This act directed OSHA to revise the bloodborne pathogens standard to establish in greater detail requirements that employers identify and make use of effective and safer medical devices.

Source: Adapted from Strader, M., & Decker, P. (1995). *Role Transition to Patient Care Management*. Norwalk, Conn.: Appleton and Lange; http://www.osha.gov/needlesticks/needlefact.html

place violence, mandatory overtime, conflict management, delegation, ethical issues, compensation, needlestick safety, latex allergies, pollution prevention, and ergonomics are all addressed within the workplace advocacy arena. For ANA information on these issues, a substantial resource is the ANA website *(http://www.nursingworld.org)*.

Programs

The primary objective of any workplace safety program is to prevent staff members from harm and to protect the organization from liability related to that harm.

The first step in development of a workplace safety program is to *recognize a potential hazard* and then take steps to control it. Based

on OSHA regulations (U.S. Department of Labor, 1995), the employer must inform staff members of any potential health hazards and provide as much protection from these hazards as possible. In many cases, initial warnings come from the CDC; NIOSH; and other federal, state, and local agencies. For example, employers must provide tuberculosis testing and hepatitis B vaccine; protective equipment such as gloves, gowns, and masks; and immediate treatment after exposure for all staff members who may have contact with blood-borne pathogens. They are expected to remove hazards, educate employees, and establish institution-wide policies and procedures to protect their employees (Herring, 1994; Roche, 1993). Nurses who are not provided with latex gloves may refuse to participate in any activities involving blood or blood products. The employee cannot be discriminated against in the workplace, and reasonable accommodations for safety against blood-borne pathogens must be provided. This may mean that the nurse with latex allergies is placed in an area where exposure to blood-borne pathogens is not an issue (Strader & Decker, 1995; U.S. Department of Labor, 1995).

The second step in a workplace safety program is a *thorough assessment of the degree of risk entailed*. Staff members, for example, may become very fearful in situations that do not warrant such fear.

Nancy Wu is the nurse manager on a busy geriatric unit. The majority of the clients require total care: bathing, feeding, positioning. She has observed that several of the staff members working on the unit use poor body mechanics when lifting and moving the clients. In the last month, several of the staff members have been referred to employee health for back pain. This week, she noticed that the clients seem to remain in the same position for long periods of time and frequently are never out of bed or are in a chair for the entire day. When she confronted the staff, the response was the same from all of them: "I have to work for a living. I can't afford to risk a back injury for someone who may not live past the end of the week." Nancy Wu was concerned about the care of the clients as well as the apparent lack of information her staff had about prevention of back injuries. She decided to seek assistance from the nurse practitioner in charge of employee health in developing a back injury prevention program.

Assessment of the workplace may require considerable data-gathering to document the incidence of the problem and consultation with experts before a plan of action is drawn up. Health care organizations often create formal committees comprised of experts from within the institution and representatives from the affected departments to assess these risks. It is important that staff members from various levels of the organization be allowed to offer input into an assessment of safety needs and risks.

The third step is to *draw up a plan* to provide optimal protection for staff members. It is not always a simple matter to protect staff members without interfering with the provision of client care. For example, some devices that can be worn to prevent transmission of tuberculosis interfere with communication with the client ("Federal agencies clash," 1993). Some attempts have been made to limit visits or withdraw home health care nurses from high-crime areas, but this leaves homebound clients without care (Nadwairski, 1992). A threat-assessment team that evaluates problems and suggests appropriate actions may reduce the incidence and severity of problems with violent behavior, but it may also increase employees' fear of violence if not handled well. Developing a safety plan includes the following:

• Consulting federal, state, and local regulations

• Distinguishing real from imagined risks

• Seeking administrative support and enforcement for the plan

• Calculating costs of a program

The final stage in developing a workplace safety program is *implementing the program*. Educating the staff, providing the necessary safety supplies and equipment, and modifying the environment contribute to an effective program. Protecting client and staff confidentiality and monitoring adherence to control and safety procedures should not be overlooked in the implementation stage (CDC, 1992; "Federal agencies clash," 1993; Jankowski, 1992).

An example of a safety program is the one for health care workers exposed to HIV instituted at the Department of Veterans Affairs Hospital, San Francisco (Armstrong, Gordon, & Santorella, 1995). An HIV exposure can be stressful for both health care workers and their loved ones. This employee assistance program includes as many as 10, 60-minute individual counseling sessions on the meaning and experience of this traumatic event. Additional counseling sessions for couples are also provided. Information about HIV and about dealing with acute stress reactions is provided. Additional counseling helps workers identify a plan to obtain assistance from their individual support systems, identify practice methods of dealing with blood-borne pathogens, and return to work.

Violence

Violence in the workplace is a contemporary social issue. Newspapers and magazines have reported on numerous violent incidents in the workplace. One of six violent crimes occurs in the workplace, and homicide is the second leading cause of workplace death (Edwards, 1999). According to the Census of Fatal Occupational Injuries, there were 674 workplace homicides in 2000, accounting for 11 percent of the total fatal work injuries in the United States (*http://www.osha.gov/ SLTC/workplaceviolence/index.html* 8/3/02). There are approximately 1000 murders and 1.5 million assaults on health care workers each year in the workplace (*http://www.osha-slc.gov/SLTC/workplaceviolence/index.html*). The rate of assaults on hospital workers is much higher than the rate of assaults for all private-sector industries (*http://www.cdc.gov/ niosh/pdfs/2002-101.pdf 8/3/02*).

The aggressor can be a disgruntled employee or employer, an unhappy significant other, or a person committing a random act of violence. Nurses have been identified as a group at risk of violence from clients, family members, and other staff members. In addition to the range of intensity of violence from minor physical injuries to death, violence may also have negative organizational outcomes. Table 11–3 identifies potential institution wide negative outcomes from workplace violence. Examples of violence can include:

TABLE 11–3
Negative Organizational Outcomes Due to Workplace Violence

- Low worker morale
- Increased job stress
- Increased worker turnover
- Reduced trust of management
- Reduced trust of coworkers
- Hostile working environment

- **Threats.** Expressions of intent to cause harm including verbal threats, threatening body language, and written threats

- **Physical assaults.** Slapping, beating, rape, homicide, and the use of weapons such as firearms, bombs, or knives

- **Muggings.** Assaults conducted by surprise with intent to rob (*http://www.cdc.gov/niosh/pdfs/ 2002-101.pdf*).

The circumstances surrounding health care work contributes to workers' susceptibility to homicide and assault (Edwards, 1999; *http://www.nursingworld.org/dlwa/ osh/wp5.htm; http://www.cdc.gov/niosh/pdfs/ 2002-101.pdf*):

- Having routine contact with the public in unrestricted areas

- Working alone or in small numbers

- Working late or until the very early morning hours

- Working in high-crime areas

- Working in buildings with poor security

- Treating weapon-carrying patients and families

- Working with inexperienced staff

- Working in units needing seclusion or restraint activities

- Transporting patients

- Patients waiting long times for service

- Having overcrowded, uncomfortable waiting areas

- Lacking staff training and policies for managing crises

Nurses must know their workplace. Start by asking yourself the following questions (*http://www/nursingworld.org/dlwa. osh/wp5.htm? 8/3/02*):

- How does violence from the surrounding community affect your workplace?

• Do services like trauma or acute psychiatric care increase the likelihood of violence?

• Does the facility's physical layout invite violence—for example, do doors open to the street or are waiting rooms cramped?

• How frequently are assaultive incidents, threats, and verbal abuse occurring? Where? Who is involved? Are incidents being reported?

• Are current emergency response systems effective?

• Is post-assaultive treatment and support available to staff?

• Are staffing patterns sufficient and is the staff experienced?

In the beginning of the chapter, we briefly discussed the nurse who was attacked and killed by a patient in April 2001. Although assaults that result in severe injury or death usually receive media coverage, most assaults on nurses by patients or coworkers are not reported. Working in a health care facility is considered to be the third most dangerous job in the United States (*http://nursingworld.org/ajn/w001/jul/ISSUES.HTM*, 8/3/02).

Ms. Jones works on the evening shift in the emergency department (ED) at a large, urban hospital. The ED frequently receives clients who have been victims of gunshot wounds, stabbings, and other gang-related incidents. Many of the clients entering the ED are high on alcohol or drugs. Ms. Jones has just interviewed a 21-year-old male client who is awaiting treatment as a result of a fight during an evening of heavy drinking. Because his injuries have been determined not to be life-threatening, he had to wait to see a doctor. "I'm tired of waiting. Let's get this show on the road," he screamed loudly as Ms. Jones walked by. "I'm sorry you have to wait, Mr. P., but the doctor is busy with another client and will get to you as soon as possible." She handed him a cup of juice she had been bringing to another client. He grabbed the cup, threw it in her face, and then grabbed her arm. Slamming her against the wall, he jumped off the stretcher and yelled obscenities at her. He continued to scream in her face until a security guard intervened.

Be aware of clues that may indicate a potential for violence (Box 11–2). These behav-

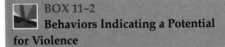

BOX 11–2
Behaviors Indicating a Potential for Violence

• History of violent behavior
• Delusional, paranoid, or suspicious speech
• Aggressive, threatening statements
• Rapid speech, angry tone of voice
• Pacing, tense posture, clenched fists, tightening jaw
• Alcohol or drug use
• Male gender, youth
• Policies that set unrealistic limits

Source: Adapted from Kinkle, S. (1993). Violence in the ED: How to stop it before it starts. *American Journal of Nursing*, 93(7), 22–24; Carroll, C., & Sheverbush, J. (September 1996). Violence assessment in hospitals provides basis for action. *American Nurse*, 18.

iors may occur in clients, family members, visitors, or even other staff members. Even clients with no history of violent behavior may react violently to medication or pain (Carroll & Sheverbush, 1996; Lanza & Carifio, 1991).

In the health care industry, violence is underreported and there is a persistent misperception that assaults are part of the job or that the victim somehow caused the assault. Causes of underreporting may be a lack of institutional reporting policies or fear on the part of employees that the assault was a result of negligence or poor job performance (U.S. Department of Labor, 1995). Table 11–4 lists some of the faulty reasoning that leads to placing blame on the victim of the assault.

Actions to address violence in the workplace include (1) identifying the factors that contribute to violence and controlling as many as possible and (2) assessing staff attitudes and knowledge regarding violence in the workplace (Carroll & Sheverbush, 1996; Collins, 1994; Mahoney, 1991).

When you begin your new job, you may want to find out what the policies and procedures related to violence in the workplace are at your institution. Preventing an incident is better than having to intervene after

TABLE 11–4
When an Assault Occurs: Placing Blame on Victims

Victim Gender

Women receive a higher degree of blame than men.

Subject Gender

Female victims receive a higher degree of blame from women than men.

Severity

The more severe the assault, the more often the victim is blamed.

Beliefs

The world is a just place and the person deserves the misfortune.

Age of Victim

The older the victim, the more he or she is held to blame.

Source: Adapted from Lanza, M.L., & Carifo, J. (1991). Blaming the victim: Complex (nonlinear) patterns of causal attribution by nurses in response to vignettes of a patient assaulting a nurse. *Journal of Emergency Nursing*, 17, 299–309.

violence has occurred. The following are suggestions to nurses about how to participate in workplace safety related to violence:

• *Participate in or initiate regular workplace assessments.* Identify unsafe areas and the factors within the organization that contribute to assaultive behavior such as inadequate staffing, high activity times of day, invasion of personal space, seclusion or restraint activities, and lack of experienced staff. Work with management to make and monitor changes.

• *Be alert for suspicious behavior* such as verbal expressions of anger and frustration, threatening body language, signs of drug or alcohol use, or presence of a weapon. Assess patients or suspicious workers, patients, and visitors for potential violence. Alert colleagues about patients or visitors with known history of assaultive behavior. Evaluate each situation for potential violence. Keep an open path for exiting.

• *Maintain behavior that helps to de-fuse anger.* Present a clam, caring attitude. Don't match threats, give orders, or present with behaviors that may be interpreted as aggressive. Acknowledge the person's feelings.

• *If you cannot defuse the situation, quickly* remove yourself from it, call security, and report the situation to management.

Box 11–3 lists some additional actions that can be taken to protect staff members and clients from violence in the workplace.

What if, in spite of all precautions, violence occurs? What should you do?

• Report to your supervisor. Report threats as well as actual violence. Include a description of the situation; names of victims, witnesses, and perpetrators; and any other pertinent information.

• Call the police. Although the assault is at work, nurses are entitled to the same rights as workers assaulted in another other setting.

BOX 11–3
Steps Toward Increasing Protection from Workplace Violence

• Security personnel and escorts
• Panic buttons in medication rooms, stairwells, activity rooms, and nursing stations
• Bulletproof glass in reception, triage, and admitting areas
• Locked or key-coded access doors
• Closed-circuit television
• Metal detectors
• Use of beepers and/or cellular car phones
• Handheld alarms or noise devices
• Lighted parking lots
• Escort or buddy system
• Enforced wearing of photo identification badges

Source: Adapted from Simonowitz, J. (1994). Violence in the workplace: You're entitled to protection. *RN*, 57(11), 61–63; *http://nursingworld.org/dlwa/osh/wp6.htm*, 5/28/02.

• Get medical attention. This includes actual medical care, counseling, and evaluation.

• Contact your collective bargaining unit or your state nurses association. Inform them if the problems persist.

• Be proactive. Get involved in policy-making

(http://nursingworld.org/ajn/2001/jul/ ISSUES.HTM 5/28/02).

◼ Sexual Harassment

A new supervisor was hired on the unit. After months of interviewing, the candidate selected was a young male nurse whom the staff members jokingly described as "a blond Tom Cruise." The new supervisor was an instant hit with the predominantly female executives and staff members. However, he soon found himself on the receiving end of sexual jokes and innuendoes. He had been trying to prove himself a competent supervisor, with hopes of eventually moving up to a higher management position. He viewed the behavior of the female staff members and supervisors as undermining his credibility, in addition to being embarrassing and annoying. He attempted to have the unwelcome conduct stopped by discussing it with his boss, a female nurse manager. She told him jokingly that it was nothing more than "good-natured fun" and besides, "men can't be harassed by women" (Outwater, 1994).

The laws that prohibit discrimination in the workplace are based on the Fifth and Fourteenth amendments to the Constitution, mandating due process and equal protection under the law. The Equal Employment Opportunity Commission (EEOC) oversees the administration and enforcement of issues related to workplace equality. Although there may be exemptions from any law, it is important that nurses recognize that there is significant legislation that prohibits employers from making workplace decisions based on race, color, sex, age, disability, religion, or national origin.

The employer may ask questions related to these issues but cannot make decisions about employment based on them. Behaviors that could be defined as sexual harassment are identified in Table 11–5. The EEOC issued a statement in 1980 that sexual harassment is a form of sex discrimination pro-

TABLE 11–5

Behaviors That Could Be Defined as Sexual Harassment

Pressure to participate in sexual activities
Asking about another person's sexual activities, fantasies, preferences
Making sexual innuendoes, jokes, comments, or suggestive facial expressions
Continuing to ask for a date after the other person has expressed disinterest
Making sexual gestures with hands or body movements or showing sexual graffiti or visuals
Making remarks about a person's gender or body

hibited by Title VII of the Civil Rights Act of 1964. Two forms of sexual harassment are identified; both are based on the premise that the action is unwelcome sexual conduct:

1 Quid pro quo. Sexual favors are given in exchange for favorable job benefits or continuation of employment. The employee must demonstrate that he or she was required to endure unwelcome sexual advances to keep the job or job benefits and that rejection of these behaviors would have resulted in deprivation of a job or benefits. Example: The administrator approaches a nurse for a date in exchange for a salary increase 3 months before the scheduled review.

2 Hostile environment. This is the most common sexual harassment claim and the most difficult to prove. The employee making the claim must prove that the harassment is based on gender and that it has affected conditions of employment or created an environment so offensive that the employee could not effectively discharge the responsibilities of the job (Outwater, 1994).

In 1993, the Supreme Court ruled that a plaintiff is not required to prove any psychological injury to establish a harassment claim. If the environment could be shown to be hostile or abusive, there was no further need to establish that it was also psychologically injurious. Although sexual harassment against women is more common, men can also be victims of sexual harassment.

Sexual harassment can cost an employer money, unfavorable publicity, expensive lawsuits, and large damage awards. Low morale caused by a hostile work environment can cause significant decreases in employee productivity, increased absenteeism, increases in sick leave and medical payments, and decreased job satisfaction.

In addition to Title VII, other legal protections include Title IX of the Education Amendments of 1972 and state fair employment statutes. Title IX of the Education Amendments of 1972 prohibits sex discrimination and sexual harassment in any educational program receiving financial assistance from the federal government. Students and employees are included in this law. Most state fair employment statutes apply to public and private employers, employment agencies, and labor organizations. Often, state workers' compensation statutes provide remedies for employees who have been injured, either physically or psychologically, by sexual harassment in the workplace. Prohibition against sexual harassment in the workplace may also be included in collective bargaining agreements (*http://nursingworld.org/readroom/position/workplac/wkharass.htm* 8/3/02).

Addressing the issue of sexual harassment in the workplace is important. As an employee, you should be familiar with the policies and procedures related to reporting sexual harassment incidents. If you supervise other employees, you should regularly review the agency's policies and procedures. Seek appropriate guidance from your human resources personnel. If an employee approaches you with a complaint, a confidential investigation of the charges should be initiated. Above all, do not dismiss any incidents or charges of sexual harassment involving yourself or others as "just having fun" or respond that "there is nothing anyone can do." Responses such as this can have serious consequences in the workplace (Outwater, 1994).

The ANA cites four tactics to fight sexual harassment (*http://www.nursingworld.org/dlwa/wpr/wp3/htm*, 9/25/99):

1 Confront. Indicate immediately and clearly to the harasser that the attention is un-wanted. If you are in a union facility, ask the nursing representative to accompany you.

2 Report. Report the incident immediately to your supervisor. If the harasser is your supervisor, report the incident to a higher authority. File a formal complaint and follow the chain of command.

3 Document. Document the incident immediately while it is fresh in your mind—what happened, when and where it occurred, and how you responded. Name any witnesses. Keep thorough records, and keep them in a safe place away from work.

4 Support. Seek support from friends, relatives, and organizations such as your state nurses association. If you are a student, seek support from a trusted faculty member or advisor.

◼ Latex Allergy

A nurse developed hives in 1987, nasal congestion in 1989, and asthma in 1992. She was diagnosed with latex allergy. Eventually, she developed severe respiratory symptoms in the health care environment even when she had no direct contact with latex. The nurse was forced to leave her occupation because of these health effects (Bauer, et al., 1993).

A midwife initially suffered hives, nasal congestion, and conjunctivitis. Within a year, she developed asthma, and 2 years later she went into shock after a routine gynecological examination during which latex gloves were used. The midwife also suffered respiratory distress in latex-containing environments when she had no direct contact with latex products. She was unable to continue working (Bauer et al., 1993).

A physician with a history of seasonal allergies, runny nose, and eczema on his hands suffered severe runny nose, shortness of breath, and collapse minutes after putting on a pair of latex gloves. A cardiac arrest team successfully resuscitated him. (Rosen, et al., 1993).

Latex products are manufactured from the milky fluid of the rubber tree. Latex allergy was first identified in the late 1970s. It has become such a major health problem in the workplace that both OSHA and the ANA have devoted websites to the problem. It is estimated that currently 8 to 12 percent of health care workers are sensitive to natural rubber latex products. Table 11–6 lists products commonly produced with latex.

TABLE 11–6
Latex Equipment

Emergency Equipment	Personal Protective Equipment	Office Supplies	Hospital Supplies
Blood pressure cuffs	Gloves	Rubber bands	Anesthesia masks
Stethoscopes	Surgical masks	Erasers	Catheters
Disposable gloves	Goggles		Wound drains
Oral and nasal airways	Respirators		Injection ports
Endotracheal tubes	Rubber aprons		Rubber tops of multidose vials
Tourniquets			Dental dams
IV tubing			Hot water bottles
Syringes			Baby bottle nipples
Electrode pads			Pacifiers

Source: Adapted from OSHA Latex allergy: *http://www/osha-slc.gov/SLTC/latexallergy/index.html*; and OSHA latex alert *http://www.cdc.gov/niosh/latexalt.html?*, 9/25/99

Since the 1987 CDC recommendations for universal precautions, the use of latex gloves has greatly increased the exposure of health care workers to natural rubber latex (NRL). The two major routes of exposure to NRL are skin and inhalation, particularly when glove powder acts as a carrier for NRL protein (OSHA latex alert at *http://www.cdc.gov/niosh/latexalt.html*, 9/25/99). Reactions range from contact dermatitis with scaling, drying, cracking, and blistering skin to allergic contact dermatitis in the form of generalized hives. More serious generalized reactions can progress to generalized urticaria, rhinitis, wheezing, swelling, shortness of breath, and anaphylaxis. According to NIOSH, the most common reaction to latex products is irritant contact dermatitis, the development of dry, itchy, irritated areas on the skin, usually the hands. This reaction is caused by irritation from wearing gloves and by exposure to the powders added to them.

Irritant contact dermatitis is not a true allergy. Allergic contact dermatitis (sometimes called *chemical sensitivity dermatitis*) results from the chemicals added to latex during harvesting, processing, or manufacturing. These chemicals can cause a skin rash similar to that of poison ivy. Neither irritant contact dermatitis nor chemical sensitivity dermatitis is a true allergy (*http://www.cdc.gov/niosh/98-113.html* 8/3/02).

Latex allergy should be suspected if an employee develops symptoms after latex exposures. A complete medical history can reveal latex sensitivity, and blood tests approved by the Food and Drug Administration are available to detect latex antibodies. Skin testing and glove-use tests are also available.

Compete latex avoidance is the most effective approach. Medications may reduce allergic symptoms, and special precautions are needed to prevent exposure during medical and dental care. Encourage employees with a latex allergy to wear a medical alert bracelet.

Decreasing the potential for development of latex allergy consists of reducing unnecessary exposure to NRL proteins for all health care workers. Many employees in a health care setting, such as food handlers or gardeners, can use alternative gloves. If an employee must use NRL gloves, gloves with a lower protein content and those that are powder-free should be considered. Good housekeeping practices should be identified to remove latex-containing dust from the workplace. Employee education programs to ensure appropriate work practices and hand washing should be encouraged. Identification of employees with increased potential for latex allergies is not possible. However, clinical evidence indicates that certain workers may be at greater risk, including those with the following histories:

- History of allergies to pollens, grasses, and certain foods or plants (avocado, banana, kiwi, chestnut)

- History of multiple surgeries

Decrease the potential for latex allergy problems *http://www.cdc.gov/niosh/ 98-113.html 8/3/02):*

- Evaluate any cases of hand dermatitis or other signs or symptoms of potential latex allergy.

- Use latex-free procedure trays and crash carts.

- Use non-latex gloves for activities that do not involve contact with infectious materials.

- Avoid using oil-based creams or lotions, which can cause glove deterioration.

- Seek ongoing training and information about the latest information related to latex allergy.

- Wash, rinse, and dry hands thoroughly after removing gloves or between glove changes.

- Use powder-free gloves.

In spite of all precautions, what do you do if you develop a latex allergy? At this point, you must never wear latex gloves. Be aware of the following precautions *http://nursingworld.org/dlwa/osh/wp7.htm 5/28/02):*

- Avoid all types of latex exposure.

- Wear a medical alert bracelet.

- Carry an EPI-kit with auto-injectible epinephrine.

- Alert employers and colleagues to your latex sensitivity.

- Carry non-latex gloves.

OSHA "Right to Know" laws require employers to inform health care workers of potentially dangerous substances in the workplace. For continuing information on latex allergies you can visit the NIOSH homepage at *http://www.cdc.gov/niosh.*

We have identified the risks of latex allergies to health care workers. Patients are also at risk and should be screened for allergies. As with the health care worker, patients with a history of hay fever, food allergies (especially to bananas, avocados, potatoes, tomatoes), asthma, or eczema can be at risk. A thorough health history is vital. Treat any indication of potential latex sensitivity seriously (Society of Gastroenterology Nurses and Associates, 2001).

◼ Needlestick Injuries

In 1997, a 27-year-old nurse, Lisa Black, attended an in-service session on postexposure prophylaxis for needlesticks. A short time later, she was attempting to aspirate blood from a patient's intravenous line. The patient, in the advanced stages of acquired immunodeficiency syndrome (AIDS), moved, and the needle went into Lisa's hand. Nine months later she tested positive for HIV and 3 months after that for hepatitis C. She continues to share her story with nurses everywhere in an effort to prevent this unfortunate accident from happening to one more nurse (Trossman, 1999a).

OSHA estimates that 5.6 million health care workers are at risk of occupational exposure to bloodborne pathogens. These exposures lead to diseases such as hepatitis B, hepatitis C, and HIV.

Health care workers suffer between 600,000 and 1 million injuries from conventional needles and sharps on an annual basis with over 80 percent of these injuries preventable by safer needleless devices. On April 18, 2001, the Needlestick Act or revised Bloodborne Pathogens Standard went into effect. The revised OSHA Bloodborne Pathogens Standard obligates employers to consider safer needle devices when they conduct their annual review of their exposure control plan. Frontline employees must be included in the annual review and updating of standards process. Stricter requirements are now in effect for annual review and updating to reflect changes in technology that eliminate or reduce exposure to bloodborne pathogens (*http://www.osha.gov/needlesticks/ needlefaq.html 8/3/02*).

Your Employer's Responsibility

According to the current OSHA requirements, your employer must provide you with the following (ANA, 1993; *http:// www.nursingworld.org/dlwa/osh/wp2.htm, 9/28/99*):

- Free hepatitis B vaccine
- Protective equipment that fits you (gloves, gowns, goggles, masks)
- Immediate, confidential medical evaluation, treatment, and follow-up if exposed
- Implementation of universal precautions institution-wide
- Adequate sharps disposal
- Removal of hazards from the workplace
- Annual employee training

Your Responsibility

What are your responsibilities related to this revised legislation? Each year your employer must review and update its bloodborne pathogen standards. You will need to take the time to learn new devices and make certain that the current safety requirements are enforced with employees. Be part of the solution—volunteer to participate in evaluation committees or work on teams testing new devices. Follow these guidelines in your daily nursing practice (ANA, 1993; Brooke, 2001; *http://www. nursingworld.org/dlwa/osh/wp2.htm, 9/28/99; Perry, 2001*):

- Always use universal precautions.
- Properly use and dispose of sharps.
- Be immunized against hepatitis B.
- Immediately wash all exposed skin with soap and water.
- Flush affected eyes or mucous membranes with saline or water.
- Report all exposures according to your facility's protocol.
- If possible, know the HIV/HBV status of your patient.

- Comply with postexposure follow-up.
- Support others who are exposed.
- Become active in the safety committee—be a change agent.
- Educate others.

◨ Ergonomic Injuries

Occupational-related back injuries affect 35 to 80 percent of nurses over the lifetime of their career. The annual cost is estimated to be as high as $16 billion annually in the United States. Injuries can become so severe that the nurse may have to leave the profession.

Back Injuries

The problem with lifting a patient is not just one of overcoming heavy weight. Size, shape, and deformities of the patient as well as balance and coordination, combativeness, uncooperativeness, and contractures must be considered. Any unpredictable movement or resistance from the patient can quickly throw the nurse off balance and result in a back injury. Environmental considerations such as space, equipment interference, and unadjustable beds, chairs, and commodes also contribute to back injury risk (Edlich, Woodard,& Haines, 2001).

This issue of back injuries and other ergonomic related injuries has become so severe that in July 2001 OSHA began to develop a comprehensive approach to ergonomics. Public forums, meetings with stakeholder groups and individuals, as well as written comments were analyzed. Out of this work, a four-pronged comprehensive approach to ergonomics was developed to include   (*http://www.osha.gov/ergonomics/ ergofact02.html 8/3/02*):

1 Task or industry specific written guidelines

2 Enforcement

3 Outreach/assistance

4 Research

Although guidelines are less legislated standards, OSHA will use the General Duty

Clause to cite employers for ergonomic hazards. Under the OSHA Act's General Duty Clause, employers must keep their workplaces free from recognized serious hazards, including ergonomic hazards. This requirement exists whether or not there are voluntary guidelines *(http://www.osha.gov/ergonomics/FAQs-external.html 8/3/02).*

Suggestions for decreasing back injuries for nurses (Trossman, 1999b; Slattery, 1998; Edlich, Woodard, & Haines, 2001):

- Participate on the safety committee as a nursing representative to develop written guidelines detailing transfer requirements.

- Work in teams if possible—don't be afraid to ask for help.

- Use transfer and lifting equipment.

- Consider environment such as size of room and proximity of beds and chair.

- Do back exercises.

Repetitive Stress Injuries

Repetitive stress injuries (RSIs) have been called the *workplace epidemic of the modern age.* RSIs usually affect people who spend long hours at computers, switchboards, and other worksites where repetitive motions are performed. The most common RSIs are carpal tunnel syndrome and mouse elbow. As technology increases in health care facilities, the use of computers increases for all health care personnel. Badly designed computer workstations present the highest risk of RSIs. Preventive measures (Krucoff, 2001):

- Keep the monitor screen straight ahead of you, about an arm's length away. Position the center of the screen where your gaze naturally falls.

- Align the keyboard so that the forearms, wrists, and hands are aligned parallel to the floor. Do not bend the hands back.

- Position the mouse directly next to you and on the same level as the keyboard.

- Keep thighs parallel to the floor as you sit on the chair. Feet should touch the floor

and the chair back should be ergonomically sound.

- Vary tasks. Avoid long sessions of sitting. Do not use excessive force when typing or clicking the mouse.

- Keep fingernails short and use fingertips when typing.

◼ Impaired Workers

Substance Abuse

Sue had been a nurse for 20 years. Current marital and family problems were affecting her at work. To ease the tension, she took a Xanax from a patient's medication drawer. This seemed to ease her tension. She continued to take medications, working her way up to narcotic analgesics.

Bill had begun weekend binge-drinking in college. Ten years later, he still continues the habit several times during the month. He does not feel he is an alcoholic because he can control his drinking. After he begins showing up at work hung-over and making medication errors, he is fired for the medication errors. At the exit interview, no mention is made of his drinking problem. The agency feared a lawsuit for defamation of character.

Mr. P., the unit manager, has noticed that Ms. J. has frequently been late for work. She arrives with a wrinkled uniform, dirty shoes, unkempt hair, and broken nails. Lately she has been overheard making terse remarks to clients such as, "Who do you think I am—your maid?" and spends longer and longer periods of time off the unit. The floor has a large number of surgical clients who receive intramuscular and oral medications for pain. Lately Ms. J.'s clients continue to complain of pain even after medication administration has been charted. Ms. J. frequently forgets to waste her intramuscular narcotics in front of another nurse. Mr. P. is concerned that Ms. J. may be an impaired nurse.

Alcohol and drug abuse continue to be major health problems in this country. Health care professionals are not immune to alcoholism or chemical dependency. In addition, various kinds of mental illnesses may also affect a nurse's ability to deliver safe, competent care. Impaired workers can adversely affect client care, staff retention, morale, and management time as team members try to pick up the slack for the impaired worker (Damrosch & Scholler-Jaquish, 1993). The most common signs of impairment are shown (Damrosch & Scholler-Jaquish, 1993):

- Witnessed consumption of alcohol or other substances on the job

• Changes in dress, appearance, posture, gestures

• Slurred speech, abusive/incoherent language

• Reports of impairment or erratic behavior from clients and/or coworkers

• Witnessed unprofessional conduct

• Significant lack of attention to detail

• Witnessed theft of controlled substances

Most employers and 37 state boards of nursing have strict guidelines related to impaired nurses. Impaired-nurse programs conducted by state boards of nursing work with the employer to assist the impaired nurse to remain licensed while receiving help for the addiction problem. It is important that you become aware of workplace issues surrounding the impaired worker, signs and symptoms of impairment, and the policies and reporting procedures concerning an impaired worker. Compassion from coworkers and supervisors is of utmost importance in assisting the impaired worker to seek help (Damrosch & Scholler-Jaquish, 1993; Sloan & Vernarec, 2001). The National Council of State Boards lists all state boards of nursing. Information on support programs for impaired nurses can be obtained from each state board (*http://www.ncsbn.org/ public/regulation/boards_of_nursing_board. htm*, 8/3/02).

Each of us has the responsibility to uphold the standards of the nursing profession. Although it is difficult to report a colleague, covering up or ignoring the problem can cause serious risks for the patient and the nurse. Most states accept anonymous reports. In many states, state law requires hospitals and health care providers to report impaired practitioners, but the law also grants immunity from civil liability if the report was made in good faith (Sloan & Vernarec, 2001).

Rotating Shifts

A recent concern regarding safety in the workplace involves nurses working rotating shifts. Nurses who work permanently at night often readjust their sleep-wake cycle. Nurses who randomly rotate shifts throw off their circadian rhythm. Fatigue, the number one complaint of these nurses, is the result of the body never getting the chance to adapt to changing sleep-wake cycles.

One of the most serious effects of rotating night shifts is the increasing number of nurses affected by coronary heart disease (CHD). Studies indicate that nurses who rotate to nights for 6 years have a 70 percent greater risk of developing CHD than nurses who never rotated shifts (Trossman, 1999b). Suggestions for nurses who rotate shifts:

• Try to schedule working the same shifts for an entire scheduling period instead of rotating different shifts in one schedule.

• Try to schedule to same days off within the schedule.

• If you become sleepy during the shift, take a walk or climb stairs.

• Limit caffeine intake, especially toward the end of the shift.

• If you work evenings or nights, do not eat a big meal at the end of the shift. This interferes with sleep.

• Try to sleep a continuous block of time instead of catching a few hours here and there.

• Make the room you are sleeping in as dark and noise-free as possible.

• Maintain good nutrition and an exercise program.

• Negotiate your schedule with your manager. If you and your colleagues feel strongly about eliminating rotating shifts, work together to make changes (Trossman, 1999b).

Mandatory Overtime

Debate is currently heating up on the topic of mandatory overtime. When nurses routinely are forced to work beyond their scheduled hours, they can suffer a range of emotional and physical effects. As patient acuity and workloads increase, working overtime puts the patient and the nurse at greater risk. Mandatory overtime is seen by nurses as a control issue. Working overtime should be a choice, not a requirement. In some facilities, nurses are being threatened with dismissal or charge of patient abandonment if they refuse to participate in mandatory overtime *(http://www.nursingworld.org/tan/98mayjun/ot.htm)*.

The ANA presented the following message to the 107th Congress, 2001. "ANA opposes the use of mandatory overtime as a staffing tool. We urge you to support legislation that would ban the use of mandatory overtime through Medicare and Medicaid law. Nurses must be given the opportunity to refuse overtime if we believe that we are too fatigued to provide quality care." *(http://www.nursingworld.org/gova/federal/legis/107/ovrtme.htm)*.

Staffing Ratios

Although some state nurses associations are calling for mandated staffing ratios, the issue is not clear-cut. At this time, there is an absence of adequate information to evaluate current standards and requirements. However, several studies have shown that understaffing, especially during peak occupancy, is associated with adverse outcomes among workers and patients. In one study, the higher rates of infection with methicillin-resistant *Staphylococcus aureus* (MRSA) were clustered during times of peak occupancy with the increased use of nurse overtime and temporary staff to meet the needs. In another study, the rate of *S. aureus* infections in a neonatal intensive care unit was 16 times higher after a period of understaffing (Lundstrom, et al., 2002).

Rather than mandate staffing ratios, the 2000 ANA House of Delegates recommended that the ANA:

1 Develop a comprehensive strategy that positions registered nurses (RNs) to safeguard cost-effective, quality care based on the recommendations of the ANA Principles for Nurse Staffing which call for:

- RNs to collaborate in staffing decisions

- Development of a product that addresses the definitions, assumptions, and methodologies of staffing to assist RNs in collaborating on staffing decisions

2 Promote the use of ANA Principles for Nurse Staffing in health care agencies.

3 Develop workplace advocacy and collective bargaining strategies that help RNs address concerns about under staffing and suboptimal care.

4 Promote the establishment and use of upwardly adjustable, minimal nurse-patient ratios to serve as a safety net when staffing tools are misused or ineffective.

5 Promote the development of nurse-patient ratios that are based on a logical system for assigning severity level or risk category, current expert knowledge, and recommendations from specialty nursing organizations.

6 Seek funding and promote research on the relationship between staffing and patient outcomes in collaboration with other organizations.

7 Advocate for mandatory reporting of nursing-sensitive structure, process, and outcome indicators in order to monitor the adequacy of staffing in all health care facilities.

8 Advocate for federal and state legislation that addresses the sufficiency of nurse staffing.

9 Identify necessary criteria and conditions to guide the appropriate use of RNs in areas other than their primary unit *(http://nursingworld.org/about/summary/sum00/staffing.htm)*.

Hospital workforce issues will continue to be influenced by economic changes, managed care and insurance issues, media forces, and the nursing shortage. Nurses voice disillusionment with nursing practice and decreased loyalty to organizations. Nursing leaders in the 21st century must demonstrate a respect and value for their nursing staff, communicate effectively with all levels of the organization, maintain visibility, and establish participative decision-making. As you move forward in your career, be part of the solution, not the problem (Ray, Turkel, & Marino, 2002).

◻ Reporting Questionable Practices

Most employers have policies that encourage the reporting of behavior that may affect the workplace environment. Behaviors to report may include (ANA, 1994):

1 Endangering a client's health or safety

2 Abusing authority

3 Violating laws, rules, regulations, or standards of professional ethics

4 Grossly wasting funds

The Code for Nurses (ANA, 2001) is very specific about nurses' responsibility to report questionable behavior that may have an impact on the welfare of a patient:

When the nurse is aware of inappropriate or questionable practice in the provision of health care, concern should be expressed to the person carrying out the questionable practice and attention called to the possible detrimental effect upon the client's welfare. When factors in the health care delivery system threaten the welfare of the client, similar action should be directed to the responsible administrative person. If indicated, the practice should then be reported to the appropriate authority within the institution, agency, or larger system. (ANA, 2001)

The sources of various federal and state guidelines governing the workplace are listed in Box 11-4.

Protection by the agency should be afforded to both the accused and the person doing the reporting. *Whistleblower* is the term used to describe an employee who reports employer violations to an outside agency. Do not assume that doing the right thing will protect you. Speaking up could get you fired unless you are protected by a union contract or other formal employment agreement. In May 1994, the U.S. Supreme Court ruled that nurses who direct the work of other employees may be considered supervisors and

therefore may not be covered by the protections guaranteed under the National Labor Relations Act. This ruling may cause nurses to have no protection from retaliation if they report illegal practices in the workplace (ANA, 1995b). The 1995 brochure from the ANA (1995a), *Protect Your Patients—Protect Your License,* stated, "Be aware that reporting quality and safety issues may result in reprisals by an employer."

Does this mean that you should never speak up? Case law, federal and state statutes, and the federal False Claims Act may afford a certain level of protection. Some states have whistleblower laws. They usually apply to only state employees or to certain types of workers. Although these laws may offer some protection, the most important point is to first work through the employer's chain of command and internal procedures.

- Gather the facts. Review relevant laws, policies, procedures, and standards of care.

BOX 11–4
Laws Governing Health Care Practices

- State nurse practice acts
- Federal and state health regulations
- State and federal pharmacy laws for controlled substances
- Occupational Safety and Health Administration (OSHA) state and federal standards and regulations
- State medical records and communicable disease laws
- Environmental laws regulating hazardous waste, air, and water quality
- Centers for Disease Control and Prevention (CDC) guidelines
- Federal and state antidiscrimination laws
- State clinical laboratory regulations
- Joint Commission on the Accreditation of Healthcare Organization (JCAHO) regulations

Source: Adapted from American Nurses Association. (1994). *Guidelines on Reporting Incompetent, Unethical, or Illegal Practices.* Washington, D.C.: ANA.

- Ask: Does the practice violate an actual law, or do you just consider it unfair?

- Know the state law requiring mandatory reporting and adhere to the process.

- Type your documentation and include day, date, time, and circumstances. Identify any witnesses. Do not copy patient records or incident reports or breach patient confidentiality in any way.

- Send a copy of your complaint to the Director of Nursing and any other department affected, and keep a copy for your records.

- Utilize your ethics committee or human resources department if appropriate (Sloan, 2002).

"Given the move toward managed care, the increased competition amongst health care organizations, and the need to cut costs in order to remain competitive, one can anticipate that the conditions which give rise to typical instances of whistleblowing will continue to get worse" (Fletcher, Sorrell,& Silva,1998, p. 1).

It is the responsibility of professional nurses to become acquainted with the state and federal regulations, standards of practice and professional performance, and agency protocols and practice guidelines governing their practice. Lack of knowledge will not protect you from ethical and legal obligations. Your state nurses' association can help you seek information related to incompetent, unethical, or illegal practices. When you join your state association, you will gain access to an organization that has input into policies and procedures designed to protect the public.

◼ Terrorismn

Since the attacks on the World Trade Center and the Pentagon, as well as the anthrax outbreaks and continued terrorist threats nationwide, concerns related to biological and chemical agents have surfaced. The CDC website {*http://www.bt.cdc.gov/*} supports ongoing updated information related to public health emergency preparedness and response. Representatives from the ANA have been serving on an American College of Emergency Physicians task force to develop strategies that will equip health care professionals with the skills and information needed to deliver care to people with injuries resulting from nuclear, biological, or chemical incidents (*http://nursingworld.org/tan/01novdec/respond.htm 8/3/02*). The ANA is also working with many other agencies under the supervision of the CDC to determine how best to provide information and support for frontline clinicians related to the diagnosis and management of bioterrorism-related infections. The ANA website *www.nursingworld.org* provides numerous links and publications related to emergency preparedness.

What can you do? You may not be serving on a national task force, but your importance in emergency readiness and bioterrorism is important. Following are some suggestions for steps that can be implemented in the workplace (*http://www.awhonn.org/HealthPolicyLegislative/BIOTERRORISM PREPAREDNESS/bioterrorism preparedness.html*):

- Know the evacuation procedures and routes in your facility.

- Develop your knowledge of the most likely and dangerous biochemical agents.

- Monitor for unusual disease patterns and notify appropriate authorities as needed.

- Know the backup systems available for communication and staffing in the event of emergencies.

◼ Enhancing the Quality of Work Life

Both the social and physical aspects of a workplace can affect the way in which people work and how they feel about their jobs. The social aspects include working relationships, a climate that allows growth and creativity, and cultural diversity.

Social Environment

Working Relationships

Many aspects of the social environment have received attention in earlier chapters. Team building, effectively communicating, and developing leadership skills are essential to the development of effective working relationships. The day-to-day interactions with one's peers and supervisors have a major impact on the quality of the workplace environment.

Support of One's Peers and Supervisors

Most employees keenly feel the difference between a supportive and a nonsupportive environment.

Ms. B. came to work already tired. Her baby was sick and had been awake most of the night. Her team expressed concern about the baby when she told them she had a difficult night. Each team member voluntarily took an extra client so that Ms. B. could have a lighter assignment that day. When Ms. B. expressed her appreciation, her team leader said, "We know you would do the same for us." Ms. B. worked in a supportive environment.

Ms. G. came to work after a sleepless night. Her young son had been diagnosed with leukemia and she was very worried about him. When she mentioned her concerns, her team leader interrupted her, saying, "Please leave your personal problems at home. We have a lot of work to do and expect you to do your share." Ms. G. worked in a nonsupportive environment.

Support from peers and supervisors involves professional concerns as well as personal ones. In a supportive environment, people are willing to make difficult decisions, take risks, and "go the extra mile" for team members and the organization. In contrast, in a nonsupportive environment, they are afraid to take risks, avoid making decisions, and usually limit their commitment.

Involvement in Decision-Making

The importance of having a voice in the decisions made about one's work and patients cannot be overstated. Empowerment is a related phenomenon. It is a sense of having both the ability and the opportunity to act effectively (Kramer & Schmalenberg, 1993).

Empowerment is the opposite of apathy and powerlessness. Many actions can be taken to empower nurses: remove barriers to their autonomy and to their participation in decision-making, publicly express confidence in their capability and value, reward initiative and assertiveness, and provide role models who demonstrate confidence and competence. The following illustrates the difference between empowerment and powerlessness:

Soon after completing orientation, nurse A heard a new nurse aide scolding a client for soiling the bed. Nurse A did not know how incidents of potential verbal abuse were handled in this institution, so she reported it to the nurse manager. The nurse manager asked nurse A several questions and thanked her for the information. The new aide was counseled immediately after their meeting. Nurse A noticed a positive change in the aide's manner with clients after this incident. Nurse A felt good about having contributed to a more effective client care team. Nurse A felt empowered and will take action again when another occasion arises.

A colleague of nurse B was an instructor at a nearby community college. This colleague asked nurse B if students would be welcome on her unit. "Of course," replied nurse B. "I'll speak with my head nurse about it." When nurse B spoke with her head nurse, the response was that the unit was too busy to accommodate students. In addition, nurse B received a verbal reprimand from the supervisor for overstepping her authority by discussing the placement of students. "All requests for student placement must be directed to the education department," she said. The supervisor directed nurse B to write a letter of apology for having made an unauthorized commitment to the community college. Nurse B was afraid to make any decisions or public statements after this incident. Nurse B felt alienated and powerless.

Professional Growth and Innovation

The difference between a climate that encourages staff growth and creativity and one that does not can be quite subtle. In fact, many people are only partly aware, if at all, of whether or not they work in an environment that fosters professional growth and learning. Yet the effect on the quality of the work done is pervasive and it is an important factor in distinguishing the merely good health care organization from the excellent health care organization.

Much of the responsibility for staff development and promotion of innovation lies with upper-level management, people who can sponsor seminars, conduct organization-wide workshops, establish educational policies, promote career mobility, develop clinical ladders, initiate innovative projects, and reward suggestions.

Some of the ways in which first-line managers can develop and support a climate of professional growth are to encourage critical thinking, provide opportunities to take advantage of educational programs, encourage new ideas and projects, and reward professional growth.

Encourage Critical Thinking

If you ever find yourself or other staff members saying, "Don't ask why; just go ahead and do it," you need to evaluate the type of climate in which you are functioning. An inquisitive frame of mind is relatively easy to suppress in a work environment. Clients and staff members quickly perceive a nurse's impatience or defensiveness when too many questions are raised. Their response will be to simply give up asking these questions.

On the other hand, if you support critical thinkers and act as a role model who adopts a questioning attitude, you can encourage others to do the same.

Seek Out Educational Opportunities

In most organizations, first-line managers do not have discretionary funds that can be allocated for educational purposes. However, they can usually support a staff member's request for educational leave or for financial support and often have a small budget that can be used for seminars or workshops.

Team leaders and nurse managers can make it either easier or more difficult for staff members to further their education. They can make things difficult for the staff member who is trying to balance work, home, and school responsibilities. Or they can pitch in and help lighten the load of the staff member who has to finish a paper or take an examination. Unsupportive supervisors have even attacked staff members who pursue further education, criticizing every minor error and

blocking their advancement. Obviously, such behavior should be dealt with quickly by upper-level management because it is a serious inhibitor of staff development.

Encourage New Ideas

The increasingly rapid accumulation of knowledge in the health care field mandates continuous learning for safe practice. Intellectual curiosity is a hallmark of the professional.

Every move up the professional ladder should bring new challenges that enrich one's work (Roedel & Nystrom, 1987). As a professional, you can be a role model for an environment in which every staff member is both challenged and rewarded for meeting these challenges. Participating in brainstorming sessions, group conferences, and discussions encourages the generation of new ideas. Although new nurses may think that they have nothing to offer, it is important to participate in activities that encourage staff members to look at fresh new ideas.

Reward Professional Growth

A primary source of discontent in the workplace is lack of recognition. Positive feedback and recognition of our contributions are important intangible rewards in the workplace. Everyone enjoys praise and recognition. A smile, a card or note, or a verbal "thank you" goes a long way with coworkers in recognizing a job well done. Staff recognition programs have also been identified as a means to increase self-esteem, social gratification, morale, and job satisfaction (Hurst, Croker, & Bell, 1994).

Cultural Diversity

Ms. V. is beginning orientation for a new staff nurse position. She has been told that part of her orientation will be a morning class on cultural diversity. She says to the human resources person in charge of orientation, "I don't think I need to attend that class. I treat all people as equal. Besides, anyone living in the United States has an obligation to learn the language and ways of those of us who were born here, not the other way around."

Mr. M. is a staff nurse on a medical-surgical unit. A young man with HIV infection has been admitted recently. He is scheduled for surgery in the morning and has requested that his significant other be present for the preoperative teaching. Mr. M. reluctantly agrees but mumbles under his breath to a coworker, "It wouldn't be so bad if they didn't throw their homosexuality around and act like an old married couple. Why can't he act like a man and get his own preop instructions?"

Diversity in health care organizations includes ethnicity, culture, gender, lifestyle, and career stages of employees. The composition of nurses in health care is changing to include more older workers, minorities, and men. Working with people who have different customs, traditions, communication styles, and beliefs can be exciting as well as challenging. Workforce diversity in terms of age, gender, culture, ethnicity, race, primary language, physical capabilities, and lifestyle presents a challenge to the workplace. An organization that fosters diversity in the workplace encourages respect and understanding of human characteristics and acceptance of the similarities and differences that make us human.

Often, when stressful situations arise, gender, age, and culture can contribute to misunderstandings. Davidhizer, Dowd, and Giger (1999) identified six important factors in their model for understanding cultural diversity:

1 Communication. Communication and culture are closely bound. Culture is transmitted through communication, and culture influences how verbal and nonverbal communication is expressed. The use of vocabulary, voice qualities, intonation, rhythm, speed, silence, touch, body postures, eye movements, and pronunciation all differ among cultural groups and even vary among persons from similar cultures. Using respect as a central core to a relationship, each one of us needs to assess personal beliefs and communication variables of others in the workplace.

2 Space. Personal space is the area that surrounds our body. The amount of personal space individuals prefer varies from person to person and from situation to situation. Cultural beliefs also influence a person's personal space comfort zone. In the workplace, an understanding of our coworkers' comfort related to personal space is important. Often, this comfort is relayed in nonverbal rather than verbal communication.

3 Social organization. In most cultures, the family is the most important social organization. For some people, the importance of family supersedes other personal, work, or national causes. Because the health care industry employs a large number of women, the value of the family becomes an important issue in the workplace. For some people, the importance of caring for a sick child overrides the importance of being on time or even coming to work, regardless of staffing needs or policies.

4 Time. Time orientation is often related to culture, environment, and family experiences. Some cultures are more past-oriented and focus on maintaining traditions, with little interest in goals. People from cultures with more of a present and future orientation may be more likely to engage in activities, such as returning to school or receiving certifications, that will enhance the future. Working with people who have different time orientations may cause difficulty in planning schedules and setting deadlines for the group.

5 Environment control. Environmental control is viewed as those activities that an individual plans to control nature. Environmental control is best understood through the psychological terms *internal* and *external locus of control*. Individuals with an external locus of control believe in fate or chance. People with an internal locus of control believe in developing plans and directing their environment. In the workplace, nurses are expected to operate from an internal locus of control. This approach may be different from what a person has grown up with or how a client deals with illness.

6 Biological variations. More and more information is available to health care workers about the variations among races in aspects such as body structure, skin color, genetic variations, susceptibility to disease, and psychological differences. The Joint Commission on the Accreditation of Healthcare Organizations (JCAHO) states that cultural factors must be assessed in developing materials for patient education.

As you begin your career, be alert to the signs of cultural diversity or insensitivity where you work. Signs that increased sensitivity and responsiveness to the needs of a culturally diverse workforce are needed on your team or in your organization may include a greater proportion of minorities or women in lower-level jobs, lower career mobility and higher turnover rates in these groups, and acceptance or even approval of insensitivity and unfairness (Malone, 1993). Observe interaction patterns, such as where people sit in the cafeteria or how they cluster during coffee breaks. Are they mixing freely, or can you see divisions by gender, race, language, or status in the organization (Moch & Diemert, 1990; Ward, 1992)? Other indications of an organization's diversity "fitness" include the following (Mitchell, 1995):

- The personnel mix reflects the current and potential population being served.

- Individual cultural preferences pertaining to issues of social distance, touching, voice volume and inflection, silence, and gestures are respected.

- There is awareness of special family and holiday celebrations important to people of different cultures.

- The organization communicates through action that people are individuals first and members of a particular culture second.

Effective management of cultural diversity requires considerable time and energy. Although organized cultural diversity programs are usually the responsibility of middle- and upper-level managers, you can play a part in raising awareness. You can be a culturally competent practitioner and a role model for others by becoming:

- Aware of and sensitive to your own culture-based preferences

- Willing to explore your own biases and values

- Knowledgeable about other cultures

- Respectful of and sensitive to diversity among individuals

- Skilled using and selecting culturally sensitive intervention strategies

Some additional do's and don'ts for managing diversity are listed in Table 11–7

Physical Environment

Attention to the physical environment of the workplace is not as well developed as the social aspect, especially in nursing. We have already discussed the increasing focus on workplace ergonomics, such as modifications to various elements of the physical environment, such as the floors, chairs, desks, beds, and workstations, to decrease the incidence of back and upper extremity injuries.. The use of lighting, colors, and music to improve the workplace environment is increasing. Computer workstations designed to promote efficiency in the client care unit are becoming commonplace. Relocation of supplies and substations closer to client rooms to reduce the number of steps, improved visual and auditory scanning of clients from the nurses' station, better light and ventilation, a unified information system, and reduced need for client transport are all possible with changes in the physical environment.

Health care pollution is a more recently identified problem. The CDC stated that less than 2 percent of all hospital waste must be

TABLE 11–7
Do's and Don'ts for Managing Diversity

DO . . .	Don't . . .
Recognize diversity	Pretend everyone is alike
Value diversity	Expect everyone to conform to the prevailing culture
Develop informal supports	Seek a quick solution
Ensure fairness	Develop different standards of performance
Make these principles an integral part of your individual philosophy	Expect one workshop to solve the problem

incinerated, yet most hospitals claim they incinerate 75 to 100 percent. Dioxin emissions, mercury, and battery waste are often not disposed of properly in the hospital environment. Disinfectants, chemicals, waste anesthesia gases, and laser plume that floats in the air are other sources of pollution exposure for nurses. Nurses have a responsibility to be aware of these potential problems and identify areas in the hospital at risk. Rethinking product choices, such as avoiding the use of polyvinyl chloride (PVC) or mercury products, providing convenient collection sites for battery and mercury waste, and making waste management education for employees mandatory are starts toward a more pollution-free environment. (Slattery, 1998).

◼ Conclusion

Workplace safety is an area of increasing concern. Staff members have a right to be informed of any potential risks in the workplace. Employers have a responsibility to provide adequate equipment and supplies to protect employees and to create programs and policies to inform employees about minimizing risks to the extent possible. Issues of workplace violence, sexual harassment, impaired workers, ergonomics, and terrorism should be addressed to protect both employees and patients. Workplace issues of mandatory overtime and staffing ratios will continue to be discussed as the nursing shortage continues.

A social environment that promotes professional growth and creativity and a physical environment that offers comfort and maximum work efficiency should be considered in improving the quality of work life. Cultural awareness, respect for the diversity of others, and increased contact between groups should be the goals of the workforce for the next century.

Many waking hours are spent in the workplace. It can offer a climate of companionship, professional growth, and excitement. You can be part of the solution if you remain aware of workplace issues.

Study Questions

1 Why is it important for nurses to understand the major federal laws enacted to protect the individual in the workplace?

2 What actions can nurses take if they believe that OSHA guidelines are not being followed in the workplace?

3 What are nurses' responsibilities in dealing with transmission of blood-borne pathogens in the workplace?

4 What information do you need to obtain from your employer related to biochemical terrorism?

5 What are your feelings about mandatory overtime and staffing ratios? What information would you need to make informed decisions about these topics?

6 Describe the difference between a supportive and a nonsupportive social environment in the workplace.

7 How can you, as a new nurse, raise awareness related to cultural diversity issues in the workplace?

Workplace Safety

Levin, P., Hewitt, J., & Misner, T. (1998) Insights of nurses about assault in hospital-based emergency departments. *Image*, 30, 249–254.

The purpose of this qualitative study was to explore nurses' opinions about factors they believe contribute to assault. Twenty-two nurses from 15 hospitals in a large U.S. metropolitan area participated in the study. No focus group had fewer than five participants. All the participants were females. Fourteen themes emerged.

1. **Types of patients.** Substance abuse, psychiatric, and dementia patients were identified as most likely to assault a nurse

2. **Geographic location.** Identified violence as endemic in urban areas related to gangs and drugs

3. **Nurse attitude and body language**

4. **Vulnerability.** Having to do one's job and worrying about assault

5. **Security.** "Having people who just stand at the door" who lack knowledge of restraining techniques and the warning signs of escalation

6. **Administrative issues.** Having the "it can't happen here" attitude

7. **Assault reporting.** Concerns reported were not addressed

8. **Safety training.** Incidents were more common when nurses and security personnel lacked aggression-management skills

9. **Societal changes.** Lack of respect for nurses and health care workers

10. **Pervasiveness of anger.** Related to health care delivery system changes, workplace, and culture

11. **Previous assault experiences.** Both verbal and physical assaults and threats from patients and families; verbal abuse from physicians was also identified

12. **Effects.** Muscle tension, loss of sleep, nightmares, and flashbacks as well as the immediate broken bones or wounds or long-term chronic pain; sadness related to a sense of professional loss

13. **Beyond control.** Types of patients admitted; geographic location of hospital

14. **Possible solutions.** Personal, departmental, and administrative solutions identified

This study indicated that personal, workplace, and environmental factors all contribute to assault. Personal strategies, such as setting boundaries, physically keeping a distance, and acknowledging that "enough is enough," were identified. Early interventions with alerting security, keeping patients and families better informed, using chemical restraints, and improving the physical layout were offered as solutions. Changes in hospital policies and ongoing training were important administrative issues.

Workplace Safety *(Continued)*

Interview one of the nurses on your unit about workplace violence. What risk factors has he or she identified? What solutions does he or she recommend? What other solutions can you add to the list?

_____

_____

_____

_____

Review the policy and procedure related to needlestick injuries at the agency where you are currently practicing. Based on the current OSHA requirements, evaluate the policy.
What needleless system is currently in place?

_____

_____

_____

_____

Review the circumstances surrounding health care workers' susceptibility to homicide and assault. Assess the clinical facility where you are currently practicing. What circumstances place this facility at risk?

_____

_____

_____

_____

What safety procedures/policies are currently in place to decrease the potential for violence?

_____

_____

_____

_____

Critical Thinking Exercise

You have been hired as a new RN on a busy pediatric unit in a large metropolitan hospital. The hospital provides services for a culturally diverse population including African American, Asian, and Hispanic people. Family members often attempt alternative healing practices specific to their culture and bring special foods from home to entice a sick child to eat. One of the more experienced nurses said to you, "We need to discourage these people from fooling with all this hocus-pocus. We are trying to get their sick kid well in the time allowed under their managed care plans, and all this medicine-man stuff is only making the kid sick longer. Besides, all this stuff stinks up the rooms and brings in bugs." You have observed how important these healing rituals and foods are to the clients and families and believe that both the families and the children have benefited from this nontraditional approach to healing.

1 What are your feelings about nontraditional healing methods?

2 How should you respond to the experienced nurse?

3 How can you be a client advocate without alienating your coworkers?

4 What could you do to assist your coworkers in becoming more culturally sensitive to their clients and families?

5 How can health care facilities incorporate both Western and nontraditional medicine? Should they do this? Why or why not?

WEBSITES

American Nurses Association (ANA): *http://www.nursingworld.org*

ANA: *http://www.nursingworld.org/dlwa/osh/wp5.htm*

ANA: *http://nursingworld.org/ajn/w001/jul/ISSUES.HTM*

ANA: *http://www.nursingworld.org/dlwa/osh/wp2.htm*

ANA: *http://nursingworld.org/readroom/position/workplac/wkharass.htm*

ANA: *http://nursingworld.org/ajn/2001/jul/ISSUES.HTM*

ANA: *http://www.nursingworld.org/dlwa/wpr/wp3/htm*

ANA: *http://nursingworld.org/dlwa/osh/wp7.htm*

ANA: *http://www.nursingworld.org/tan/98mayjun/ot.htm*

ANA: *http://www.nursingworld.org/gova/federal/legis/107/ovrtme.htm*

ANA: *http://nursingworld.org/about/summary/sum00/staffing.htm*

ANA: *http://www.nursingworld.org/dlwa/osh/wp2.htm.*

AWHONN: *http://www.awhonn.org/HealthPolicyLegislative/BIOTERRORISM PREPAREDNESS/bioterrorism preparedness.html*

Centers for Disease Control and Prevention (CDC): *http://www.cdc.gov/*

CDC: *http://www.cdc.gov/health/diseases.htm*

CDC: *http://www.cdc.gov/niosh/about.html*

CDC: *http://www.cdc.gov/niosh/pdfs/2002-101.pdf*

CDC: *http://www.cdc.gov/niosh/98-113.html*

CDC: *http://www.bt.cdc.gov/*

CDC: *http://nursingworld.org/tan/01novdec/respond.htm*

National Council State Boards of Nursing:

http://www.ncsbn.org/public/regulation/boards_of_nursing_board.htm

National Institute for Occupational Safety and Health Homepage: *http://www.cdc.gov/niosh*

OSHA: *http://www.osha.gov*

OSHA: Latex allergy: *http://www/oshaslc.gov/SLTC/latex-allergy/index.html.*

OSHA: Latex alert: *http://www.cdc.gov/niosh/latexalt.html/*

OSHA: National News Release: *http://www.osha.gov/media;oshnews/sept98/needles.html.*

OSHA: *http://www.osha.gov/SLTC/needlestick/index.html*

OSHA: *http://www.osha.gov/needlesticks/needlefaq.html*

OSHA: *http://www.osha.gov/needlesticks/needlefact.html*

OSHA: *http://www.osha.gov/SLTC/workplaceviolence/index.html*

OSHA: *http://www.osha.gov/ergonomics/ergofact02.html*

OSHA: *http://www.osha.gov/ergonomics/FAQs-external.html*

OSHA: *http://www.osha.gove/SLTC/healthcarefacilities/harzards.html*

OSHA: *http://www/osha-slc.gov/SLTC/latexallergy/index.html*

OSHA: *alerthttp://www.cdc.gov/niosh/latexalt.html*

REFERENCES

American Nurses Association (ANA). (2001). *Code for Nurses.* Washington, D.C.: ANA.

ANA. (1993). *HIV, Hepatitis-B, Hepatitis-C: Blood-Borne Diseases.* Washington, D.C.: ANA.

ANA. (1994). *Guidelines on Reporting Incompetent, Unethical, or Illegal Practices.* Washington, D.C.: ANA.

ANA. (1995a). *Protect Your Patients—Protect Your License.* Washington, D.C.: ANA.

ANA. (1995b). *The Supreme Court Has Issued the Ultimate Gag Order for Nurses.* Washington, D.C.: ANA.

Armstrong, K., Gordon, R., & Santorella, G. (1995). Occupational exposure of healthcare workers to HIV. *Social Work in Health Care, 21*(3), 61–80.

Arbury, S. (2002). Healthcare workers at risk. *Job Safety and Health Care Quarterly, 13*(2), 30–31.

Bauer, X., Ammon, J., Chen Z., Beckman, W., & Czuppon, A.B. (1993). Health risk in hospitals through airborne allergens for patients pre-sensitized to latex. *Lancet, 342,* 1148–1149.

Brooke, P. (2001). The legal realities of HIV exposure. *RN, 64*(12), 71–73.

Carroll, C., & Sheverbush, J. (September 1996). Violence assessment in hospitals provides basis for action. *American Nurse,* 18.

Centers for Disease Control and Prevention (CDC). (1992). Surveillance for occupationally acquired HIV infection—United States, 1981–1992. *MMWR, 41*(43), 823–825.

Chisholm, R.F. (1992). Quality of working life: A crucial management perspective for the year 2000. *Journal of Health and Human Resources Administration, 15*(1), 6–34.

Collins, J. (1994). Nurses' attitudes toward aggressive behavior following attendance at "The Prevention and Management of Aggressive Behavior Programme." *Journal of Advanced Nursing, 20,* 117–131.

Damrosch, S., & Scholler-Jaquish, A. (1993). Nurses' experiences with impaired nurse coworkers. *Applied Nursing Research, 6*(4), 154–160.

Davidhizar, R., Dowd, S., Giger, J. (1999). Managing diversity in the healthcare workplace. *Health Care Supervisor, 17*(3), 51–62.

Edlich, R., Woodard, C. & Haines, M. (2001). Disabling back injuries in nursing personnel. *Journal of Emergency Nursing, 27*(2), 150–155.

Edwards, R. (1999). Prevention of workplace violence. *Aspen's Advisor for Nurse Executives, 14*(8), 8–12.

Federal agencies clash as TB workplace safety debate rages. (1993). *The Nation's Health, 23*(1), 1, 24.

Fletcher, J., Sorrell, J. & Silva, M. (1998). Whistleblowing as a failure of organizational ethics. *http://nursingworld.org/ojin/topic8/toic8_3htm*

Herring, L.H. (1994). *Infection Control.* New York: National League for Nursing.

Himali, U. (1995). Caring for the caregivers. *American Nurse, 27*(6), 8.

Hurst, K.L., Croker, P.A., & Bell, S.K. (1994). How about a lollipop? A peer recognition program. *Nursing Management, 25*(9), 68–73.

Jankowski, C.B. (1992). Radiation protection for nurses: Regulations and guidelines. *Journal of Nursing Administration, 22*(22), 30–34.

Kinkle, S. (1993). Violence in the ED: How to stop it before it starts. *American Journal of Nursing, 93*(7), 22–24;

Kramer, M., & Schmalenberg, C. (1993). Learning from success: Autonomy and empowerment. *Nursing Management, 24*(5), 58–64.

Krucoff, M. (2001). How to prevent repetitive stress injury in the workplace? *American Fitness, 19*(1), 31.

Lanza, M.L., & Carifio, J. (1991). Blaming the victim: Complex (nonlinear) patterns of casual attribution by nurses in response to vignettes of a patient assaulting a nurse. *Journal of Emergency Nursing, 17*(5), 299–309.

Levin, P., Hewitt, J., & Misner, T. (1998) Insights of nurses about assault in hospital-based emergency departments. *Image, 30,* 249–254.

Lundstrom, T., Pugliese, G., Bartley, J., Cox, J., & Guither, C. (2002). Organizational and environmental factors that affect worker health and safety and patient outcomes. *American Journal of Infection Control,* 30(2), 93–106.

Mahoney, B. (1991). The extent, nature, and response to victimization of emergency nurses in Pennsylvania. *Journal of Emergency Nursing,* 17, 282–292.

Malone, B.L. (1993). Caring for culturally diverse racial groups: An administrative matter. *Nursing Administration Quarterly,* 17(2), 21–29.

Mitchell, A. (1995). Cultural diversity: The future, the market, and the rewards. *Caring,* 14(12), 44–48.

Moch, S.D., & Diemert, C.A. (1987). Health promotion within the nursing work environment. *Nursing Administration Quarterly,* 11(3), 9–12.

Nadwairski, J.A. (1992). Inner-city safety for home care providers. *Journal of Nursing Administration,* 22(9), 42–47.

National Safety Council (1992). *Accident Prevention Manual for Business and Industry.* Chicago: National Safety Council.

OSHA. (1989, January 26). OSHA's Safety and Health Program Management Guidelines. *Federal Register* 54(16), 3904–3916.

Outwater, L.C. (1994). Sexual harassment issues. *Caring,* 13(5), 54–56, 58, 60.

Pennsylvania Bar Institute. (1996). Legal Definition of Sexual Harassment: *http://www.de.psu.edu/harass/legal/define.htm.*

Perry, J. (2001). Attention all nurses!: New legislation puts safer sharps in your hands. *American Journal of Nursing,* 101(9), 24AA–24CC.

Ray, M., Turkel, M., & Marino, F. (2002). The transformative process for nursing in workforce redevelopment. *Nursing Administration Quarterly,* 26(2), 1–14.

Roche, E. (23 February 1993). Nurses' risks and their rights. *Vital Signs,* p 3.

Roedel, R.S., & Nystrom, P.C. (1987). Clinical ladders and job enrichment. *Hospital Topics,* 65(2), 22–24.

Rosen, A., Isaacson, D., Brady, M., & Corey J.P. (1993). Hypersensitivity to latex in health care workers: Report of five cases. *Otolaryngology—Head and Neck Surgery,* 109, 731–734.

Simonowitz, J. (1994). Violence in the workplace: You're entitled to protection. *RN,* 57(11), 61–63

Slattery, M. (September/October 1998). Caring for ourselves to care for our patients. *American Nurse,* 12–13.

Sloan, A. (2002). Legally speaking: Whistleblowing: Proceed with caution. *RN,* 65(1), 67–68, 70, 80–81.

Sloan, A., & Vernarec, E. (2001). Impaired nurses: Reclaiming careers. *Medical Economics,* 64(2), 58–64.

Society of Gastroenterology Nurses and Associates. (2001). Guidelines for preventing sensitivity and allergic reactions to natural rubber latex in the workplace. *Gastroenterology Nursing,* 24(2), 88–94.

Strader, M.K., & Decker, P.J. (1995). *Role Transition to Patient Care Management.* Norwalk, Conn.: Appleton & Lange.

Trossman, S. (May/June 1999a). When workplace threats become a reality. *American Nurse,* 1, 12.

Trossman, S. (September/October 1999b). Working 'round the clock. *American Nurse,* 1–2.

U.S. Department of Labor (OSHA). (1995). *Employee Workplace Rights and Responsibilities.* OSHA 95-35.

Ward, L.B. (27 December 1992). In culturally diverse work place, language may alienate. *Miami Herald.*

UNIT III

Professional Issues

12 Nursing Practice and the Law

13 Questions of Values and Ethics

14 Historical Leaders in Nursing

15 Your Nursing Career

16 Nursing Today

17 Looking to the Future

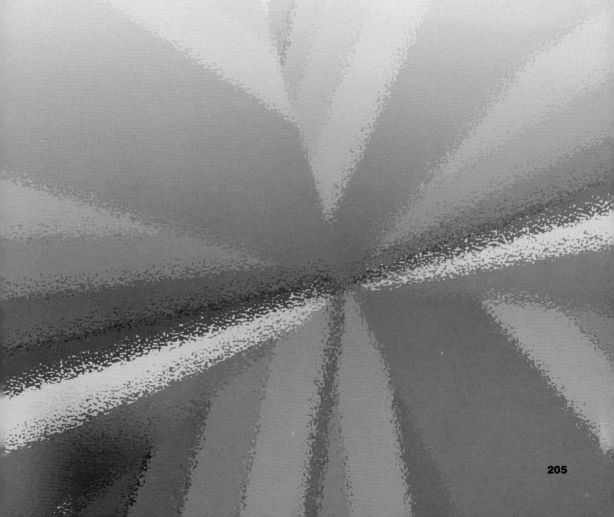

CHAPTER 12

Nursing Practice and the Law

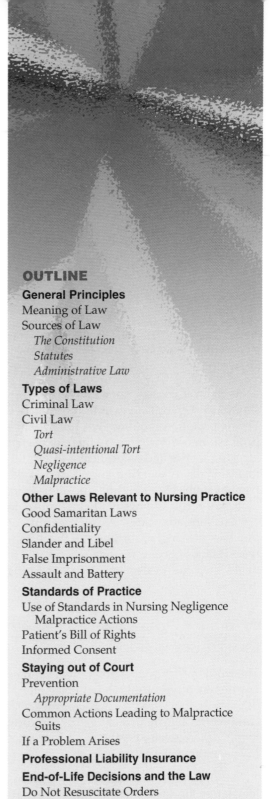

OBJECTIVES

After reading this chapter, the student should be able to:

- Identify three major sources of laws.

- Explain the differences between various types of laws.

- Differentiate between negligence and malpractice.

- Explain the difference between an intentional and an unintentional tort.

- Explain how standards of care are used in determining negligence and malpractice.

- Explain the difference between internal standards and external standards.

- Discuss advance directives and how they pertain to clients' rights.

OUTLINE

General Principles
Meaning of Law
Sources of Law
   The Constitution
   Statutes
   Administrative Law

Types of Laws
Criminal Law
Civil Law
   Tort
   Quasi-intentional Tort
   Negligence
   Malpractice

Other Laws Relevant to Nursing Practice
Good Samaritan Laws
Confidentiality
Slander and Libel
False Imprisonment
Assault and Battery

Standards of Practice
Use of Standards in Nursing Negligence
   Malpractice Actions
Patient's Bill of Rights
Informed Consent

Staying out of Court
Prevention
   Appropriate Documentation
Common Actions Leading to Malpractice
   Suits
If a Problem Arises

Professional Liability Insurance

End-of-Life Decisions and the Law
Do Not Resuscitate Orders
Advance Directives
   Living Will and Durable Power of Attorney
     for Health Care (Health Care Surrogate)
Nursing Implications

Conclusion

The courtroom was cold and sterile. Scanning her surroundings with nervous eyes, Marie decided she knew how Alice must have felt when the Queen of Hearts screamed for her head. The image of the White Rabbit running through the woods, looking at his watch, yelling, "I'm late! I'm late!" flashed before her eyes. For a few moments, she indulged herself in thoughts of being able to turn back the clock and rewrite the past. The future certainly looked grim at that moment.

The calling of her name broke her reverie. Mr. Jefferson, the attorney for the plaintiff, wanted her undivided attention regarding the fateful day when she injected a client with 40 mEq of potassium chloride in error. That day, the client died following cardiac arrest because Marie failed to check the appropriate dosage and route for the medication. She had administered 40 mEq of potassium chloride by intravenous (IV) push. Her 15 years of nursing experience meant little to the court. Because she had not followed hospital protocol and had violated an important standard of practice, Marie stood alone. She was being sued for malpractice.

As client advocates, nurses have a responsibility to deliver safe care to their clients. This expectation requires that nurses have professional knowledge at their expected level of practice and be proficient in technological skills. A working knowledge of the legal system, client rights, and behaviors that may result in lawsuits helps nurses to act as client advocates. As long as nurses practice nursing according to the established standards of care, they will be able to avoid the kind of day in court that Marie experienced.

◼ General Principles

Meaning of Law

The word *law* has several different meanings. For the purposes of this chapter, *law* means those rules that prescribe and control social conduct in a formal and legally binding manner (Bernzweig, 1994). Laws are created in one of three ways:

1 *Statutory laws* are created by various legislative bodies, such as state legislatures or the Congress. Some examples of federal statutes include the Patient Self-Determination Act of 1990 and the Americans with Disabilities Act. State statutes include the state Nurse Practice Act, the State Board of Nursing, and the Good Samaritan Act. Laws that govern nursing practice are statutory laws.

2 *Common law* develops within the court system as judicial decisions are made in various cases and precedents for future cases are set. In this way, a decision made in one case can affect decisions made in later cases of a similar nature. This portion of American law is based on the English tradition of case law. This is "judge-made law" (Black, 1957). Many times a judge in a subsequent case will follow the reasoning of a judge in a previous case. Therefore, one case sets a precedent for another.

3 *Administrative law* is established through the authority given to government agencies, such as a state board of nursing, by a legislative body. It is then the duty of these governing boards to meet the intent of the law or statute.

Sources of Law

The Constitution

The Constitution is the foundation of American law. The Bill of Rights, comprising the first 10 amendments to the U.S. Constitution, is the basis for protection of individual rights. These laws define and limit the power of the government and protect citizens' freedom of speech, freedom of assembly, freedom of religion, freedom of the press, and freedom from unwarranted intrusion by government into personal choices. State constitutions can expand individual rights but cannot deprive people of rights guaranteed by the U.S. Constitution.

Constitutional law evolves. As individuals or groups bring suit to challenge interpretations of the Constitution, decisions are made concerning application of the law to that particular event. An example is the protection of freedom of speech. Are obscenities protected? Can one person threaten or criticize another person? The freedom to criticize is protected; threats are not protected. The definition of what constitutes obscenity is often debated and has not been fully clarified by the courts.

Statutes

Localities, state legislatures, and the U.S. Congress create statutes. These can be found in multivolume sets of books.

At the federal level, conference committees comprising representatives of both Houses of Congress negotiate the resolution of any differences between the Houses on wording of the final bill before it becomes law. If the bill does not meet with the approval of the executive branch of government, the president can veto it. If that occurs, the legislative branch must have enough votes to override the veto or the bill will not become law.

Nurses have an opportunity to influence the development of statutory law both as citizens and as health care providers. Writing to or meeting with state legislators or members of Congress is a way to demonstrate interest in such issues and their outcomes in terms of the laws passed. Passage of a new law is often a long process that includes compromise of all interested individuals.

Administrative Law

The Department of Health and Human Services, the Department of Labor, and the Department of Education are federal agencies that have been given the responsibility for administering health care–related laws. At the state level are departments of health and mental health and licensing boards. Administrative agencies are staffed with professionals who develop the specific rules and regulations that direct the implementation of statutory law. These rules must be reasonable and consistent with the existing statutory law and the intent of the legislature. Usually, they go into effect only after review and comment by affected persons or groups. For example, the state nursing board receives the authority to issue and revoke licenses from specific statutory laws, which means that each board of nursing has the responsibility to oversee the professional nurse's competence.

◗ Types of Laws

Another way to look at the legal system is to divide it into two categories: criminal law and civil law.

Criminal Law

Criminal laws were developed to protect society from actions that threaten its existence. Criminal acts, although directed toward individuals, are considered offenses against the state. The perpetrator of the act is punished, and the victim receives no compensation for injury or damages. There are three categories of criminal law:

1 Felony. The most serious category, this includes such acts as homicide, grand larceny, and a nurse practice act violation

2 Misdemeanor. Includes lesser offenses such as traffic violations or shoplifting of a small dollar amount

3 Juvenile. Crimes carried out by individuals under the age of 18; specific age varies by state and crime

There are occasions when a nurse breaks a law and is tried in criminal court. A nurse who illegally distributes controlled substances, either for personal use or for the use of others, for example, is violating the law. Falsification of records of controlled substances is also a criminal action. In some states, altering a client record may be a misdemeanor (Northrop & Kelly, 1987). For example:

Nurse V. needed to administer a blood transfusion. Because she was in a hurry, she did not properly check the paperwork and violated the standard of practice established for blood administration. Because the nurse failed to follow the designated protocol, the patient was transfused with incompatible blood, suffered from a transfusion reaction, and died. Nurse V. attempted to conceal her conduct and falsified the records. She was found guilty of manslaughter. (Northrop & Kelly, 1987)

Civil Law

Civil laws usually involve the violation of one person's rights by another person. Areas of civil law that particularly affect nurses are tort law, contract law, antitrust law, employment discrimination, and labor laws.

Tort

The remainder of this chapter focuses primarily on tort law. A *tort* is "a legal or civil wrong committed by one person against the person or property of another" (Black, 1957, p. 1660). Tort law recognizes that individuals in their relationships with each other have a general duty not to harm others (Cushing, 1988). For example, as drivers of automobiles, each of us has a duty to drive safely so that others will not be harmed. A roofer has a duty to install a roof properly so that it will not collapse and injure individuals within the structure. Nurses have a duty to deliver care in such a manner that the consumers of care are not harmed. These legal duties of care may be violated intentionally or unintentionally.

Quasi-intentional Tort

A *quasi-intentional tort* is a combination of an unintentional and an intentional tort. It is defined as "a voluntary act that directly causes injury or distress without intent to injure or to cause distress" (Catalano, 1996, p. 298). The elements of cause and desire are present, but the element of intent is missing. Quasi-intentional torts usually involve problems in communication that result in damage to a person's reputation, violation of personal privacy, or infringement of an individual's civil rights.

Negligence

Negligence is the unintentional tort of acting or failing to act as an ordinary, reasonable, prudent person, resulting in harm to the person to whom the duty of care is owed (Black, 1957). The legal elements of negligence consist of duty, breach of duty, causation, and harm or injury (Cushing, 1988). All four elements must be present in the determination. For example, if a nurse administers the wrong medication to a client but the client is not injured, the element of harm has not been met. However, if a nurse administers appropriate pain medication but fails to put up the side rails and the client falls and breaks a hip, all four elements have been satisfied. The duty of care is the standard of care. The law defines *standard of care* as that which a reasonable, prudent practitioner with similar education and experience would do or not do in similar circumstances (Prosser & Keeton, 1984).

Malpractice

Malpractice is the term used for professional negligence. When fulfillment of duties requires specialized education, the term *malpractice* is used.

An important principle in understanding negligence is *respondeat superior,* or the captain of the ship doctrine. Translated literally, this phrase means, "let the master speak." The doctrine of *respondeat superior* holds employers liable for any negligence by their employees when the employees were acting within the realm of employment and when the alleged negligent acts happened during employment (Prosser & Keeton, 1984). Consider the following scenario:

A nursing instructor on a clinical unit in a busy metropolitan hospital instructed his students not to administer any medications unless he was present. Luis, a second-level student, was unable to find his instructor, so he decided to administer digoxin to his client without supervision. The dose was 0.125 mg. The unit dose came as digoxin 0.5 mg/mL. Luis administered the entire amount without checking the digoxin dose or the client's blood and potassium levels. The client became toxic, developed a dysrhythmia, and was transferred to the intensive care unit (ICU). The family sued the hospital and the nursing school for malpractice. The nursing instructor was sued under the principle of *respondeat superior,* even though specific instructions to the contrary had been given to the students.

■ Other Laws Relevant to Nursing Practice

Good Samaritan Laws

In the past, fear of being sued often prevented trained professionals from assisting during an emergency. To encourage physicians and nurses to respond to emergencies, many states developed what are now known as the Good Samaritan laws. When administering emergency care, nurses and physicians are protected from civil liability by Good Samaritan laws as long as they behave in the same manner as an ordinary, reasonable, and prudent professional would have in the same or similar circumstances (Prosser & Keeton, 1984). In other words, when assisting during an emergency, nurses must still observe professional standards of care.

Confidentiality

It is possible for nurses to be involved in lawsuits other than those involving negligence. For example, clients have the right to confidentiality, and it is the duty of the professional nurse to ensure this right. This assures the client that information obtained by a nurse while giving him or her care will not be communicated to anyone who does not have a need to know (Cushing, 1988). For example:

Leonard was admitted for pneumonia. With Leonard's permission, an HIV test was performed and the result was positive. Several nurses were discussing the situation in the cafeteria and were overheard by one of Leonard's coworkers, who had come to visit him. This individual reported the test results to Leonard's supervisor. When Leonard returned to work, he was fired for "poor job performance," although he had had superior job evaluations. In the process of filing a discrimination suit against his employer, Leonard discovered that the information on his health status had come from a group of nurses. A lawsuit was filed against the hospital and the nurses involved based on a breach of confidentiality.

Slander and Libel

Nurses rarely think of themselves as being guilty of slander or libel. The term *slander* refers to the spoken word and *libel* to the written word. Making a false statement about a client's condition that may result in an injury to that client is considered slander. Putting a false statement into writing is libel. For example, stating that a client who had blood drawn for drug testing has a substance abuse problem, when in fact the client does not carry that diagnosis, could be considered a slanderous statement. Such a statement could result in harm or injury if the client is fired from his or her job because it was overheard and repeated (remember Leonard).

Slander and libel also refer to statements made about coworkers or other individuals that you may encounter in both your professional and educational life. Think before you speak and write. Sometimes what may appear to be harmless to you, such as a complaint, may contain statements that damage another person's credibility personally and professionally. Consider this example:

Several nurses on a unit were having difficulty with the nurse manager. Rather than approach the manager or follow the chain of command, they decided to send a written statement to the chief executive officer (CEO) of the hospital. In this letter, they embellished some of the incidents that occurred and took out of context statements the nurse manager had made, changing the meanings of the remarks. The nurse manager was called to the CEO's office and reprimanded for these events and statements, which in reality had not occurred. The nurse manager sued the nurses for slander and libel based on the premise that her personal and professional reputation had been tainted.

False Imprisonment

False imprisonment is confining an individual against his or her will by either physical (restraining) or verbal (detaining) means. The following examples fall within the definition of false imprisonment:

- Using restraints on individuals without the appropriate written consent

- Restraining mentally handicapped individuals who do not represent a threat to themselves or others

- Detaining unwilling clients in an institution when they desire to leave

- Keeping persons who are medically cleared for discharge for an unreasonable amount of time

- Removing the clothing of clients to prevent them from leaving the institution

- Threatening clients with some form of physical, emotional, or legal action if they insist on leaving

Sometimes clients are a danger to themselves and to others. Nurses often need to decide on the appropriateness of restraints as a protective measure. Nurses should try to obtain the cooperation of the client before applying any type of restraints. The first step is to attempt to identify a reason for the risky behavior and resolve the problem. If this fails, document the need for restraints, consult with the physician, and carefully follow the institution's policies and standards of practice. Failure to follow these guidelines may result in greater harm to the client and possibly a lawsuit for the staff. Consider the following:

Mr. Harrison, who is 87 years old, was admitted through the emergency department with severe lower abdominal pain of 3 days' duration. Physical assessment revealed severe dehydration in a man in acute distress. A surgeon was called, and an abdominal laparotomy was performed, revealing a ruptured appendix. Surgery was successful, and the client was sent to the ICU for 24 hours. On transfer to the surgical floor the next day, Mr. Harrison was in stable condition. Later that night, he became confused, irritable, and anxious. He attempted to climb out of bed and pulled out his indwelling urinary catheter. The nurse restrained him. The next day, his irritability and confusion continued. Mr. Harrison's nurse placed him in a chair, tying him in and restraining his hands. Three hours later he was found in cardiopulmonary arrest.

A lawsuit of wrongful death and false imprisonment was brought against the nurse manager, the nurses caring for Mr. Harrison, and the institution. During discovery, it was determined that the primary cause of Mr. Harrison's behavior was hypoxemia. A violation of law occurred with the failure of the nursing staff to notify the physician of the client's condition and to follow the institution's standard of practice on the use of restraints.

To protect themselves against charges of negligence or false imprisonment in such cases, nurses should discuss safety needs with patients, their families, or other members of the health care team. Careful assessment and documentation of client status are also imperative; confusion, irritability, and anxiety often have metabolic causes that need correction, not restraint.

There are also statutes and case laws specific to the admission of clients to psychiatric institutions. Most states have guidelines for emergency involuntary hospitalization for a specific time period. Involuntary admission is considered necessary when clients are a danger to themselves or others. Specific procedures must be followed. A determination by a judge or administrative agency or certification by a specified number of physicians that a person's mental health justifies detention and treatment may be required. Once admitted, these clients may not be restrained unless the guidelines established by state law and the institution's policies are followed. Clients who voluntarily admit themselves to psychiatric institutions are also protected against false imprisonment. Nurses need to make themselves aware of the policies of their state and employing institution.

Assault and Battery

Assault is a threat to harm. *Battery* is touching another person without their consent. Most medical treatments, particularly surgery, would be battery if it were not for informed consent from the client. The significance of an assault is in the threat. "If you don't stop pushing that call bell, I'll give you this injection with the biggest needle I can find" is considered an assaultive statement. Battery would occur if the injection were given when it was refused, even if medical personnel deemed it was for the "client's good." Holding down a violent client against his or her will and injecting a sedative is battery. With few exceptions, clients have a right to refuse treatment.

◼ Standards of Practice

Concern for the quality of care is a major part of nursing's responsibility to the public. Therefore, the nursing profession is accountable to the consumer for the quality of its services. One of the defining characteristics of a profession is the ability to set its own standards. Nursing standards were established as guidelines for the profession to ensure acceptable quality of care (Beckman, 1995). Standards of practice are also used as criteria to determine whether appropriate care has been delivered. In practice, they represent the minimum acceptable level of care. Nurses are judged on generally accepted standards of practice for their level of education, experience, position, and specialty area. Standards of the profession take many forms. Some are written and may be included in recommendations by professional organizations, job descriptions, agency policies and procedures, and textbooks. Others, which may be intrinsic to the custom of practice, are not found in writing (Beckman, 1995).

State boards of nursing and professional organizations vary by role and responsibility in relation to standards of development and implementation (ANA, 1998). Statutes, professional organizations, and health care institutions establish standards of practice. The Nurse Practice Acts of individual states define the boundaries of nursing practice within the state. The courts have upheld the authority of boards of nursing to regulate standards. The boards accomplish this through direct or delegated statutory language (ANA, 1998). The American Nurses Association also has specific standards of practice in general and in several clinical areas (see Appendix 2).

Internal standards of practice are those that institutions develop. They are usually explained in a specific institutional policy, and the institution includes these standards in policy and procedure manuals. For example, guidelines for the appropriate administration of a specific chemotherapeutic agent or agents are included in an institutional policy and procedure manual. The guidelines are based on the current literature and research. It is the nurse's responsibility to maintain currency with an institution's standards of practice. It is the institution's responsibility to notify the health care personnel of any changes and instruct the personnel about the changes. Institutions may accomplish this task through written memos or meetings and inservice education.

With the expansion of advanced nursing practice, it has become particularly important to clarify the legal distinction between nursing and medical practice. It is impor-

tant to be aware of the boundaries between these professional domains because crossing them can result in legal consequences and disciplinary action. The Nurse Practice Act and related regulations developed by most state legislatures and state boards of nursing help to clarify nursing roles at the various levels of practice.

Use of Standards in Nursing Negligence Malpractice Actions

When omission of prudent care or acts committed by a nurse or those under his or her supervision cause harm to a client, standards are used as a guide to determine whether appropriate care was administered. Many nurses assume that the standards of nursing practice are the only ones used to determine whether malpractice or negligence exists. Other standards may be used. These may include, but are not limited to (ANA, 1998):

- State, local, or national standards

- Institutional policies that alter or adhere to the nursing standards of care

- Expert opinions on the appropriate standard of care at the time

- Available literature and research that substantiates a standard of care or changes in the standard

Patient's Bill of Rights

In 1973, the American Hospital Association approved a statement called "A Patient's Bill of Rights." These standards were derived from the ethical principle of autonomy.

Informed Consent

Without consent, many of the procedures performed on clients in a health care setting may be considered battery or unwarranted touching. When clients consent to treatment, they give health care personnel the right to deliver care and perform specific treatments without fear of prosecution. Although physicians are responsible for obtaining informed consent, nurses often find themselves involved in the process. It is also the physician's responsibility to give information to a client about a specific treatment or medical intervention (*Giese v. Stice*, 1997). The individual institution does not hold responsibility for obtaining the informed consent unless (1) the physician or practitioner is employed by the institution, or (2) the institution was aware or should have been aware of the lack of informed consent and did not act on this fact (Guido, 2001). Some institutions require the physician or independent practitioner to obtain his or her own informed consent by obtaining the client's signature at the time the explanation for treatment is given.

The informed consent form should contain all the possible negative outcomes as well as the positive. Nurses may be asked to obtain the signatures on this form. The following are some criteria to help ensure that a client has actually given an informed consent (Guido, 2001; Kozier, Erb, Blais, & Wilkinson, 1995; Northrop & Kelly, 1987):

- A mentally competent adult has voluntarily given the consent.

- The client understands exactly to what he or she is consenting.

- The consent includes the risks involved in the procedure, alternative treatments that may be available, and the possible outcome if the treatment is refused.

- The consent is written.

- A minor's parent or guardian usually gives consent for treatment.

Ideally, a nurse should be present when the physician is explaining the treatment to the client. Before obtaining the client's signature, the nurse asks the client to recall exactly what the physician has told him or her about the treatment. If at any point the nurse thinks that the client does not understand the treatment or the expected outcome, the nurse must notify the physician of this fact. To give informed consent, the client must be fully in-

formed. Clients have the right to refuse treatment, and nurses must respect this right. If a client refuses the recommended treatment, a client must be informed of the possible consequences of this decision.

Implied consent is a form of consent in which the consent is assumed. This may be an issue in an emergency when an individual is unable to give consent, as in the following scenario:

An elderly woman is involved in a car accident on a major highway. The paramedics called to the scene find her unresponsive and in acute respiratory distress; her vital signs are unstable. The paramedics immediately intubate her and begin treating her cardiac dysrhythmias. Because she is unconscious and unable to give her verbal consent, there is an implied consent for treatment.

◼ Staying out of Court

Prevention

Unfortunately, the public's trust in the medical profession has declined over recent years. Consumers are better informed and more assertive in their approach to health care. They demand good and responsible care. If clients and their families feel that behaviors are uncaring or that attitudes are impersonal, they are more likely to sue for what they view as errors in treatment. The same applies to nurses. If nurses demonstrate an interest in and caring behaviors toward clients, a relationship develops. Individuals do not sue those they view as "caring friends." The potential to change the attitudes of health care consumers is within the power of health care personnel. Demonstrating care and concern and making clients and families aware of choices and methods can help decrease liability. Nurses who involve clients and their families in decisions about care reduce the likelihood of a lawsuit. Tips to prevent legal problems are listed in Box 12–1.

All health care personnel are accountable for their own actions and adherence to the accepted standards of health care. Most negligence and malpractice cases arise from a violation of the accepted standards of prac-

BOX 12–1
Tips to Avoid Legal Problems

- Keep yourself informed regarding new research findings related to your area of practice.
- Insist that the health care institution keep personnel apprised of all changes in policies and procedures and in the management of new technological equipment.
- Always follow the standards of care or practice for the institution.
- Delegate tasks and procedures only to appropriate personnel.
- Identify patients at risk for problems such as falls or the development of decubiti.
- Establish and maintain a safe environment.
- Document precisely and carefully.
- Write detailed incident reports and file them with the appropriate personnel or department.
- Recognize certain patient behaviors that may indicate the possibility of a lawsuit.

tice and the policies of the employing institution. Common causes of negligence are listed in Table 12–1. Expert witnesses on both sides are called to cite the accepted standards and assist attorneys in formulating the legal strategies pertaining to those standards. For example, most medication errors can be traced back to a violation of the accepted standard of medication administration, the *five rights* (Kozier et al., 1995), which have been amended to include a sixth right (Iyer & Comp, 1999):

1 Right drug

2 Right dose

3 Right route

4 Right time

5 Right patient

6 Right documentation

Appropriate Documentation

The adage "not documented, not done" holds true in nursing. According to the law, if something is not documented, then the responsible party did not do whatever needed to be done. If a nurse does not do something, that leaves the nurse open to negligence or malpractice charges.

TABLE 12–1
Common Causes of Negligence

Problem	Prevention
Client falls	Identify clients at risk. Place notices instituting fall precautions. Follow institutional policies on the use of restraints. Always be sure beds are in their lowest positions. Use siderails appropriately.
Equipment injuries	Check thermostats and temperature in equipment used for heat or cold application. Check wiring on all electrical equipment.
Failure to monitor	Observe IV infusion sites as directed by institutional policy. Obtain and record vital signs, urinary output, cardiac status, etc. as directed by institutional policy and more often if client condition dictates. Check pertinent laboratory values.
Failure to communicate	Report pertinent changes in client status to appropriate personnel. Document changes accurately. Document communication with appropriate source.
Medication errors	Follow the Six Rights. Monitor client responses. Check client medications for multiple drugs for the same actions.

Nursing documentation needs to be legally credible. Legally credible documentation is an accurate accounting of the care the client received. It also indicates the competence of the individual who delivered the care.

Charting by exception creates defense difficulties. When this method of documentation is used, investigators need to review the entire client record in an attempt to reconstruct the care given to the client. Clear, concise, and accurate documentation helps nurses when they are named in lawsuits. Often, this documentation clears the individual of any negligence or malpractice. Documentation is credible when it is:

- **Contemporaneous.** Documenting at the time care was provided

- **Accurate.** Documenting exactly what you did

- **Truthful.** Documenting only what you actually did or observed

- **Appropriate.** Documenting only what you would be comfortable discussing in a public setting

Box 12–2 lists some documentation tips.

In the case of Luis, the nursing student violated the *right dose* principle and therefore made a medication error. When a nurse signs off on medications for all clients for the shift before the medications are administered, he

---

BOX 12–2
Some Documentation Guidelines

- Medications
  Always chart the time, route, dose, and response.
  Always chart prn medications and the client response.
  Always chart when a medication was not given, the reason (client in radiology, physical therapy, etc.; do not chart that the medication was not on the floor), and the nursing intervention.
  Chart all medication refusals and report them to the appropriate source.
- Physician communication
  Document each time a call is made to a physician, even if he or she is not reached. Include the exact time of the call. If the physician is reached, document the details of the message and the physician's response.
  Read verbal orders back to the physician and confirm the client's identity as written on the chart. Chart only verbal orders that you have heard from the source, not those told to you by another nurse or unit personnel.
- Formal issues in charting
  Before writing on the chart, check to be sure you have the correct client record.
  Check to make sure each page has the client's name and the current date stamped in the appropriate area.
  If you forgot to make an entry, chart "late entry" and place the date and time at the entry.
  Correct all charting mistakes according to the policy and procedures of your institution.
  Chart in an organized fashion following the nursing process.
  Write legibly and concisely and avoid subjective statements.
  Write specific and accurate descriptions.
  When charting a symptom or situation, chart the interventions taken and the client response.
  Document your own observations, not those that were told to you by another party.
  Chart frequently to demonstrate ongoing care, and chart routine activities.
  Chart client and family teaching and the response.

or she is left open to charges of medication error.

In the case of Mr. Harrison, the institutional personnel were found negligent because of a direct violation of the institution's standards regarding the application of restraints.

Nursing units are busy and often understaffed. These realities exist but should not be allowed to interfere with the safe delivery of health care. Clients have a right to safe and effective health care, and nurses have an obligation to deliver this care.

Common Actions Leading to Malpractice Suits

- Failure to appropriately assess a client
- Failure to report changes in client status to the appropriate personnel
- Failure to document in the client record
- Altering or falsifying a client record
- Failure to obtain informed consent
- Failure to report a coworker's negligence or poor practice
- Failure to provide appropriate education to a client and/or family members
- Violation of internal or external standards of practice

If a Problem Arises

When served with a summons or complaint, people often panic, allowing fear to overcome reason and sanity. First of all, you are required to answer the complaint. Failure to do this may result in a default judgment, causing greater distress and difficulties.

In addition, you can do many things to protect yourself if you are named in a lawsuit. You may want to obtain legal representation to protect personal property. Never sign any documents without consulting with your malpractice insurance carrier or your legal representative. If you are personally covered by malpractice insurance, notify the company immediately and follow their in-

structions carefully. Institutions usually have lawyers to defend themselves and their employees. Whether or not you are personally insured, contact the legal department of the institution where the act took place. You need to keep a file of all papers, proceedings, meetings, and telephone conversations about the case. Although a pending or ongoing legal case should not be discussed with coworkers or friends, do not withhold any information you have from your attorneys, even if you believe that it may be harmful to you. Let the attorneys and the insurance company help you decide how to handle the difficult situation. They are in charge of damage control. Concealing information usually causes more damage than disclosing it.

Sometimes, nurses feel that they are not being adequately protected or represented by the attorneys from their employing institution. If this happens, consider hiring a personal attorney who is experienced in malpractice. This information can be obtained through either the State Bar Association or the local Trial Lawyer's Association.

◘ Professional Liability Insurance

Various forms of professional liability insurance are available to nurses. These policies have been developed to protect nurses against personal financial losses if they are involved in a medical malpractice suit. If a nurse is charged with malpractice and found guilty, the employing institution has the right to sue the nurse to reclaim damages. Professional malpractice insurance protects the nurse in these situations.

◘ End-of-Life Decisions and the Law

When a heart ceases to beat, a client is in a state of cardiac arrest. Both in modern health care institutions and in the community, it is common to begin cardiopulmonary resuscitation (CPR) when cardiac arrest occurs. In health care institutions, an elaborate mechanism is put into action when a client "codes." Much controversy exists concerning when these mechanisms should be used and whether individuals who have no chance of regaining full viability should be resuscitated.

Do Not Resuscitate Orders

A do not resuscitate (DNR) order is a specific directive to health care personnel not to initiate CPR measures. Only a physician can write a DNR order, usually after consulting with the client or family. Other members of the health care team are expected to comply with the order. Clients have the right to request a DNR order. However, they may make this request without a full understanding of what it really means. Take the following example:

When Mrs. Vincent, 58 years old, was admitted to the hospital for a hysterectomy, she explicitly stated, "I want to be made a DNR." The nurse, rather concerned by the statement, questioned Mrs. Vincent's understanding of a DNR order. The nurse asked her, "Do you mean that if you are walking down the hall after your surgery and your heart stops beating, you do not want the nurses or physicians to do anything? You want us to just let you die?" Mrs. Vincent responded with a resounding, "No, that is not what I mean. I mean if something happens to me and I won't be able to be the way I am now, I want to be a DNR!" The nurse then explained the concept of a DNR order.

New York state has one of the most complete laws regarding DNR orders in both acute and long-term care facilities. The New York law sets up a hierarchy of surrogates that may ask for a DNR status for incompetent clients. The state has also ordered that all health care facilities ask clients their wishes regarding resuscitation (Guido, 2001.) The American Nurses Association advocates that every facility have a written policy regarding the initiation of such orders (ANA, 1992). The client or, if the client is unable to speak for himself or herself, a family member or guardian, should make clear the client's preference for either having as much as possible done or withholding treatment (see the next section, Advance Directives). Elements to include in a DNR order are listed in Box 12–3.

Advance Directives

The legal dilemmas that may arise in relation to DNR orders often require court decisions. For this reason, in 1990 Senator John Danforth of Missouri and Senator Daniel Moynihan of New York introduced the Patient Self-Determination Act to address questions regarding life-sustaining treatment. The act was created to allow people the opportunity to make decisions about treatment in advance of a time when they might become unable to participate in the decision-making process. Through this mechanism, families can be spared the burden of having to decide what the family member would have wanted.

Federal law requires that health care institutions that receive federal money (from Medicare, for example) inform clients of their right to create advance directives. The Patient Self-Determination Act provides guidelines for developing advance directives concerning what will be done for individuals if they no longer are able to actively participate in making decisions about care options. The Patient Self-Determination Act (S.R. 13566) states that institutions must do several things:

> **BOX 12–3**
> **Elements to Include in a Do Not Resuscitate (DNR) Order**
>
> - Statement of the policy of the institution that resuscitation will be initiated unless there is a specific order to withhold resuscitative measures
> - Statement from the client regarding specific desires
> - Description of the client's medical condition to justify a DNR order
> - Statement about the role of the family members or significant others
> - Definition of the scope of the DNR order
> - Delineation of the roles of various caregivers
>
> Source: American Nurses Association. (1992). *Position Statement on Nursing Care and Do Not Resuscitate Decisions.* Washington, D.C.: ANA.

• **Provide information to every client.** On admission, all clients must be informed in writing of their rights under state law to accept or refuse medical treatment while they are competent to make decisions about their care. This includes the right to execute advance directives.

• **Document.** All clients must be asked whether they have a living will or have chosen a durable power of attorney for health care (also known as a *health care surrogate*). The response must be indicated on the medical record and a copy of the documents, if available, should be placed on the client's chart.

• **Educate.** Nurses, other health care personnel, and the community need to understand what the Patient Self-Determination Act requires, as well as the state laws regarding advance directives.

• **Be respectful of clients' rights.** All clients are to be treated with respectful care regardless of their decision regarding life-prolonging treatments.

Living Will and Durable Power of Attorney for Health Care (Health Care Surrogate)

The two most common forms of advance directives are living wills and durable power of attorney for health care (health care surrogate).

A living will is a legally executed document that states an individual's wishes regarding the use of life-prolonging medical treatment in the event that he or she is no longer competent to make informed treatment decisions on his or her own behalf and is suffering from a terminal condition (Catalano, 2000; Flarey, 1991). A condition is considered terminal when, to a reasonable degree of medical certainty, there is little likelihood of recovery or the condition is expected to cause death. It may also refer to a persistent vegetative state characterized by a permanent and irreversible condition of unconsciousness in which there is (1) absence of voluntary action or cognitive behavior of any kind and (2) an inability to communicate

or interact purposefully with the environment (Marshall, Marshall, Vos, & Chestnut, 1990).

Another form of advance directive is the appointment of a health care surrogate. Chosen by the client, the health care surrogate is usually a family member or close personal friend. The role of the health care surrogate is to make the client's wishes known to medical and nursing personnel. Imperative in the designation of a health care surrogate is a clear understanding of an individual's wishes should the need arise to know them.

In some situations, clients are unable to adequately or competently express themselves although they are not terminally ill. For example, clients with advanced Alzheimer's disease or other forms of dementia cannot communicate their wishes, clients under anesthesia are temporarily unable to communicate effectively, and the condition of comatose clients does not allow for expression of health care wishes. In these situations, the health care surrogate can make treatment decisions on the behalf of the client. However, when a client regains the ability to make his or her own decisions and is capable of expressing them effectively, he or she resumes control of all decision-making pertaining to medical treatment (Reigle, 1992). Nurses and physicians may be held accountable when they go against a client's wishes regarding DNR orders and advance directives.

In the case *Wendland v. Sparks* (1998), the physician and nurses were sued for "not initiating CPR." In this particular case, the client had been in the hospital for more than 2 months for lung disease and multiple myeloma. Although improving at the time, during the hospitalization she had experienced three cardiac arrests. Even after this, the client had not requested to be made a DNR. Her family had not discussed this either. After one of the arrests, the client's husband had told the physician that he wanted his wife placed on artificial life support if it was necessary (Guido, 2001). The client had a fourth cardiac arrest. One nurse went to obtain the crash cart, and another to get the physician who happened to be in the area. The physician checked the heart rate, pupils, and respirations and stated, "I just cannot do it to her." (Guido, 2001, p. 158). She ordered the nurses to stop the resuscitation and the physician pronounced the client. The nurses stated that if they had not been given a direct order they would have continued their attempts at resuscitation. "The court ruled that the physician's judgment was faulty and that the family had the right to sue the physician for wrongful death" (Guido, 2001, p. 158). The nurses were cleared in this case because they were following a physician order.

Nursing Implications

The Patient Self-Determination Act does not specify who should discuss treatment decisions or advance directives with clients. Because directives are often implemented on nursing units, however, nurses need to be knowledgeable about living wills and health care surrogates and be prepared to answer questions that clients may have about directives and the forms used by the health care institution.

As client advocates, the responsibility for creating an awareness of individual rights often falls on nurses. It is the responsibility of the health care institution to educate personnel about the policies of the institution so that nurses and others involved in client care can inform health care consumers of their choices. Nurses who are unsure of the policies in their health care institution should contact the appropriate department.

■ Conclusion

Nurses need to understand the legalities involved in the delivery of safe health care. It is important to know the standards of care established within your institution because these will be the standards to which you will be held accountable. Health care consumers have a right to quality care, and nurses have an obligation to deliver it. Caring for clients safely and avoiding legal difficulties require nurses to adhere to the expected standards of care and carefully document changes in client status.

Study Questions

1. How do federal laws, court decisions, and state boards of nursing affect nursing practice? Give an example of each.

2. The next time you are on your clinical unit, look at the nursing documentation done by several different staff members. Do you believe it is adequate? Explain your rationale.

3. How does your institution handle medication errors?

4. If a nurse is found to be less than proficient in the delivery of safe care, how should the nurse manager remedy the situation?

5. Describe the areas that should be accessed in determining standards of care. Explain whether each is an example of an internal or external standard of care.

6. Explain the importance of federal agencies in setting standards of care in health care institutions.

7. What is the difference between consent and informed consent?

8. Look at the forms for advance directives and DNR policies in your institution. Do they follow the guidelines of the Patient Self-Determination Act?

9. What should a practicing nurse do to stay out of court? What should a nurse not do?

Critical Thinking Exercise

Mr. Evans, 40 years old, was admitted to the medical-surgical unit from the emergency department with a diagnosis of acute abdomen. He had a 20-year history of Crohn's disease and had been on prednisone, 20 mg, every day for the past year. Because he was allowed nothing by mouth (NPO), total parenteral nutrition was started through a triple-lumen central venous catheter line, and his steroids were changed to Solu-Medrol, 60 mg by IV push q6h. He was also receiving several IV antibiotics and medication for pain and nausea. Over the next several days, his condition worsened. He was in severe pain and needed more analgesics. One evening at 9 P.M., it was discovered that his central venous catheter line was out. The registered nurse notified the physician, who stated that a surgeon would come in the morning to replace it. The nurse failed to ask the physician what to do about the IV steroids, antibiotics, and fluid replacement because the patient was still NPO. At 7 A.M., the night nurse noted that the client had had no urinary output since 11 P.M. the night before. She failed to report this information to the day shift.

The client's physician made rounds at 9 A.M. The nurse for Mr. Evans did not discuss the fact that the client had not voided since 11 P.M. the previous night, nor did she request orders for alternative delivery of the steroids and antibiotics. At 5 P.M. that evening, while Mr. Evans was having a computed tomography scan, his blood pressure dropped to 70 mm Hg, and because no one was in the scan room with him, he coded. He was transported to the ICU and intubated. He developed sepsis and acute respiratory distress syndrome.

1 List all the problems you can find with the nursing care in this case.

2 What were the nursing responsibilities in reporting information?

3 What do you think was the possible cause of the drop in Mr. Evan's blood pressure and his subsequent code?

4 If you worked in risk management, how would you discuss this situation with the nurse manager and the staff?

Student Activities

1 Make arrangements to attend a court case regarding negligence or malpractice.

2 Interview the risk manager at your clinical institution.

3 Review three charts on your clinical unit. Identify documentation issues that could possibly lead to legal problems.

4 Develop an in-service program to help the nurses on your clinical unit avoid possible legal issues with documentation.

REFERENCES

American Nurses Association (ANA). (1992). *Position Statement on Nursing Care and Do Not Resuscitate Decisions.* Washington, D.C.: ANA.

American Nurses Association (ANA). (1998). *Legal Aspects of Standards and Guidelines for Clinical Nursing Practice.* Washington, D.C.: ANA.

Beckman, J.P. (1995). Nursing Malpractice: Implications for Clinical Practice and Nursing Education. Seattle: Washington University Press.

Bernzweig, E.P. (1994). *The Nurse's Liability for Malpractice.* New York: McGraw-Hill.

Black, H.C. (1957). *Black's Law Dictionary.* St. Paul, Minn.: West Publishing.

Catalano, J.T. (2000). *Nursing Now! Today's Issue, Tomorrow's Trends,* 2nd ed. Philadelphia: F.A. Davis.

Catalano, J.T. (1996). *Contemporary Professional Nursing.* Philadelphia: F.A. Davis.

Cushing, M. (1988). *Nursing Jurisprudence.* Norwalk, Conn.: Appleton & Lange.

Flarey, D. (1991). Advanced directives: In search of self-determination. *Journal of Nursing Administration,* 21(11), 17.

Giese v. Stice, 567 NW 2d 156 (Nebraska, 1997).

Guido, G.W. (2001). *Legal and Ethical Issues in Nursing,* 3rd ed. Upper Saddle River, N.J.: Prentice-Hall.

Iyer, P., & Comp, N. (1999). *Documentation: A Nursing Process Approach,* 3rd ed. St. Louis, Mo.: Mosby-Year Book.

Kozier, B., Erb, G., Blais, K., & Wilkinson, J.M. (1995). *Fundamentals of Nursing: Concepts, Process and Practice,* 15th ed. Menlo Park, Calif.: Addison-Wesley.

Marshall, S.B., Marshall, L.F., Vos, H.R., & Chestnut, R.M. (1990). *Neuroscience Critical Care: Pathophysiology and Patient Management.* Philadelphia: W.B. Saunders.

Northrop, C.E., & Kelly, M.E. (1987). State of New Jersey v. Winter. In *Legal Issues in Nursing.* St. Louis, Mo.: C.V. Mosby.

Patient Self-Care Determination Act. (1989). S.R. 13566, Congressional Record.

Prosser, W.L., & Keeton, D. (1984). *The Law of Torts,* 5th ed. St. Paul, Minn.: West Publishing.

Reigle, J. (1992). Preserving patient self-determination through advance directives. *Heart Lung,* 21(2), 196–198.

Wendland v. Sparks. (1998). 574 N.W. 2d 327 (Iowa, 1998).

CHAPTER 13

Questions of Values and Ethics

OBJECTIVES

After reading this chapter, the student should be able to:

- Discuss the way values are formed.

- Differentiate between personal ethics and professional ethics.

- Compare and contrast various ethical theories

- Apply the seven basic ethical principles to an ethical issue

- Identify an ethical dilemma in the clinical setting.

- Discuss current ethical issues in health care and possible solutions.

OUTLINE

Values
Value Systems
How Values Are Developed
Values Clarification

Belief Systems

Morals and Ethics
Morals
Ethics
Ethical Theories
Ethical Principles
　Autonomy
　Nonmaleficence
　Beneficence
　Justice
　Confidentiality
　Veracity
　Accountability
Ethical Codes
Ethical Dilemmas

Resolving Ethical Dilemmas Faced by Nurses
Assessment
Planning
Implementation
Evaluation
Current Ethical Issues
Practice Issues Related to Technology
　Genetics and the Limitations of Technology
　Professional Dilemmas

Conclusion

It is 1961. In a large metropolitan hospital, 10 health care professionals are meeting to consider the cases of three different individuals. Ironically, the cases have something in common. Larry Jones, age 66, Irma Kolnick, age 31, and Nancy Roberts, age 10, are all suffering from chronic renal failure and are in need of hemodialysis. Equipment is scarce, the cost of the treatment is prohibitive, and it is doubtful that treatment will be covered by health insurance. The hospital is able to provide this treatment to only one of these individuals. Who shall live, and who shall die? In a novel of the same name, Noah Gordon called this decision-making group the *Death Committee* (Gordon, 1963). Today, such groups are referred to as ethics committees.

In previous centuries, we had neither the knowledge nor the technology to prolong life. The main role of nurses and physicians was supporting patients through times of illness, helping them toward recovery, or keeping them comfortable until death. There were few "who shall live, and who shall die?" decisions.

The polio epidemic that raged through Europe and the United States during 1947–1948 initiated the development of units for patients on manual ventilation (the "iron lung"). At this time, Danish physicians invented a method of manual ventilation by using a tube placed in the trachea of polio patients. This was the beginning of mechanical ventilation as we know it today.

During the 1950s, the development of mechanical ventilation required more intense nursing care and patient observation. The care and monitoring of these patients proved to be more efficient when the patients were kept in a single patient care area, hence the term *intensive care*. The late 1960s brought greater technological advances, especially in the care of seriously ill patients with cardiovascular disease. These new therapies and monitoring methods made the intensive care unit possible (*www.aacn.org*, 2002).

Health care can now keep alive people who would die without intervention. The development of new drugs and advances in biomechanical technology permit physicians and nurses to challenge nature. This progress also brings new, perplexing questions. The ability to prolong life has created some heartbreaking situations for families and terrible ethical dilemmas for health care professionals. How is the decision made of when to turn off the life support machines that are keeping alive someone's beloved son or daughter after, for example, an auto accident? Families and professionals alike are faced with some of the most difficult ethical decisions at times like this. How do we define death? How do we know when it has occurred? Perhaps we also need to ask, "What is life? Is there ever a time when life is no longer worth living?"

Health care professionals have looked to philosophy, especially the branch that deals with human behavior, for resolution of these issues. The field of biomedical ethics (or simply bioethics), a subdiscipline of the area known as ethics—or the philosophical study of morality—has evolved. In essence, bioethics is the study of medical morality, the moral and social implications of health care and science in human life (Mappes & Zembaty, 1991).

To understand biomedical ethics, we need to first consider the basic concepts of values, belief systems, ethical theories, and morality. We will then discuss the resolution of ethical dilemmas in health care.

◼ Values

Webster's New World Dictionary (2000) defines *values* as the "estimated or appraised worth of something, or that quality of a thing that makes it more or less desirable, useful." Values, then, are judgments about the importance or unimportance of objects, ideas, attitudes, and attributes. They become a part of a person's conscience and worldview. Values provide a frame of reference and act as pilots to guide behaviors and assist people in making choices.

Value Systems

A value system is a set of related values. For example, one person may value (believe to be important) material things, such as money, objects, and social status. Another person may value more abstract concepts, such as kindness, charity, and caring. Values may vary significantly based on an individual's culture. An individual's system of values frequently affects how he or she makes decisions. For example, one person may base a decision on cost, and another person placed in the same situation may base the decision on a more abstract quality, such as kindness. There are different categories of values:

- *Intrinsic values* are those related to sustaining life, such as food and water (Steele & Harmon, 1983).

- *Extrinsic values* are not essential to life. Things, people, and ideas such as kindness, understanding, and material items are extrinsically valuable.

- *Personal values* are qualities that people consider valuable in their private lives. Such things as strong family ties and acceptance by others are personal values.

- *Professional values* are qualities considered important by a professional group. Autonomy, integrity, and commitment are examples of professional values.

People's behaviors are motivated by values. Individuals take risks, relinquish their own comfort and security, and generate extraordinary efforts because of their values (Edge & Groves, 1994). Traumatic brain injury patients may overcome tremendous barriers because they value independence. Racecar drivers may risk death or other serious injury because they value competition and winning.

Values also generate the standards by which people judge others. For example, if you value work over leisure activities, you will look unfavorably on the coworker who refuses to work over the weekend. If you believe that health is more important than wealth, you would approve of spending money on a relaxing vacation or perhaps joining a health club, rather than putting it in the bank. Often people adopt the values of individuals they admire. For example, a nursing student may begin to value humor after observing it used effectively with clients. You can see that values provide a guide for decision-making and give addi-

tional meaning to life. Individuals develop a sense of satisfaction when they work toward achieving values they believe are important.

How Values are Developed

Values are learned (Wright, 1987). Values can be taught directly, incorporated through societal norms, or modeled through behavior. Children learn by watching their parents, friends, teachers, and religious leaders. Through continuous reinforcement, children eventually learn about and then adopt values as their own. Because of the values they hold dear, people often make great demands on themselves, ignoring the personal cost. Here is an example:

David grew up in a family in which educational achievement was highly valued. Not surprisingly, he adopted this as one of his own values. At school, he worked very hard because some of the subjects did not come easily to him. When his grades did not reflect his great effort, he felt as though he had disappointed his family as well as himself. By the time David reached the age of 15, he had developed severe migraine headaches.

Values change with experience and maturity. For example, young children often value objects, such as a favorite blanket or stuffed animal. Older children are more likely to value a particular event, such as a scouting expedition. As they enter adolescence, they may value peer opinion over the opinions of their parents. Young adults often value certain ideals, such as beauty and heroism. The values of adults are formed from all of these experiences as well as from learning and thought.

The number of values that people hold is not as important as what values they consider to be important. Choices are influenced by values. The way people use their own time and money, choose friends, and pursue a career are all influenced by values.

Values Clarification

Values clarification is deciding what you believe is important. It is the process that helps people become aware of their own values. Values play an important role in everyday decision-making. For this reason, nurses need to be aware of what they value and what they do not. This process helps them to behave in a manner that is consistent with their values. Both personal and professional values can affect nurses' decisions. Understanding your values simplifies solving problems, making decisions, and developing better relationships with others when you begin to realize how they develop their values. Raths, Harmon, and Simmons (1979) suggested using a three-step model of choosing, prizing, and acting, with seven substeps, to identify your own values (Table 13–1).

You may have used this method when making the decision to go to nursing school. Today, many career options are available. For some people, nursing is a first career; for others, it may be a second career. Using the model in Table 13–1, let's analyze the valuing process:

1 Choosing. After researching alternative career options, you freely chose nursing school from a whole range of options. This choice was most likely influenced by factors such as educational achievement and abilities, finances, support and encouragement from others, time, and feelings about people.

TABLE 13–1
Values Clarification

Choosing

1 Free choice
2 Choosing from alternatives
3 Deciding after giving consideration to the consequences of each alternative

Prizing

4 Being satisfied about the choice
5 Being willing to declare the choice to others

Acting

6 Making the choice a part of one's world view and incorporating it into behavior
7 Repeating the choice

Source: Adapted from Raths L.E., Harmon, M., & Simmons, S.B. (1979). *Values and Teaching.* New York: Charles E. Merrill.

2 Prizing. Once the choice was made, you were satisfied with it and told your friends about it.

3 Acting. *You* have entered school and begun the journey to your new career. Later in your career, you may decide to return to school for a bachelor's or master's degree in nursing.

As you have progressed through school, you have probably begun to develop a new set of values—your professional values. Professional values are those established as being important in your practice, such as caring, quality of care, and ethical behaviors.

◼ Belief Systems

Belief systems are an organized way of thinking about why people exist within the universe. The purpose of belief systems is to explain such mysteries as life and death, good and evil, and health and illness. Usually these systems include an ethical code that specifies appropriate behavior. People may have a personal belief system, may participate in a religion that provides such a system, or both.

Members of primitive societies worshiped events in nature. Unable to understand the science of weather, for example, early civilizations believed these things to be under the control of someone or something that needed to be appeased, and they developed rituals and ceremonies to appease these unknown entities. They called these entities gods and believed that certain behaviors either pleased or angered the gods. Because these societies associated certain behaviors with specific outcomes, they created a belief system that enabled them to function as a group.

As higher civilizations evolved, belief systems became more complex. Archeology has provided us with evidence of the religious practices of ancient civilizations (Wack, 1992). The Aztec, Mayan, Incan, and Polynesian cultures each had a religious belief system comprised of many gods and goddesses for the same functions. The Greek, Roman, Egyptian, and Scandinavian societies believed in a hierarchy of gods as well as individual gods and goddesses. Interestingly, although given different names by different cultures, most of the deities had similar purposes. For example, Zeus was the Greek king of the gods, and Thor was the Norse god of thunder. Both used a thunderbolt as their symbol. Sociologists believe that these religions developed to explain what was then unexplainable. Human beings have a deep need to create order from chaos and to have logical explanations for events. Religion explains theologically what objective science cannot.

Along with the creation of rites and rituals, religions also developed codes of behaviors, or ethical codes. These codes contribute to the social order. There are rules regarding how to treat family members, neighbors, the young, and the old. Many religions have also developed rules regarding marriage, sexual practices, business practices, property ownership, and inheritance.

The advancement of science certainly has not made belief systems any less important. In fact, the technology explosion has created an even greater need for these systems. Technological advances often place people in situations that justify religious convictions rather than oppose them. Many religions, particularly Christianity, focus on the will of a supreme being, and technology, for example, is considered a gift that allows health care personnel to maintain the life of a loved one. Other religions, such as certain branches of Judaism, focus on free choice or free will, leaving such decisions in the hands of humankind. Many Jewish leaders believe that if genetic testing indicates, for instance, that an infant will be born with a disease such as Tay-Sachs, which causes severe suffering and ultimately death, an abortion may be an acceptable option.

Belief systems often help survivors in making decisions and living with them afterward. So far, more questions than answers have emerged from these technological advances. As science explains more and more previously unexplainable phenomena, we need beliefs and values to guide our use of this new knowledge.

Morals and Ethics

Morals

Although the terms *morals* and *ethics* are often used interchangeably, *ethics* usually refers to a standardized code as a guide to behaviors, whereas *morals* usually refers to an individual's own code for acceptable behavior. Morals arise from an individual's conscience. They act as a guide for individual behavior and are learned through instruction and socialization. You may find, for example, that you and your clients disagree on the acceptability of certain behaviors, such as premarital sex, drug use, or gambling. Even in your nursing class, you will probably encounter some disagreements because each of you has developed a personal code that defines acceptable behavior.

Ethics

Ethics is the part of philosophy that deals with the rightness or wrongness of human behavior. It is also concerned with the motives behind behaviors. *Bioethics*, specifically, is the application of ethics to issues that pertain to life and death. The implication is that judgments can be made about the rightness or goodness of health care practices.

Ethical Theories

Several ethical theories have emerged to justify moral principles (Guido, 2001). *Deontological theories* take their norms and rules from the duties individuals owe each other by goodness of the commitments they make and the roles they take upon themselves. The term *deontological* comes from the Greek word, *deon,* or duty. This theory is attributed to the 18th century philosopher, Immanuel Kant (Kant, 1949). Deontological ethics considers the intention of the action, not the consequences of the action. In other words, it is the individual's good intentions or good will (Kant, 1949) that determine the worthiness or goodness of the action.

Teleological theories take their norms or rules for behaviors from the consequences of the action. This theory is also referred to as *utilitarianism.* According to this concept, what makes an action right or wrong is its utility or usefulness. Usefulness is considered to be the amount of happiness the action carries. "Right" encompasses actions that have good outcomes, whereas "wrong" is composed of actions that result in bad outcomes. This theory had its origins with David Hume, a Scottish philosopher. According to Hume's approach, "Reason is and ought to be the slave of the passions" (Hume, 1978, p. 212). Based on this idea, ethics depend on what people want and desire. The passions determine what is right or wrong. However, individuals who hold follow teleological theory disagree on how to decide on the "rightness" or "wrongness" of an action (Guido, 2001) because individual passions differ.

Principalism is an arising theory receiving a great deal of attention in the biomedical ethics community. This theory integrates existing ethical principles and tries to resolve conflicts by relating one or more of these principles to a given situation. Ethical principles actually influence professional decision-making more than ethical theories.

Ethical Principles

Ethical codes are based on principles that can be used to judge behavior. Ethical principles assist decision-making because they are a standard for measuring actions. They may be the basis for laws, but they themselves are not laws. *Laws* are rules created by a governing body. Laws can operate because the government has the power to enforce them. They are usually quite specific, as are the punishments for disobeying them. Ethical principles are not confined to specific behaviors. They act as guides for appropriate behaviors. They also take into account the situation in which a decision must be made. You might say that ethical principles speak to the essence or fundamentals of the law, rather than to the exactness of the law (Macklin, 1987). Here is an example:

Mrs. Van Gruen, 82 years old, was admitted to the hospital in acute respiratory distress. She was diagnosed with aspiration pneumonia and soon became septic, developing adult respiratory distress syndrome. She had a living will, and her attorney was her designated health care surrogate. Her competence to make decisions was uncertain because of her illness. The physician presented the situation to the attorney, indicating that without a feeding tube and tracheostomy, Mrs. Van Gruen would die. According to the laws governing living wills and health care surrogates, the attorney could have made the decision to withhold all treatments. However, he felt he had an ethical obligation to still discuss the situation with his client. The client requested that the tracheostomy and the feeding tube be inserted, which were done.

In some situations, two or more principles may conflict with each other. Making a decision under these circumstances is very difficult. We now consider several of the ethical principles that are most important to nursing practice—autonomy, nonmaleficence, beneficence, justice, confidentiality, veracity, and accountability—and then look at some of the ethical dilemmas nurses encounter in clinical practice.

Autonomy

Autonomy is the freedom to make decisions for oneself. This ethical principle requires that nurses respect clients' rights to make their own choices about treatment. Informed consent before treatment, surgery, or participation in research is an example. To be able to make an autonomous choice, individuals need to be informed of the purpose, benefits, and risks of the procedures to which they are agreeing. Nurses accomplish this by providing information and supporting clients' choices.

Nurses are often in a position to protect a client's autonomy. They do this by ensuring that others do not interfere with the client's right to proceed with a decision. If a nurse observes that a client has insufficient information to make an appropriate choice, is being forced into a decision, or is unable to understand the consequences of the choice, then the nurse may act as a client advocate to ensure the principle of autonomy.

Sometimes nurses have difficulty with the principle of autonomy because it also requires respecting another's choice even if you disagree with it. According to the principle of autonomy, a nurse cannot replace a client's decision with his or her own, even when the nurse honestly believes that the client has made the wrong choice. A nurse can, however, discuss concerns with clients and make sure they have thought about the consequences of the decision they are about to make.

Nonmaleficence

The ethical principle of *nonmaleficence* requires that no harm be done, either deliberately or unintentionally. This rather complicated word comes from Latin roots: *non*, which means *not*; *male*, which means *bad*; and *facere*, which means *to do*.

The principle of nonmaleficence also requires that nurses protect from danger individuals who are unable to protect themselves because of their physical or mental condition. An infant, a person under anesthesia, and a person with Alzheimer's disease are examples of people with limited ability to protect themselves. We are ethically obligated to protect our clients when they are unable to protect themselves.

This obligation to do no harm extends to the nurse who for some reason is not functioning at an optimal level. For example, a nurse who is impaired by alcohol or drugs is knowingly placing clients at risk. Other nurses who observe such behavior have an ethical obligation to protect the client according to the principle of nonmaleficence.

Beneficence

The word *beneficence* also comes from Latin roots: *bene*, which means *well*, *facere*, which means *to do*.

The principle of beneficence demands that good be done for the benefit of others. For nurses, this means more than delivering competent physical or technical care. It requires helping clients meet all their needs, whether physical, social, or emotional. *Beneficence* is caring in the truest sense, and caring fuses thought, feeling, and action. It requires knowing and being truly understanding of the situation and the thoughts and ideas of the individual (Benner & Wrubel, 1989).

Sometimes physicians, nurses, and families withhold information from clients for the sake of beneficence. The problem with doing this is that it does not allow competent individuals to make their own decisions based on all available information. In an attempt to be beneficent, the principle of autonomy is violated. This is just one of many examples of the ethical dilemmas encountered in nursing practice. For instance:

Mrs. Gonzalez has just been admitted to the oncology unit with ovarian cancer. She is scheduled to begin chemotherapy treatment. Her two children and her husband have requested that the physician ensure that Mrs. Gonzalez not be told her diagnosis because they feel she would not be able to deal with it. The information is communicated to the nursing staff.

After the first treatment, Mrs. Gonzalez becomes very ill. She refuses the next treatment, stating that she didn't feel sick until she came to the hospital. She asks the nurse what could possibly be wrong with her that she needs a medicine that makes her sick when she doesn't feel sick. Only people who get cancer medicine get this sick! Mrs. Gonzalez then asks the nurse, "Do I have cancer?"

As the nurse, you understand the order that the client is not to be told her diagnosis. You also understand your role as a patient advocate.

1 To whom do you owe your duty: the family or the client?

2 How do you think you may be able to be a client advocate in this situation?

3 What information would you communicate to the family, and how can you assist them in dealing with their mother's concerns?

Justice

The principle of *justice* obliges nurses and other health care professionals to treat every person equally regardless of gender, sexual orientation, religion, ethnicity, disease, or social standing (Edge & Groves, 1994). This principle also applies in the work and educational setting. Everyone should be treated and judged by the same criteria according to this principle. Here is an example:

Found on the street by the police, Mr. Johnson was admitted through the emergency room to a medical unit.

He was in deplorable condition: his clothes are dirty and ragged, he is unshaven, and he is covered with blood. His diagnosis is chronic alcoholism, complicated by esophageal varices and end-stage liver disease. Several nursing students overheard the staff discussing Mr. Johnson. The essence of the conversation was that no one wanted to care for him because he was dirty, smelly, and brought this condition on himself. The students, upset by what they heard, went to their instructor about the situation. The instructor explained that every individual has a right to good care despite his or her economic or social position. This is the principle of justice.

Confidentiality

The principle of *confidentiality* states that anything said to nurses and other health care providers by their clients must be held in the strictest confidence. Exceptions exist only when clients give permission for the release of information or when the law requires the release of specific information. Sometimes, just sharing information without revealing an individual's name can be a breach in confidentiality if the situation and the individual are identifiable. It is important to realize that what seems like a harmless statement can become harmful if other people can piece together bits of information and identify the client.

Nurses come into contact with people from different walks of life. When working within communities, people are bound to know other people, who know other people, and so on. Individuals have lost families, jobs, and insurance coverage because nurses have shared confidential information and others have acted on that knowledge (AIDS Update Conference, 1995).

In today's electronic environment, the principle of confidentiality has become a major concern. Many health care institutions, insurance companies, and businesses use electronic media to transfer information. These institutions store sensitive and confidential information in computer databases. These databases need to have security safeguards to prevent unauthorized access. Health care institutions have addressed the situation through the use of limited access, authorization passwords, and security tracking systems. It is important to remember that even the most secure system developed is vulnerable and can be accessed by an individual who understands the complexities of computer systems.

Veracity

Veracity requires nurses to be truthful. Truth is fundamental to building a trusting relationship. Intentionally deceiving or misleading a client is a violation of this principle. Deliberately omitting a part of the truth is deception and violates the principle of veracity. This principle often creates ethical dilemmas. When is it all right to lie? Some ethicists believe it is never appropriate to deceive another individual. Others think that if another ethical principle overrides veracity, then lying is permissible. Consider this situation:

Ms. Allen has just been told that her father has Alzheimer's disease. The nurse practitioner wants to come into the home to discuss treatment. Ms. Allen refuses, saying that the nurse practitioner should under no circumstances tell her father the diagnosis. She explains to the practitioner that she is sure he will kill himself if he learns that he has Alzheimer's disease. She bases this concern on statements he has made regarding this disease.

The nurse practitioner replies that a medication is available that might help her father. However, it is available only through a research study being conducted at a nearby university. To participate in the research, the client must be informed of the purpose of the study, the medication to be given, its side effects, and follow-up procedures. Ms. Allen continues to refuse to allow her father to be told his diagnosis because she is positive he will commit suicide.

The nurse practitioner faces a dilemma: does he abide by Ms. Allen's wishes based on the principle of beneficence, or does he abide by the principle of veracity and inform his client of the diagnosis. What would you do?

Accountability

Accountability means accepting responsibility for one's actions. Nurses are accountable to their clients and to their colleagues. When providing care to clients, nurses are responsible for their own actions, good and not so good. If something was not done, do not chart or tell a colleague that it was. An example of violating accountability is the story of Anna:

Anna was a registered nurse who worked nights on an acute care unit. She was an excellent nurse, but as the acuity of the clients' conditions increased, she was unable to keep up with both clients' needs and the technology, particularly intravenous lines (IVs). She began to chart that all the IVs were infusing as they should, even when they were not. Each morning, the day shift would find that the actual infused amount did not agree with what the paperwork showed. One night, Anna allowed an entire liter to be infused in 2 hours into a client with congestive heart failure. When the day staff came on duty, they found the client expired, the bag empty, and the tubing filled with blood. Anna's IV sheet showed 800 mL left in the bag. It was not until a lawsuit was filed that Anna took responsibility for her behavior.

The idea of a standard of care evolves from the principle of accountability. Standards of care provide a ruler for measuring nursing actions.

Ethical Codes

A *code of ethics* is a formal statement of the rules of ethical behavior for a particular group of individuals. A code of ethics is one of the hallmarks of a profession. This code makes clear the behavior expected of its members.

The Code of Ethics for Nurses with Interpretive Statements provides values, standards, and principles to help nursing function as a profession. The original code was developed in 1985. In 1995, the American Nurses Association Board of Directors and the Congress on Nursing Practice initiated the *Code of Ethics Project* (ANA, 2002). The code may be viewed online at *http://www.nursingworld.org*.

Ethical codes are dynamic. They reflect the values of the profession and the society for which they were developed. Changes occur as society and technology evolve. For example, years ago no thought was ever given to do not resuscitate orders or withholding food and fluids. These things were not issues then, but the technological advances that have made it possible to keep people in a kind of twilight life, comatose and unable to participate in living in any way, have made these very important issues in health care.

It is not the purpose of ethical codes to change with every little breeze but to maintain a steady course, evolving as needed, but continuing to emphasize the basic ethical principles. Technology has increased our knowledge and skills, but our ability to make decisions regarding ourselves and those we care for is still guided by the principles of autonomy, nonmaleficence, beneficence, justice, confidentiality, veracity, and accountability.

Ethical Dilemmas

What is a dilemma? The word *dilemma* is of Greek derivation. A lemma was an animal resembling a ram and having two horns. Thus came the saying "stuck on the horns of a dilemma." The story of Hugo illustrates a hypothetical life-or-death dilemma with a touch of humor:

One day, Hugo, dressed in a bright red cape, walked through his village into the countryside. The wind caught the corners of the cape, and it was being whipped in all directions. As he walked down the dusty road, Hugo happened to pass by a lemma. Hugo's bright red cape caught the lemma's attention.

Lowering its head with its two horns poised in attack position, the animal began to chase poor Hugo down the road. Panting and exhausted, Hugo reached the end of the road to find himself blocked by a huge stone wall. He turned to face the lemma, which was ready to charge. A decision needed to be made, and Hugo's life depended on this decision. If he moved to the left, the lemma would gore his heart. If he moved to the right, the lemma would gore his liver. Alas, no matter what his decision, our friend Hugo would be "stuck on the horns of da lemma."

Like Hugo, nurses are often faced with difficult dilemmas. Also, as Hugo found, an ethical dilemma can be a choice between two unpleasant alternatives.

An ethical dilemma occurs when a problem exists that forces a choice between two or more ethical principles. Deciding in favor of one principle will violate the other. Both sides have goodness and badness to them, but neither decision satisfies all the criteria that apply. Ethical dilemmas also have the added burden of emotions. Feelings of anger, frustration, and fear often override rationality in the decision-making process. Consider the case of Mr. Sussman:

Mr. Sussman, 80 years old, was admitted to the neuro-science unit after suffering left hemispheric bleeding. He had total right hemiplegia and was completely non-responsive, with a Glasgow Coma Scale score of 8. He had been on IV fluids for 4 days, and the question of placing a percutaneous endoscopic gastrostomy (PEG) tube for enteral feedings was raised. The elder of the two children asked what the chances of recovery were. The physician explained that Mr. Sussman's current state was probably the best he could attain but that miracles happen every day and stated that tests could help in determining the prognosis. The family asked that these be performed.

After the results were in, the physician explained that the prognosis was grave, but that IV fluids were insufficient to sustain life. The PEG tube would be a necessity if the family wished to continue with food and fluids.

As the physician went down the hall, the family pulled in the nurse, Gail, who had been with Mr. Sussman during the previous 3 days and asked, "If this were your father, what would you do?" This situation became an ethical dilemma for Gail as well. If you were Gail, what would you say? Depending on your answer, what would be the possible principles that you might violate?

◻ Resolving Ethical Dilemmas Faced by Nurses

Ethical dilemmas can occur in any aspect of our lives, personal or professional. Here we focus on the resolution of professional dilemmas. The various models for resolving ethical dilemmas consist of 5 to 14 sequential steps. Each step begins with the complete understanding of the dilemma and concludes with the evaluation of the implemented decision.

The nursing process provides a helpful mechanism for finding solutions to ethical dilemmas. The first step is assessment, including identification of the problem. The simplest way to do this is to create a statement that summarizes the issue. The remainder of the process evolves from this statement (Box 13–1).

Assessment

Ask yourself, "Am I directly involved in this dilemma?" An issue is not an ethical dilemma for nurses unless they are directly involved or have been asked for their opinion about a situation. Some nurses involve themselves in situations when their opinion

> **BOX 13–1**
> **Questions to Help Resolve Ethical Dilemmas**
>
> - What are the medical facts?
> - What are the psychosocial facts?
> - What are the patients' wishes?
> - What values are in conflict?

has not been solicited. This is generally unwarranted unless the issue is a violation of the professional code of ethics.

Nurses are frequently in the position of hearing both sides of an ethical dilemma. Often, all that is asked for is an empathetic listener. At other times, when guidance is requested, we can help people work through the decision-making process (remember the principle of autonomy).

Collecting data from all the decision makers helps identify the reasoning process being used by these individuals as they struggle with the issue. The following questions assist in the information-gathering process:

- *What are the medical facts?* Find out how the physicians, physical and occupational therapists, dietitians, and your fellow nurses view the client's condition and treatment options. Speak with the client if possible, and determine his or her understanding of the situation.

- *What are the psychosocial facts?* In what emotional state is the client right now? The client's family? What kind of relationship exists between the client and his or her family? What are the client's living conditions? Who are the individuals who form the client's support system? How are they involved in the client's care? What is the client's ability to make medical decisions about his or her care? Do financial considerations need to be taken into account? What concepts or things does the client value? What does the client's family value? The answers to these questions will give you a better understanding of the situation. You may also find yourself asking more questions to complete the picture. The social facts of a situation also include institutional policies, legal aspects, and economic factors. The personal belief systems of physicians and other health care professionals also influence this aspect.

• *What are the client's wishes?* Remember the ethical principle of autonomy. With very few exceptions, if the client is competent, his or her decisions take precedence. Too often, the family's or physician's worldview and belief system overshadow that of the client. Nurses can assist by maintaining the focus on the client. If the client is unable to communicate, try to discover whether the individual has discussed the issue in the past. If the client has completed a living will or designated a health care surrogate, this will also help determine the client's wishes. By interviewing family members, the nurse often can learn about conversations in which the client voiced his or her feelings about treatment decisions. Through guided interviewing, the nurse can encourage the family to tell anecdotes that provide relevant insights into what the client's values and beliefs are.

• *What values are in conflict?* To assess values, begin by listing each person involved in the situation. Then identify the values represented by each person. You can do this by asking questions such as, "What do you feel is the most pressing issue here?" and "Tell me more about your feelings regarding this situation." In some cases, you may find little disagreement among the people involved, just a different way of expressing their beliefs. In others, however, you may discover a serious value conflict.

Planning

For planning to be successful, everyone involved in the decision must be included in the process. Thompson and Thompson (1985) listed three very specific but integrated phases of this planning:

1 *Determine the goals of treatment.* Is cure a goal, or is the goal to keep the client comfortable? Is the goal life at any cost, or is it a peaceful death at home? These goals need to be client focused, reality centered, and attainable. They should be consistent with current medical treatment and, if possible, be measurable according to an established timeframe.

2 *Identify the decision makers.* As mentioned earlier, nurses may or may not be decision makers in these health-related ethical dilemmas. It is important to know who the decision makers are and what their belief systems are. When the client is a capable participant, this task is much easier. However, people who are ill are often too exhausted to speak up for themselves or to ensure that their voices are heard. When this happens, the client needs an advocate. Family, friends, spiritual advisers, and nurses often act as advocates for clients. If the client is unable to speak for himself or herself, then someone else must speak for him or her. A family member may need to be designated as the primary decision maker, a role often called the *health care surrogate.*

The creation of living wills, establishment of advance directives, and appointment of a health care surrogate while a person is still healthy often ease the burden for the decision makers during a later crisis. Clients can exercise autonomy through these mechanisms, even though they may no longer be able to directly communicate their wishes. When these documents are not available, the information gathered during the assessment of social factors helps identify those individuals who may be able to act in the client's best interest.

3 *List and rank all the options.* Performing this task involves all the decision makers. It is sometimes helpful to begin with the least desired choice and methodically work toward the preferred treatment choice that is most likely to lead to the desired outcome. Asking all participating parties to discuss what they believe are reasonable outcomes to be attained with the use of available medical treatment often helps in the decision process. By listening to others in a controlled situation, family members and health care professionals discover that they actually want the same thing as the client and just had different ideas about how to achieve their goal.

Implementation

During the implementation phase, the client or the surrogate (substitute) decision makers and members of the health care team reach a mutually acceptable decision. This occurs through open discussion and sometimes negotiation. An example of negotiation follows:

Elena's mother has metastatic ovarian cancer. She and Elena have discussed treatment options. Her physician suggested the use of a new chemotherapeutic agent that has demonstrated success in many cases. But Elena's mother emphatically states that she has had enough and would just like to spend her remaining time doing whatever she chooses. Elena would like her mother to try the drug.

To resolve the dilemma, the oncology nurse practitioner and the physician sit down to talk with Elena and her mother. Everyone reviews the facts and expresses their feelings about the situation. Seeing Elena's distress over her decision, Elena's mother says, "OK, I will try the Taxol for 1 month. If there is no improvement after this time, I want to stop all treatment and live out the time I have with my daughter and her family." All agreed that this is a reasonable decision.

The role of the nurse during the implementation phase is to ensure that communication does not break down. Ethical dilemmas are often emotional issues, filled with guilt, sorrow, anger, and other strong emotions. These strong feelings can cause communication failures among decision makers. Remind yourself, "I am here to do what is best for this client."

Keep in mind that an ethical dilemma is not always a choice between two attractive alternatives. Many are between two unattractive, even unpleasant choices. Elena's mother's options did not include the choice she really wanted: good health and a long life.

Once an agreement is reached, the decision makers must live with it. Sometimes, an agreement is not reached because the parties cannot reconcile their conflicting belief systems or values. At other times, caregivers are unable to recognize the worth of the client's point of view. Occasionally, the client or the surrogate may make a request that is not institutionally or legally possible. In some cases, a different institution or physician may be able to honor the request. In other cases, the client or surrogate may request information from the nurse regarding illegal acts. When this happens, the nurse should sit down with the client and family and ask them to consider the consequences of their proposed actions. It may be necessary to bring other counselors into the discussion (with the client's permission) to negotiate an agreement.

Evaluation

As in the nursing process, the purpose of evaluation in resolving ethical dilemmas is to determine whether the desired outcomes have occurred. In the case of Mr. Sussman, some of the questions that could be posed by Gail to the family are as follows:

- "I have noticed the amount of time you have been spending with your father. Have you observed any changes in his condition?"

- "I see Dr. Washburn spoke to you about the test results and your father's prognosis. How do you feel about the situation?"

- "Now that Dr. Washburn has spoken to you about your father's condition, have you considered future alternatives?"

Changes in client status, availability of medical treatment, and social facts may call for reevaluation of a situation. The course of treatment may need to be altered. Continued communication and cooperation among the decision makers are essential.

Another model, the MORAL model created by Thiroux (1977) and refined for nursing by Halloran (1982), is gaining popularity at the bedside. The MORAL acronym reminds nurses of the sequential steps needed for resolving an ethical dilemma. This ethical decision-making model is easily implemented in all client care settings (Box 13–2).

Current Ethical Issues

During the fall of 1998, the well-known Dr. Jack Kevorkian (sometimes called *Dr. Death* in the press) openly admitted that at the patient's request, he gave the patient a lethal dose of medication causing the individual's death. His statement raised the consciousness of the American people and the health care system about the issues of euthanasia and assisted suicide. Do individuals have the right to consciously end their own lives when they are suffering from terminal conditions? If they are unable to perform the act themselves, should others assist them in ending their lives? Should assisted suicide be legal? We do not have answers to these difficult questions, yet clients and their families across the country face these same questions every day.

The primary goal of nursing and other health care professions is to keep people alive and well or, if we cannot do this, to help them live with their problems and die peacefully. To accomplish this end, we struggle to improve our knowledge and skills so that we can care for our clients, provide them with some quality of life, and bring them back to the state known as wellness. The costs involved in achieving this goal can be astronomical.

Questions are being raised more and more often about who should receive the benefits of this technology. Managed care and the competition for resources are also creating ethical dilemmas. Other difficult questions, such as who should pay for care when the illness may have been due to poor health care practices such as smoking or substance abuse, are also being debated.

BOX 13–2
The MORAL Model

- M   Massage the dilemma
- O   Outline the options
- R   Resolve the dilemma
- A   Act by applying the chosen option
- L   Look back and evaluate the complete process, including the actions taken

Practice Issues Related to Technology

Genetics and the Limitations of Technology

When facing issues of technology, the principles of beneficence and nonmaleficence may be in conflict. A specific technology administered with the intention of "doing good" may result in enormous suffering. Causing this type of torment is in direct conflict with the idea of "do no harm" (Burkhardt & Nathaniel, 1998). At times, this is an accepted consequence, such as the use of chemotherapy. However, the ultimate outcome in this case is that recovery is expected. In situations in which little or no improvement is expected, the issue of whether the good outweighs the bad prevails. Suffering induced by technology may include physical, spiritual, and emotional components for both the client and the families.

Today, many low birth weight infants and infants with birth defects who not so long ago would have been considered incompatible with life are maintained on machines in highly sophisticated neonatal units. This process may keep babies alive only to die several months later or may leave them with severe chronic disabilities. Children with chronic disabilities require additional medical, educational, and social services. These services are expensive and often require families to travel long distances to obtain them (Urbano, 1992).

Genetic diagnosis and gene therapy present new ethical issues for nursing. *Genetic diagnosis* is a process that involves analyzing parents or an embryo for a genetic disorder. This is usually done before in vitro fertilization with couples who have a high risk of conceiving a child with a genetic disorder. The embryos are tested and only those that are free of genetic flaws are implanted.

Genetic screening is used only as a tool to determine whether couples hold the possibility of giving birth to a genetically impaired infant. For example, in older couples it is commonplace to test for Down syndrome. In other cases, say, if a couple has one child with a genetic disorder, genetic specialists test the parents or the fetus for the presence of the gene. This leads to issues pertaining to reproductive rights. It also opens new issues: What is a disability versus a disorder, and who decides this? Is a disability a disease and does it need to be cured or prevented? The technology is also used to determine whether individuals are predisposed to certain diseases, such as breast cancer or Huntington's chorea.

Genetic engineering is the ability to change the genetic structure of an organism. Through this process, researchers have created more disease-resistant fruits and vegetables and certain medications, such as insulin. This process theoretically allows for the genetic alteration of embryos, eliminating genetic flaws and creating healthier babies. This technology enables researchers to make a brown-haired individual blonde, to change brown eyes to blue, and make a short person taller. Imagine being able to "engineer" your child. Imagine, as Aldous Huxley did in *Brave New World* (1932), being able to create a society of perfect individuals: "We also predestine and condition. We decant our babies as socialized human beings, as Alphas or Epsilons, as future sewage workers or future . . . he was going to say future World controllers but correcting himself said future directors of Hatcheries, instead" (p. 12).

The ethical implications pertaining to genetic technology are profound. For example, some questions recently raised by the Human Genome Project relate to:

• Fairness in the use of the genetic information

• Privacy and confidentiality of obtained genetic information

• Genetic testing of an individual for a specific condition due to family history:

○ Should testing be performed if no treatment is available?

○ Should parents have the right to have minors tested for adult-onset diseases?

○ Should parents have the right to use gene therapy for genetic enhancement?

The Human Genome Project is dedicated to mapping and identifying the genetic composition of humans. Scientists hope to identify and eradicate many of the genetic disorders affecting individuals. Initiated in 1990, the Human Genome Project was projected to be a 13-year effort coordinated by the U.S. Department of Energy and the National Institutes of Health. The project originally was slated to take 15 years; however, the swift technological advances accelerated the timeframe, and in February 2001, the scientists announced that they had cracked the human genetic code and accomplished the following goals (Human Genome Project Information, 2002):

• Identified all of the genes in human DNA

• Determined the sequences of the 3 billion chemical bases that make up human DNA

• Stored this information in databases

• Developed tools for data analysis

• Addressed the ethical, legal, and social issues that may arise from the project

Rapid advances in the science of genetics and its applications present new and complex ethical and policy issues for individuals, health care personnel, and society. Economics come into play because currently only those who can afford the technology have access to it. Efforts need to be directed toward creating standards that identify the uses for genetic data and the protection of human rights and confidentiality. This is truly the new frontier.

A primary responsibility of nursing is to help clients and families cope with the purposes, benefits, and limitations of the new technologies. Hospice nurses and critical care nurses help clients and their families with end-of-life decisions. Nurses will need to have knowledge about the new genetic technologies because they will fill the roles of counselors and advisers in these areas. Many nurses now work in the areas of in vitro fertilization and genetic counseling.

Professional Dilemmas

Most of this chapter has dealt with client issues, but ethical problems may involve leadership and management issues as well. What
do you do about an impaired coworker? Personal loyalties often cause conflict with professional ethics, creating an ethical dilemma.
For this reason, most nurse practice acts
address this problem today and require the
reporting of impaired professionals and providing rehabilitation for them.

Other professional dilemmas may involve
working with incompetent personnel. This
may be frustrating for both staff and management. Regulations created to protect individuals from unjustified loss of position and
the enormous amounts of paperwork, remediation, and time that must be exercised to
terminate an incompetent health care worker
often make management look the other way.

Employing institutions that provide nursing services have an obligation to establish a
process for the reporting and handling of
practices that jeopardize client safety (ANA,
1994). The behaviors of incompetent staff
place both clients and other staff members in
jeopardy, and, eventually, the incompetency
may lead to legal action that may have been
avoidable if a different approach had been
taken.

◼ Conclusion

Ethical dilemmas are becoming more common in the changing health care environment. More questions are being raised, and
fewer answers are available. New guidelines
need to be developed to assist in finding
more answers. Technology has given us
enormous power to alter the human organism and to keep the human organism alive,
but economics may force us to answer the
questions of what living is and when people
should be allowed to die. Will our society become the *Brave New World* of Aldous Huxley? Again and again the question is raised,
"Who shall live, and who shall die?" What is
your answer?

Study Question

1   What is the difference between intrinsic and extrinsic values? Make a list of
    your intrinsic values.

2   Consider a decision you made recently that was based on your values. How did
    you make your choice?

3   Describe how you could use the valuing process of choosing, prizing, and act-
    ing in making the decision considered in question 2.

4   Which of your personal values would be primary if you were assigned to care
    for a microcephalic infant whose parents have decided to withhold all food and
    fluids?

5   Consider this issue: The parents of the microcephalic infant confront you and
    ask you, "What would you do if this were your baby?" What do you think
    would be the most important thing to consider in responding to them?

Study Question *(Continued)*

6 Your friend is single and feels that her "biological clock" is ticking. She decides to undergo in vitro fertilization using donor sperm. She tells you that she has researched the donors' backgrounds extensively and wants to show you the "template" for her child. She asks for your professional opinion about this situation. How would you respond? Identify the ethical principles involved.

7 Over the past several weeks you have noticed that your closest friend, Jimmy, has not been himself at work. He is erratic and has been making poor client-care decisions. On two separate occasions you quietly intervened and "fixed" his errors. You have also noticed that he volunteers to give the pain medications to other nurses' clients, and you see him standing very close to other nurses when they remove controlled substances from the Medication Distribution Center. Today you watched him go to the Medication Distribution Center immediately after another colleague and then see him go into the men's room. Within about 20 minutes his behavior has completely changed. You suspect that he may be taking controlled substances. You and Jimmy have been friends for more than 20 years. You grew up together and went to nursing school together. You realize that if you approach him, you may jeopardize this close friendship that means a great deal to you.

Using the MORAL ethical decision-making model, devise a plan to resolve this dilemma.

Critical Thinking Exercise

Andy is employed in a hospital where nurses are now responsible for giving respiratory therapy treatments. To save money, his nurse manager has decided that they will wash out the suction traps and reuse them on other clients. All suction tubing will be fresh. Andy realizes that this is a breach of universal precautions.

1 To whom should Andy speak about this problem?

2 If Andy gets no response from the selected individual or individuals, where does he go next?

3 Which, if any, ethical principles have been violated?

4 What is Andy's responsibility in this situation?

Student Activities

1 In your clinical setting identify a possible ethical dilemma.
  ○ Describe the situation.
  ○ Identify the individuals involved.
  ○ Identify the ethical principles involved. Which ones are in conflict?

○ Choose an ethical decision-making model and map the process for implementing a resolution to the dilemma.

2 Make arrangements to attend a meeting of the hospital ethics committee.

○ Who is on the committee?

○ Are family members or clients allowed to attend the meeting?

○ Was an ethical decision-making model applied to the resolution of the issues?

○ Was the outcome what you expected? Explain your answer.

REFERENCES

AIDS Update Conference. (1995). Hollywood Memorial Hospital, Hollywood, Fla.

American Nurses Association (ANA). (2002). *Code of Ethics Project.* Washington, D.C.: ANA.

American Nurses Association (ANA). (1994). *Guidelines on Reporting Incompetent, Unethical, or Illegal Practices.* Washington, D.C.: ANA.

Benner, P., & Wrubel, J. (1989). *The Primacy of Caring: Stress and Coping in Health and Illness.* Menlo Park, Calif.: Addison Wesley.

Burkhardt, M.A., & Nathaniel, A.K. (1998). *Ethics and Issues in Contemporary Nursing.* Albany, N.Y.: Delmar.

Edge, R.S., & Groves, J.R. (1994). *The Ethics of Healthcare: A Guide for Clinical Practice.* Albany, N.Y.: Delmar.

Gordon, N. (1963). *The Death Committee.* New York: Fawcett Crest.

Guido, G.W. (2001). *Legal and Ethical Issues in Nursing,* 3rd ed. Saddle River, N.J.: Prentice- Hall.

Halloran, M.C. (1982). Rational ethical judgments utilizing a decision-making tool. *Heart and Lung,* 11(6), 566–570.

Human Genome Project. *http://www.ornl.gov/hgmis/about.html,* July 19, 2002.

Hume, D. (1978). A treatise of human nature. In Johnson, O.A. *Ethics,* 4th ed. New York: Holt, Rinehart, and Winston, p 212.

Huxley, A. (1932). *Brave New World.* New York: Harper Row Publishers.

Kant, I. (1949). *Fundamental Principles of the Metaphysics of Morals.* New York: Liberal Arts.

Macklin, R. (1987). *Mortal Choices: Ethical Dilemmas in Modern Medicine.* Boston: Houghton Mifflin.

Mappes, T.A., & Zembaty, J.S. (1991). *Biomedical Ethics,* 3rd ed. St. Louis, Mo.: McGraw-Hill.

Raths, L.E., Harmon, M., & Simmons, S.B. (1979). *Values and Teaching.* New York: Charles E. Merrill.

Steele, S.M., & Harmon, V. (1983). *Values Clarification in Nursing.* New York: Appleton-Century-Crofts.

Thiroux, J. (1977). *Ethics: Theory and Practice.* Philadelphia: MacMillan.

Thompson, J., & Thompson, H. (1985). *Bioethical Decision Making for Nurses.* New York: Appleton-Century-Crofts.

Urbano, M.T. (1992). *Preschool Children with Special Health Care Needs.* San Diego: Singular Publishing.

Wack, J. (1992). *Sociology of Religion.* Chicago: University of Chicago Press.

Webster's New World Dictionary. (2000). New York: Simon & Schuster.

Wright, R.A. (1987). *Human Values in Health Care.* St. Louis, Mo.: McGraw-Hill.

www.aacn.org/AACN/mrkt.nsf (December 26, 2002).

CHAPTER 14

Historic Leaders in Nursing

OBJECTIVES

After reading this chapter, the student should be able to:

- Discuss Florence Nightingale's contribution to the development of modern nursing.

- Describe the effect Lillian Wald and the Henry Street Settlement had on community health care.

- Describe the contributions that Margaret Sanger made to women's health and social reform.

- Discuss Mary Mahoney's contributions to the advancement of black nurses.

- Describe Adelaide Nutting's contributions to nursing education.

- Discuss the role of Mildred Montag and the development of associate degree nursing programs.

- Discuss the contributions made by Virginia Henderson to modern nursing.

- Discuss the common characteristics of these historic leaders in nursing.

- Discuss the history of men in nursing.

- Analyze how men have changed the face of modern nursing.

- Explain how nursing theory contributes to the advancement of nursing practice.

- Discuss some of the issues faced by the nursing profession over the past 100 years.

OUTLINE

Florence Nightingale
Background
Becoming a Nurse
The Need for Reform
The Crimean War
A School for Nurses
Health Care Reform
Nightingale's Contributions

Lillian Wald
Background
Turning Point
The Visiting Nurses
The Henry Street Settlement House
Other Accomplishments

Margaret Sanger
Background
Labor Reformer
A New Concern for Sanger
Contraception Reform

Mary Eliza Mahoney
Background
Nursing Education
Contribution to Nursing

Adelaide Nutting
Background
Nursing Education
Higher Education
Other Interests

Mildred Montag
Background

Virginia Henderson
Background
Contributions to 20th Century Nursing

Men in Nursing

Nursing Theory
Nursing Theory as a Basis for Practice

Conclusion

In its history, the nursing profession has had many great leaders. From these, we have chosen just seven who not only demonstrated the strengths of our historic leaders but also reflect some of the most important issues that the profession has had to face over the past 100 years or so. Each of these leaders initiated change within the social environment of her time using the theories of change and conflict resolution discussed earlier in the text.

Florence Nightingale is probably the best known of the seven. She is considered the founder of modern nursing. Nightingale changed the care of soldiers, the keeping of hospital records, the status of nurses, and even the profession itself. Her concepts of nursing care became the basis of modern theory development in nursing.

Lillian Wald, founder of the Henry Street Settlement, is a role model for contemporary community health nursing. Ms. Wald developed a model for bringing health care to the people. Her social conscience and determination to make changes in health care are a model for the modern-day health care revolution.

Margaret Sanger, a political activist like the others, is best known for her courageous fight to make birth control information available to everyone who needed or wanted it. Her fight to make Congress aware of the plight of children in the labor force is less well known but led to important changes in the child labor laws. Sanger was perhaps the first nurse lobbyist.

Mary Eliza Mahoney became the first black graduate nurse in the United States. Her professional attitude helped to change the status of black nurses in this country.

Adelaide Nutting is probably the best known example of the early leaders in nursing education in the United States.

Mildred Montag proposed two levels of nursing, and developed an associate's degree nursing program at Adelphi University.

Virginia Henderson, the last nursing leader discussed in this chapter, represents an example of the 20th century Florence Nightingale. Henderson wrote the nursing textbook used by nurse educators throughout the country for most of the 20th century.

The final section of this chapter introduces you to nursing theory: what it is, and why it is important to nursing as a profession. Nursing theory has helped nursing evolve into the scientifically based profession it is today.

As you read this chapter, you will see how each of these famous women exemplifies leadership in the nursing profession. Many of their characteristics—intelligence, courage, and foresight—are the same ones needed in today's nursing leaders.

Florence Nightingale

Background

Florence Nightingale, an English noble woman, was born in the city for which she was named, Florence, Italy, on May 12, 1820. She was the second daughter of William and Frances Nightingale. Her father was a well-educated, wealthy man who put considerable effort into the education of his two daughters (Donahue, 1985). Florence Nightingale learned French, German, and Italian in addition to her native English. Mr. Nightingale personally instructed her in mathematics, classical art, and literature. The family made extended visits to London every year, which provided opportunities for contact with people in the highest social circles. These contacts were very valuable to Ms. Nightingale in later years.

Despite her family's ability to shelter her from the meaner side of life, Nightingale had always shown an interest in the welfare of those less fortunate than herself. It seems that she was never quite content with herself, as she was described as a "sensitive, introspective, and somewhat morbid child" (Schuyler, 1992). She was driven to improve herself and the world around her. When she expressed an interest in becoming a nurse, her parents objected strenuously. They wanted her to assume the traditional role of well-to-do women of the time: marry, have children, and take her "rightful" place in society.

Becoming a Nurse

In the fall of 1847, Nightingale left England for a tour of Europe with family friends. In

Italy, she entered a convent for a retreat. This strengthened her religious beliefs, although she never converted from the Church of England to Catholicism. After this retreat, she felt that she had been called by God to help others. This experience made her more determined than ever to pursue nursing.

In 1851, Nightingale insisted on going to Kaiserswerth, Germany to obtain training in nursing. Her family gave her their permission on the condition that no one would know where she was. When she returned from Kaiserswerth, she began to work on her plan to make an impact in the health care field.

Nightingale soon left for France to work with several Catholic nursing sisters. While in France, she received an offer from the committee that regulated the Establishment for Gentlewomen During Illness, a nursing home in London for governesses who became ill. She was appointed superintendent of the home and soon had it well organized, although she did have some difficulties with the committee.

Because of her knowledge of hospitals, Nightingale was often consulted by social reformers and by physicians who also recognized the need for this new type of nurse. Nightingale was offered a position as superintendent of nurses at King's College Hospital, but her family objected so strongly that she remained at home instead, until she went to the Crimea.

The Need for Reform

Fortunately for Nightingale, it was fashionable to become involved in the reform of medical and social institutions in the middle of the 19th century. After completing the reorganization of the nursing home, she began visiting hospitals and collecting information about nurses' working conditions. In the course of doing this, she realized that to improve nurses' working conditions, she would first have to improve the nurses.

Up to this time, the guiding principle of nursing had revolved around charity. Nursing services in Europe were provided primarily by the family or by members of religious orders. These Catholic organizations experienced a decline during the Reformation, when the government closed churches and monasteries. Hospitals were no longer run for charitable reasons but because of social necessity.

Nursing lost its social standing when the religious orders declined. Nurses were no longer recruited from the respectable classes but from the lower classes of society. Women who needed to earn their keep entered domestic service, and nursing was considered a form of domestic service. Other women who could no longer earn a living by gambling or selling themselves also turned to nursing. Many came from the criminal classes. They lacked the spirit of self-sacrifice found in the religious orders, and they often abused clients. Many consoled themselves with alcohol and snuff.

The duties of a nurse in those days were to take care of the physical needs of clients and to make sure they were reasonably clean. The conditions under which they had to accomplish these tasks were less than ideal. Hospitals were dirty and unventilated. They were contaminated with infection and actually spread diseases instead of preventing them. The same bedsheets were used for several clients. The nurses dealt with people suffering from unrelenting pain, hemorrhage, infections, and gangrene (Kalisch & Kalisch, 1986).

To accomplish the needed reforms, Nightingale realized that she had to recruit her nurses from higher strata of society, as had been done in the past, and then educate them well. She concluded that this could be accomplished only by organizing a school to prepare reliable, qualified nurses.

The Crimean War

A letter written by war correspondent W.H. Russell comparing the nursing care in the British army unfavorably with that given to the French army created a tremendous stir in England. There was demand for change. In response, the secretary of war, Sir Sidney Herbert, commissioned Nightingale to go to the Crimea (a peninsula in southeastern Ukraine) to investigate conditions there and make improvements.

On October 21, 1854, Nightingale left for the Crimea with a group of nurses on the steamer *Vectis* (Griffith & Griffith, 1965). They found a disaster when they arrived. The hospital that had been built to accommodate 1700 soldiers was filled with more than 3000 wounded and critically ill men. There were no plumbing or sewage disposal facilities. The mattresses, walls, and floors were wet with human waste. Rats, lice, and maggots thrived in this filthy environment (Kalisch & Kalisch, 1986).

The nurses went right to work. They set up a kitchen, rented a house and converted it into a laundry, and hired soldiers' wives to do the laundry. Money was difficult to obtain, so Nightingale used the *Times* relief fund and her own personal funds to purchase medical supplies, food, and equipment. After the hospital had been cleaned and organized, she began to set up social services for the soldiers.

Nightingale rarely slept. She spent hours giving nursing care, wrote letters to families, prepared requests for more supplies, and reported back to London on the conditions that she had found and improved. At night, she made rounds accompanied by an 11-year-old boy who held her lamp when she sat by a dying soldier or assisted during emergency surgery. This is how she earned the title "The Lady with the Lamp" from the poet Longfellow (1868).

Despite their strenuous efforts and enormous accomplishments, the physicians and army officers resented the nurses. They regarded these nurses as intruders who interfered with their work and undermined their authority. There was also some conflict between Nightingale and Dr. John Hall, the chief of the medical staff. At one time, after Dr. Hall had been awarded the K.C.B. (Knight Commander of the Order of the Bath), Nightingale sarcastically referred to him as "Dr. Hall, K.C.B., Knight of the Crimean Burial Grounds." When Nightingale contracted Crimean fever, Hall used this as an excuse to send her back to England. However, Nightingale thwarted his resistance and eventually won over the medical staff by creating an operating room and supplying the instruments with her own resources. Although she returned to duty, she never fully recovered from the fever. She returned to England in 1865 a national heroine but remained a semi-invalid for the rest of her life.

A School for Nurses

After her return from the Crimea, Nightingale pursued two goals: reform of military health care and establishment of an official training school for nurses. The British public contributed more than $220,000 to the Nightingale Fund for the purpose of establishing the school.

Although opposed by most of the physicians in Britain, Nightingale continued her efforts, and the Nightingale Training School for Nurses opened in 1860. The school was an independent educational institution financed by the Nightingale Fund. Fifteen probationers were admitted to the first class. Their training lasted 1 year.

Although Nightingale was not an instructor at the school, she was consulted about all of the details of student selection, instruction, and organization. Her book *Notes on Nursing: What It Is and What It Is Not* established the fundamental principles of nursing. The following is an example of her writing:

On What Nursing Ought To Do
    I use the word nursing for want of a better. It has been limited to signify little more than the administration of medicines and the application of poultices. It ought to signify the proper use of air, light, warmth, cleanliness, quiet and the proper selection and administration of diet—all at the least expense of vital power to the patient. (Nightingale, 1859)

This book was one of the first nursing textbooks and is still widely quoted today. Many nursing theorists have used Nightingale's thoughts as a basis for constructing their view of nursing.

The basic principles on which the Nightingale school was founded are the following:

1 Nurses should be technically trained in schools organized for that purpose.

2 Nurses should come from homes that are of good moral standing.

Nightingale believed that schools of nursing must be independent institutions and that women who were selected to attend the schools should be from the higher levels of society. Many of Nightingale's beliefs about nursing education are still applicable today, particularly those involved with the progress of students, the use of diaries kept by students, and the need for integrating theory into clinical practice (Roberts, 1937).

The Nightingale school served as a model for nursing education. Its graduates were sought after worldwide. Many established other schools and became matrons (superintendents) in hospitals in other parts of England, the Commonwealth, and the United States. However, very few schools were able to remain financially independent of the hospitals, and therefore they lost much of their autonomy. This was in contradiction to Nightingale's philosophy that the training schools were educational institutions, not part of any service agency.

Health Care Reform

Nightingale's other goal was the improvement of military health care. As a result of her documentation of the conditions in the Crimea and the nurses' efforts to improve them, reforms were undertaken. Her work marked the beginning of modern military nursing.

Nightingale's statistics were so accurate and clearly reported that she was elected a member of the British Statistical Society, the first woman to hold this position. At their conference in 1860, she presented a paper entitled, "Miss Nightingale's Scheme for Uniform Hospital Statistics." Before this paper was written, each hospital had used its own names and classification systems for diseases.

Nightingale's continuous efforts to study and improve health care made her an expert in her day. Her opinions on these subjects were constantly solicited. This led to another publication, *Notes on Hospitals*.

For more than 40 years, Nightingale played an influential part in most of the important health care reforms of her time. At the turn of the 20th century, however, her energies had waned, and she spent most of the next 10 years confined to her home on South Street in London. She died in her sleep on August 13, 1910.

Nightingale's Contributions

Nightingale is believed to have been in error in only two areas. First, she did not believe in or appreciate the significance of the germ theory of infection, although her insistence on fresh air, physical hygiene, and environmental cleanliness certainly did a great deal to decrease the transmission of infectious diseases. Second, she did not support a central registry or testing for nurses similar to what was in place for physicians. She was convinced that this would undermine the profession and that a letter of recommendation from the school matron was sufficient to attest to the skill and character of the nurse.

Florence Nightingale was a woman of vision and determination. Her strong belief in herself and her abilities allowed her to pursue and achieve her goals. She was a political activist and a revolutionary in her time. Her accomplishments went beyond the scope of nursing and nursing education, penetrating into all aspects of health care and social reform.

Although many memorials have been established in honor of Florence Nightingale, it is the legacy she has left to all of us who follow in her footsteps that perpetuates her name. Through today's nurses, Nightingale's spirit and determination remain alive. She has handed her lamp to each of us, and we have become the keepers of the lamp.

Lillian Wald

Background

Born in Cincinnati, Ohio in 1867, Lillian Wald moved to Rochester, New York, where she spent most of her childhood. She received her education at Miss Crittenden's English and French Boarding and Day School for

Young Ladies and Little Girls. Her relatives were physicians and had a tremendous influence on her. They encouraged her to choose nursing as a career.

Wald attended the New York Hospital School of Nursing. After graduation, she worked as a nurse in the New York Juvenile Asylum. She felt a need for more medically oriented knowledge, so she entered Women's Medical College in New York.

Turning Point

During this time, Wald and a colleague, Mary Brewster, were asked to go to New York's Lower East Side to give a lecture to immigrant mothers on care of the sick. They were shocked by what they discovered there.

While showing a group of mothers how to make a bed, a child came up to Wald and asked for help. The boy took her to a squalid tenement apartment where nine poorly nourished people were living in two rooms. A woman lay on a bed. Although she was seriously ill, it was apparent that no one had attended to her needs for several days (Kalisch & Kalisch, 1986). Miss Crittenden's School had not prepared Wald for this, but she went right to work anyway. She bathed the woman, washed and changed the bedclothes, sent for a physician, and cleaned the room.

This incident was a turning point in her life. Wald left medical school and began a career as an advocate and helper of the poor and sick, joined by her friend Mary Brewster. They soon found that there were thousands of cases similar to the first, in just one small neighborhood.

The Visiting Nurses

Wald and Brewster established a settlement house in 1893 in a rented tenement apartment in a poor section of New York's Lower East Side. To be closer to their clients, they gave up their comfortable living quarters and moved into a smaller, upper-floor apartment there.

It did not take long for the women to build up a nursing practice. At first, they had to seek out the sick, but within weeks calls came to them by the hundreds. The people of the neighborhood trusted them and relied on them for help. Gradually, they also developed a reputation among the physicians and hospitals in the area, and requests to see clients came from these sources as well.

Lillian Wald and her nursing colleagues brought basic nursing care to the people in their home environments. These nurses were independent practitioners who made their own decisions and followed up on their own assessments of families' needs. Like Nightingale, they were very aware of the effect of the environment on the health of their clients and worked hard to improve their surroundings.

Wald was convinced that many illnesses resulted from causes outside individual control and that treatment needed to be holistic. She claimed that she chose the title *public health nurse* to emphasize the value of the nurse whose work was built on an understanding of the social and economic problems that inevitably accompanied the clients' ills (Bueheler-Wilkerson, 1993).

Because she had the freedom to explore alternatives for care during numerous births, illnesses, and deaths, Wald began to organize an impressive group of offerings, ranging from private relief to services from the medical establishment. She developed cooperative relationships with various organizations, which allowed her access to goods and jobs for her clients. News of her successes spread. Private physicians sought her out and referred their clients to her for service.

The Henry Street Settlement House

Within 2 years, the nurses had outgrown their original quarters. They needed larger facilities and more nurses. With the help of Jacob Schiff, a banker and philanthropist, they moved to a larger building at 265 Henry Street. This became known as the Henry Street Settlement House (Mayer, 1994). Nine graduate nurses moved in soon after.

By 1909, the Henry Street Settlement House had grown into a well-organized social services system with many departments. The staff included 37 nurses, 5 of whom were managers, and other men and women involved in carrying out the many activities of the settlement house.

Other Accomplishments

Wald is also credited with the development of school health nursing. Health conditions were so bad in the New York City schools that 15 to 20 children per school were sent home every day. These ill children were returned to school by their parents in the same condition. As a result, illnesses spread from child to child. Ringworm, scabies, and pediculosis were common.

To prove her point about the value of community health nurses, Wald set up an experiment using one nurse for 1 month in one school. During that time, the number of children dismissed from classes dropped from more than 10,000 to 1100. The New York Board of Health was so impressed that they hired nurses to continue the original nurse's work. Wald's nurses treated illnesses, explained the modes of transmission, and explained the reasons that some children had to be excluded from class and why others did not. The nurses also followed up on the children at home to prevent the recurrence of illnesses.

Wald was also responsible for organizing the Children's Bureau, the Nursing Service Division of the Metropolitan Life Insurance Company, and the Town and Country Nursing Service of the American Red Cross. Her dreams of expanding public health nursing, obtaining insurance coverage for home-based preventive care, and developing a national health nursing service have not become a reality. However, in view of today's health care demands, she was a visionary who believed that health care belongs in the community and that nurses have a vital role to play in community-based care. She died in 1940 and is remembered as one of the foremost leaders in public health nursing.

◼ Margaret Sanger

Background

Margaret Higgins was born in Corning, New York, on September 14, 1879. After recovering from tuberculosis, which she contracted while caring for her mother, she attended nursing school at the White Plains Hospital School of Nursing. In her autobiography, she described the school as rigid and at times inhuman; perhaps this gives us an indication of where her future interests would take her (Sanger, 1938). During her affiliation at the Manhattan Eye and Ear Hospital, she met William Sanger. They married and moved to a suburb of New York, where she stayed at home to raise their three children.

Labor Reformer

Sanger was very concerned about the working conditions faced by people living in poverty. Many workers were paid barely enough to buy food for themselves and their families. At that time, the income for a family with two working parents was about $12 to $14 a week. If only the father worked, earnings dropped to $8 a week. Obviously, when only the mother worked, the family income was even lower. A portion of this income was paid back to the company as rent for company housing. Food was often purchased through a company store, and very little was left for other expenses, including health care.

A major strike of industrial workers in Lawrence, Massachusetts, marked the beginning of Sanger's career as an advocate and social reformer. The workers had attempted a strike for better conditions before but conceded because of threatening starvation. If the workers went on strike, there was no money for food. Strike sympathizers in New York offered to help the workers and to take the children from Lawrence into their homes. Because of her interest in the situation of the underpaid workers and her involvement with New York laborers, Sanger was asked to assist in the evacuation of children from the unsettled and sometimes violent conditions in Lawrence. Following an outbreak of serious rioting, she was called to Washington to testify before the House Committee on Rules about the condition of the children. She testified that the children were poorly nourished, ill, ragged, and living in worse conditions than those seen in impoverished city slums.

Two months later, the owners of the mills sat down to talk with the workers and gave in to their demands. Sanger's interventions on behalf of the children had brought the workers' plight to the attention of the public and the people in Washington.

A New Concern for Sanger

In the spring of 1912, Sanger returned to work as a public health nurse. She was assigned to maternity cases on New York City's Lower East Side. One case she encountered became a turning point in her life. Sanger was caring for a 28-year-old mother of three children who had attempted to self-abort. This woman and her husband were already struggling to feed and clothe the children they had and could not afford any more. After 3 weeks, the woman had regained her health. However, during the physician's final visit to her home, he told the young woman that she had been lucky to survive this time but that if she tried to self-abort again, she would not need his services but those of a funeral director. The young woman pleaded with him for a way to prevent another pregnancy. The doctor replied, "Tell your husband to sleep on the roof" (Sanger, 1938). The young woman turned then to Sanger, who remained silent.

Three months later, Sanger was called to the same home. This time, the woman was in a coma and died within minutes of Sanger's arrival. At that moment, Sanger dedicated herself to learning about and disseminating information about birth control.

Contraception Reform

This task turned out to be far more difficult than Margaret Sanger had expected. The Comstock Act of 1873 classified birth control information as obscene. Unrewarding research at the Boston Public Library, the Library of Congress, and the New York Academy of Medicine only heightened her frustration. Very little information about birth control was available anywhere in the United States at that time.

But contraception was widely practiced in many European countries, so Sanger went to Europe. She studied methods of birth control in France, and when she returned to the United States, she began to publish a journal called *The Woman Rebel*. This journal carried articles about contraception, family planning, and other matters related to women's rights.

The first birth control clinic in the United States opened at 46 Amboy Street in Brooklyn in 1916. Sanger operated the clinic with her sister, Ethel Byrne, and another nurse, Fania Mindell. On the first day, more than 150 women asked them for help. Everything went smoothly until a policewoman masquerading as a client arrested the three women and recorded the names of all the by-now-frightened clients. To bring attention to their plight and to the closing of the clinic, Sanger refused to ride in the police wagon. Instead, she walked the mile to the courthouse.

Several weeks later, Sanger returned to a courthouse overflowing with friends and supporters to face the charges that had been filed against her. The public found it difficult to believe that this attractive mother, flanked by her two sons, was either demented or oversexed, as her adversaries had claimed. She did not deny the charges of disseminating birth control information, but she did challenge the law that made this information illegal. Because she refused to abide by that law, the judge sentenced her to 30 days in the workhouse.

After completing her 30 days, Sanger continued her work for many years. She solicited the support of wealthy women and used their help to gain financial backing to continue her fight. She delivered talks and organized meetings. In 1921, she organized the Birth Control Conference in New York (Kalisch & Kalisch, 1986). In 1928, she established the National Committee on Federal Legislation for Birth Control, which eventually became the Planned Parenthood Foundation. Sanger was also an accomplished author, writing *What Every Girl Should Know, What Every Mother Should Know,* and *Motherhood in Bondage.*

Conservative religious and political groups were the most vocal in their opposition to Sanger's work. In the end, however, Sanger won. Planned Parenthood is a thriving organization, and birth control information is available to anyone who seeks it, although some groups oppose its availability on religious or political grounds.

Sanger could fairly be labeled an early example of the liberated woman. She was independent and assertive during a time when it was considered politically incorrect for a woman to behave in such a manner. Perhaps her most important contributions to the community at large were her tenacity and her ability to bring to society's attention the needs of the poor and not just the favored few who had sufficient money. As a nurse, she represented that part of caring that operates in the political arena to bring about change to improve people's health and save lives.

◘ Mary Eliza Mahoney

Background

Mary Eliza Mahoney was the first African American registered nurse in the United States. She was born free on May 7, 1845 in Dorchester, Massachusetts; however, an unverified paper reports the official date as April 16 of the same year. She spent her growing up years living in Roxbury with her parents. She showed an interest in nursing during her adolescence. She worked for 15 years at the New England Hospital for Women and Children (now Dimock Community Health Center). She was a cook, a janitor, a washerwoman, and an unofficial nurse's assistant.

Nursing Education

In 1878, at the age of 33, she applied to the hospital's nursing program and was accepted as a student. She spent her training days washing and ironing and cleaning and scrubbing, expected competencies of that time. Sixteen months later, of the 43 who began the rigorous course, Mary and four white students were the only ones who completed it. After graduation she worked mostly as a private duty nurse. She ended her nursing career as director of an orphanage in Long Island, New York, a position she had held for a decade. She never married.

Contribution to Nursing

Mahoney recognized the need for nurses to work together to advance the status of black nurses within the profession. In 1896, Mahoney became one of the original members of a predominately white Nurses Associated Alumnae of the United States and Canada (later known as the American Nurses Association or ANA). She co-founded the National Association of Colored Graduate Nurses (NACGN). Mahoney delivered the welcoming speech at the first convention of the NACGN. She served as the association's national chaplain. Mary Eliza Mahoney died January 4, 1926. She is buried in the Woodlawn Cemetery in Everett, Massachusetts.

In 1936, the NACGN created an award in honor of Mahoney for women who contributed to racial integration in nursing. After the NACGN was dissolved in 1951, the ANA continued to offer this award to deserving black women. In 1976, 50 years after her death, Mary Eliza Mahoney was inducted into the Nursing Hall of Fame.

When she entered nurse's training, Mary Mahoney never envisioned how her simple act of becoming a nurse would change the status of black nurses and help them to attain leadership positions within the profession. Her dedication and untiring will to inspire future generations has been an inspiration to many men and women of color who remain dedicated members of the nursing profession.

◘ Adelaide Nutting

Background

Adelaide Nutting was born on November 1, 1858, in Frost Village, Quebec, Canada. She was the first graduate of the Johns Hopkins School of Nursing. During her student days, the journal *Trained Nurse* offered a $10 prize for an essay on a typhoid fever case. Nutting submitted her essay and won the prize. Her essay was printed in the March 1910 issue, but that was just the beginning for this dynamic nurse leader.

Nutting was a close friend of Isabel Hampton, the director of the Johns Hopkins School of Nursing, which Nutting attended. When Hampton resigned her position, Nutting, in 1894, became the superintendent of nurses and the principal of the School of Nursing at the Johns Hopkins Hospital in Baltimore, Maryland.

Nursing Education

Nutting established the 3-year, 8-hour per day program that became the prototype for diploma school education in nursing. She later came to believe that more background in the basic sciences was a necessity and developed a 6-month course that also became a model for other schools. Although associated with a hospital school of nursing, Nutting was convinced that nursing education would advance only if the profession developed more autonomy. Like Nightingale, Nutting believed that schools of nursing should be independent of hospital control or ownership.

Higher Education

Nutting is probably best known for her work in the creation of the Department of Nursing and Health at Teachers College of Columbia University. After leaving Johns Hopkins in 1907 to take the first chair in nursing at Columbia University, she became the first professor of nursing in the world. She held this position until 1925, when she was succeeded by Isabel Stewart, a former student and colleague.

Other Interests

Nutting was interested in many aspects of nursing. In 1918, she approached the Rockefeller Foundation to request funds for her alma mater, Johns Hopkins. During the in-

terview, she stressed the need for improvement in the education of public health nurses. This meeting led to the formation of a blue-ribbon committee that studied the situation and released a report that emphasized the need for university education of nurses.

Nutting also recognized the importance of cultivating benefactors for nursing. For example, she became very close to Frances Payne Bolton, a wealthy and influential citizen of Cleveland, Ohio. She convinced Bolton to fund an Army Nurse Training School at a time when women were being trained as aides rather than as professional nurses. Nutting opposed their training as aides because she believed that soldiers with war wounds needed professionals to care for them. The three major nursing organizations of the time supported the establishment of the school, but the U.S. War Department rejected the idea. In response, Frances Payne Bolton went to Washington to persuade the War Department to prepare the women as nurses. The Frances Payne Bolton School of Nursing at Case Western Reserve University in Cleveland, Ohio, is named after this supporter of nursing.

Nutting was committed to the promotion of nursing and nursing education. She was in the forefront of educational reform, first by establishing standards of diploma education and later by supporting the move to the university setting. One of her greatest achievements was improvement in the preparation of teachers of nursing. She realized early that the quality of nurses is greatly influenced by the quality of the teachers of nursing students.

◼ Mildred Montag

Background

During World War II, a nursing shortage became evident. To meet the demands for nurses, Congress enacted the Bolton Act of 1943. This created the United States Cadet Nurse Corps. According to the Bolton Act, nurses could be educated in less than 3 years and perform nursing duties and responsibilities as well as their counterparts from the traditional 3-year diploma schools (Applegate, 1988). Mildred Montag developed this program at Adelphi University.

After the war, the federal funds were withdrawn and the numbers of nursing graduates declined. The acute nursing shortage continued. In 1952, however, a project aimed at developing nursing education programs in junior and community colleges was discussed. Mildred Montag, now an assistant professor of nursing at Columbia Teacher's College, was appointed the project coordinator.

The timing for a change in nursing education had come. The post-war era created other job opportunities for women, and hospital-based diploma school was not a popular career choice. The health care delivery system was disease oriented, and patient-centered. New technologies had entered the field of health care (does any of this sound familiar?) requiring nurses to have a stronger background in the sciences and be able to use these technologies at the bedside.

Montag proposed two levels of nursing. She described a curriculum that would educate what she referred to as the *technical nurse.* This nurse would provide direct, safe nursing care under the supervision of the professional nurse in an acute care setting (Haase, 1990).

Associate degree nursing education has exerted a profound impact on nursing education. Today the associate degree in nursing is the primary model for the basic registered nurse education. These programs produce the majority of the nurse workforce. Montag's major achievement with this innovation in nursing education was to shift nursing education from the hospital, service-based institutions to the institutions of higher learning. The curriculum included general education courses needed to prepare the nurse for social and personal competency, as well as skill competency.

◨ Virginia Henderson

Background

Virginia Henderson was born November 30, 1897, in Kansas City, Missouri. She attended the U.S. Army School of Nursing during World War 1. Her mentor was Annie Goodrich, head of the Army School. Goodrich later became the first dean of the Yale School of Nursing. After the war, she continued her nursing career in public health in New York City and Washington, D.C.

Henderson decided to enter the realm of nursing education and took her first faculty position at the Norfolk Virginia Protestant Hospital School of Nursing. In 1929, she returned to New York and enrolled in Columbia Teacher's College to further her nursing education. Here she earned her bachelor's and master's degrees. In 1934, she joined the faculty of Columbia Teacher's College. She taught nursing at Columbia from 1934 to 1948.

In 1953, she joined the faculty of the Yale School of Nursing in New Haven, Connecticut, as a research associate and spent the last four decades of her life at this renowned institution of higher learning. While at Yale, she began a 19-year project to review nursing literature, and at Yale she published the four-volume *Nursing Studies Index*, which indexed the English-language nursing literature from 1900 through 1960.

Contributions to 20th Century Nursing

Virginia Henderson pioneered the work that is the essence of modern nursing. Her most important writing, *Principles and Practice of Nursing,* is considered the 20th century's equivalent to Nightingale's *Notes on Nursing.* Nightingale emphasized nature as the primary healer. With the advent of antibiotic therapy and other technological advances, Nightingale's work became dated (Henderson, 1955).

In her textbook revision in 1955, Henderson first offered her description of nursing: "I say that the nurse does for others what they would do for themselves if they had the strength, the will and the knowledge. But I go on to say that the nurse makes the patient independent of him or her as soon as possible" (Henderson, 1955). Henderson wrote three editions of this textbook. Unlike other nursing textbooks, this one emphasized the importance of nursing research, and not just routine nursing techniques. Nurse educators continued using the book throughout most of the 20th century.

As a nursing professional, Henderson actively participated in nursing organizations. She founded the Interagency Council on Information Resources for Nursing. She was a member of the ANA and acted as a consultant to the National Library of Medicine and the American Journal of Nursing Company. Henderson received many awards for her work and efforts to increase the status of the nursing profession. The Sigma Theta Tau International Nurses Honor Society named its library in honor of her outstanding contributions to nursing.

Henderson believed that nursing complemented the patient by giving him or her what was needed in "will or strength" to perform the daily activities and carry out the physician's treatment. She believed strongly in "getting inside the skin" of her patients as a way of knowing what he or she needed. As she said, "The nurse is temporarily the consciousness of the unconscious, the love of life for the suicidal, the leg of the amputee, the eyes of the newly blind, a means of locomotion for the infant and the knowledge and confidence of the new mother" (Henderson, 1955).

Henderson's beginnings were in public health, and this contributed to her definition of nursing. Because of this background, Henderson was a proponent of publicly financed, universally accessible health care services. Understanding that nurses maintained roots in the communities where they lived, she believed that nursing belonged in the forefront of health care reform. She also believed that nurses should take this opportunity to advance the profession by becoming leaders in developing plans for implementing accessible health care.

Today, Virginia Henderson is recognized as the "First Lady of Nursing" and is thought by many to be the most important nursing figure in the 20th century. Her colleagues refer to her as the 20th century Florence Nightingale (*http://www.ualberta.ca/~jmorris/nt/henderson.htm, 2000*). She represents the essence and the spirit of nursing in the 20th century to all of us.

Men in Nursing

Men's participation in nursing did not begin in the latter part of the 20th century. Early Egyptian priests practiced nursing. The priests who served the goddess Sekhmet held high social rank. The first nursing school in the world started in India in about 250 B.C., and only men were considered pure enough for admission.

During the Byzantine Empire, nursing was practiced primarily by men and was a separate profession (Kalisch & Kalisch, 1995). In every plague that swept through Europe, men risked their lives to provide nursing care. In 300 A.D. the Parabolani, a group of men, started a hospital to care for victims of the black plague. Two hundred years later, St. Benedict founded the Benedictine Nursing Order (Kalisch & Kalisch, 1995). Throughout the Middle Ages military, religious, and lay orders of men continued to provide nursing care.

Before the Civil War, male and female slaves were identified as "nurses." During the Civil War, the Union used mainly female nurse volunteers, although some men also filled this responsibility. Walt Whitman, for example, served as a volunteer nurse in the Union Army. The Confederate Army took a more formal stand and identified 30 men in each regiment to serve as military nurses. Charged with this responsibility, these men tended to the ill on the battlefields (Clay, 1928). During this war, more men died than in any other war in U.S. history.

The Alexian Brothers, named after St. Alexis, a 5th century nurse, were first organized in the 1300s to provide nursing care to those afflicted with the black death. In 1863, the Alexian Brothers opened their first hospital in this country to educate men as nurses. The Mills School for Nursing and St. Vincent's School for men were organized in

New York in 1888. At that time, men did not attend female nursing schools.

Nursing continued to develop as a predominantly female profession, excluding men from entering into schools of nursing and its professional organization. The Nurses Associated Alumnae of the United States and Canada held its first annual meeting in Baltimore in 1897. This organization developed into the ANA in 1911 and continued to exclude men until 1930. One of the early accomplishments of the organization was to prevent men from practicing as nurses in the military.

The Army Nurse Corps, created in 1901, barred men from serving as nurses (Kalisch & Kalisch, 1995). The U.S. military changed from predominantly male nurses to female. At the conclusion of the Korean War, the armed services permitted men to serve as military nurses (Brown, 1942).

Once men entered the military as nurses, their numbers increased in civilian nursing as well. Nursing schools admitted men into the classroom. The numbers of men in nursing gradually increased. Today, although still a comparatively small group, the number of men pursing nursing careers continues to rise. Men are attaining graduate degrees and specialty certifications in the profession. The face of nursing is changing as men continue to enhance the profession by resuming their historical role as caring, nurturing nurses.

Nursing Theory

The word *theory* comes from the Greek word *theoria*, which means to contemplate (Johnson & Webber, 2001) or think about. It provides an explanation of why something happens the way it does. Because individuals may have different thoughts as to why some things happen, often several theories about the same phenomenon may exist.

Throughout your nursing education you have come in contact with several theories, particularly those of human development. Maslow's Theory of Human Motivation is one such theory. His theory suggests that basic needs must be met before higher level needs become important. Nursing education often uses this theory to teach students priority setting in patient care.

Two other familiar theories to most nursing students are Freud's Theory of Psychosexual Development and Erickson's Psychosocial Stages of Development. Both these theories look at the same phenomenon, human development, but explain it differently. This is an example of how two individuals look at the same phenomenon, but view it differently.

Nurses use theory to help them think critically and make decisions supported by scientific principles. Nursing theory provides a knowledge base for nurses to use in decision-making. Throughout history, most of nursing care has been built on tradition and intuition and not necessarily scientific principles (Upton, 1999). For this reason, many consumers do not understand what nursing really is and what nurses really do. To establish a strong scientific nursing foundation, nurses need to conduct research to validate nursing actions.

Over the years, many nurse theorists have attempted to explain the relationship nursing has to individuals, the environment in which they live, and the concept of health. Presently, no one theory seems to be able to include the entirety of nursing.

Nursing Theory as a Basis for Practice

In the middle of the 20th century, nurses felt that theories from other disciplines could enhance nursing practice but could not effectively describe nursing practice. During this time an interest in defining nursing knowledge increased, and with more nurses receiving graduate degrees, nurse theorists evolved. These nurses started creating philosophies, or systems of basic principles, and conceptual models, picture representations of ideas and their relationships to one another, to explain nursing. As more nurses obtained doctoral degrees, research methods and data collection increased. This research supported the theoretical propositions in the nursing theories.

Defining nursing as a profession requires nurses to conduct research to increase the existing knowledge base, create new knowledge, and validate nursing theories. Original nursing research was based on the scientific method and modeled after the natural and physical sciences. Nursing theories have allowed nurses to examine human experiences and behavior responses more closely.

Although nursing research may be conducted by advanced practice nurses, practicing nurses play a major part in identifying researchable patient problems. They also help in gathering data for on-going research. It is important for practicing nurses to understand the necessity for nursing research and what part they may play in the research process.

■ Conclusion

As nursing moves forward in the 21st century, the need for courageous and innovative nurse leaders is greater than ever. Society's demand for high-quality health care at an affordable cost is a contemporary force for change. Nursing has become as diversified as the populations we serve. We began in hospitals, moved to the community, moved back into the hospitals, and are now seeing a move back to the community. Men were the earliest nurses, then left the profession and have now returned, bringing with them new ideas and leadership abilities. Nursing research has laid new foundations for nursing knowledge and nursing practice. We will be the Nightingales, Walds, Sangers, Mahoneys, Nuttings, Montags, and Hendersons of the future; the creativity and dedication of these nurses are part of all of us.

Study Questions

1   Read *Notes on Nursing: What It Is and What It Is Not* by Florence Nightingale. How much of its content is still true today?

2   If Margaret Sanger were alive today, how do you think she would view the issue of teaching schoolchildren about AIDS?

3   What do you think Lillian Wald would say about the status of hospitals and health care today?

4   How do you think Florence Nightingale would deal with a physician who is verbally abusive to the nursing staff?

5   If you had been Margaret Sanger, would you have decided to stop teaching women about birth control? Explain your answer.

6   If Adelaide Nutting visited your nursing school, what do you think she would say about it? What advice do you think she would give to your graduating class?

7   What is your definition of nursing? How does it compare to or contrast with Virginia Henderson's definition?

8   Would you define Florence Nightingale's view of nursing as an early theory? Explain your answer.

Critical Thinking Exercise

Alina went to nursing school on an Air Force scholarship. She has now received her assignment, which is to establish a comprehensive primary care and health promotion program clinic on board NASA's newest international space station. The crew is to remain on board the station for 6 months at a time. The crew will consist of all professional military men and women.

1 What medical and nursing equipment should Alina plan to have in this center?

2 What would the physical environment on board need to have to satisfy Florence Nightingale and Lillian Wald?

3 How do you believe Virginia Henderson would describe the role of the nurse in this environment?

4 How would a background in a nursing theory help her to plan for the possible interactions that may occur among the concepts of health, person, environment, and nursing?

5 Develop a possible nursing research topic for study in this situation.

Student Activities

1 Identify a researchable issue on your clinical unit. Describe the problem.

2 How would you go about researching this problem?

REFERENCES

Applegate, M. (1988). Associate degree nursing and health care. In *Perspectives of Nursing 1987–1989*. 207–219.

Brown, D. (1942). Men nurses in the U.S. Navy. *American Journal of Nursing*, 42, 499–501.

Bueheler-Wilkerson, K. (1993). Bring care to the people: Lillian Wald's legacy to public health nursing. *American Journal of Public Health*, 83, 1778–1785.

Clay, V. (1928). Home life of a Southern lady. In Albert B. Hart (ed.). *American History Told by Contemporaries*, Vol. 4. New York: Macmillan, 244.

Donahue, H.P. (1985). *Nursing, the Oldest Art*. St. Louis, Mo.: C.V. Mosby.

Griffith, G.J., & Griffith, H.J. (1965). *Jensen's History and Trends in Professional Nursing*, 5th ed. St. Louis, Mo.: C.V. Mosby.

Haase, P. (1990). The origins and rise of associate degree nursing education. Durham, N.C.: Duke University Press.

Henderson, V. (1955). *http://www.ualberta.ca/-jmorris/nt/henderson.htm*, accessed May 9, 2000. *http://www.unc.edu/ehallora/henderson.htm*, accessed May 9, 2000.

Johnson, B. M. & Webber, P.B. (2001). *An Introduction to Theory and Reasoning in Nursing*. Philadelphia: Lippincott.

Kalisch, P.A., & Kalisch, B.J. (1986). *The Advance of American Nursing*. Boston: Little, Brown.

Kalisch, P.A., & Kalish, B.J. (1995). *The Advance of American Nursing*, ed. 2. Boston: Little, Brown.

Longfellow, H.W. (1868). The lady with the lamp. In Williams, M. (1975). *How Does a Poem Mean?* Boston: Houghton Mifflin.

Mayer, S. (1994). Amelia Greenwald: Pioneer in international public health nursing. *Nursing and Health Care,* 15(2), 74–78.

Nightingale, F. (1859). *Notes on Nursing: What It Is and What It Is Not.* Reprinted 1992. Philadelphia: J.B. Lippincott.

Roberts, M. (1937). Florence Nightingale as a nurse educator. *American Journal of Nursing, 37*, 775.

Sanger, M. (1938). *Margaret Sanger: An Autobiography.* New York: W.W. Norton.

Schuyler, C.B. (1992). Florence Nightingale. In *Notes on Nursing: What It Is and What It Is Not.* Philadelphia: J.B. Lippincott.

Upton, D. (1999). How can we achieve evidence-based practice if we have a theory-practice gap in nursing today? *Journal of Advanced Nursing* 29(3), 549–555.

CHAPTER 15

Your Nursing Career

OBJECTIVES

After reading this chapter, the student should be able to:

- Evaluate personal strengths, weaknesses, opportunities, and threats using a SWOT analysis.

- Develop a résumé including objectives, qualifications, skills experience, work history, education, and training.

- Compose job search letters including cover letter, thank-you letter, and acceptance and rejection letters.

- Discuss components of the interview process.

- Discuss the factors involved in selecting the right position.

- Explain why the first year is critical to the planning of a career.

OUTLINE

Getting Started
SWOT Analysis
  Strengths
  Weaknesses
  Opportunities
  Threats
Beginning the Search
  Oral and Written Communication Skills
Researching Your Potential Employer
Writing a Résumé
Essentials of a Résumé
How to Begin
Education

OUTLINE (*Continued*)

Your Objective
Skills and Experience
Job Search Letters
Cover Letter
Thank-You Letter
Acceptance Letter
Rejection Letter
Using the Internet
The Interview Process
Initial Interview
Answering Questions
  Background Questions
  Professional Questions
  Personal Questions
Additional Points about the Interview
  Appearance
  Handshake
  Eye Contact
  Posture and Listening Skills
Asking Questions
After the Interview
The Second Interview
Making the Right Choice
Job Content
Development
Direction
Work Climate
Compensation
I Can't Find a Job (or I Moved)
The Critical First Year
Attitude and Expectations
Impressions and Relationships
Organizational Savvy
Skills and Knowledge
Advancing Your Career
Conclusion

Health care is one of the largest and fastest growing industries in the United States. By the year 2008 health services employment is projected to increase to 13,600,00 with over 2,800,000 new jobs. (Zedlitz, 2003, p. vii)

By now, you have invested considerable time, expense, and emotion into preparing for your new career. Your educational preparation, technical and clinical expertise, interpersonal and management skills, personal interests and needs, and commitment to the nursing profession will all contribute to meeting your career goals. Changes in technology and the anticipated lengthy nursing shortage will continue to affect the way in which nursing care is delivered. However, as these changes eventually work out, we believe that nurses will continue to play a major role in the delivery of health care. Successful nurses view nursing as a lifetime pursuit, not as an occupational stepping stone. As a professional nurse, you will find that the sky is the limit in terms of the opportunities and challenges.

What steps are important in strategizing your career path? This chapter deals with a most important endeavor: finding and keeping your first nursing position. The chapter begins with planning your initial search; developing a strengths, weaknesses, opportunities, and threats (SWOT) analysis; searching for available positions; and researching organizations. Also included is a section on writing a résumé and employment-related information about the interview process and selecting the first position.

■ Getting Started

Many students attending college today are adults with family, work, and personal responsibilities. On graduating with an associate degree in nursing, you may still have student loans and continued responsibilities for supporting a family. If this is so, you may be so focused on job security and a steady source of income that the idea of career planning has not even entered your mind. Besides, isn't the idea just to "get the first job"? Not exactly. The idea is to find the job that fits you and that is a good first step on the path to a lifelong career in nursing.

Searching for a job is a consideration of not only who will hire you for the first position but also what career path you will pursue. Yes, you do need to prepare for the first job but in doing so you also need to prepare yourself for your future as a professional nurse. Doing this first will decrease your chances of burnout and dissatisfaction with your chosen profession.

SWOT Analysis

Many students assume that their first position will be as a staff nurse on a medical-surgical floor. They see themselves as "putting in their year" and then moving on to what they really want to do. However, as the health care system continues to evolve and reallocate resources, this may no longer be the automatic first step for new graduates. Instead, the new graduate should focus on long-term career goals and the different avenues by which they can be reached.

Many times, your past experiences will be an asset in presenting your abilities for a particular position. A SWOT analysis plan, borrowed from the corporate world, can guide you through your own internal strengths and weaknesses, and an analysis of external opportunities and threats that may help or hinder your job search and career planning. The SWOT analysis is really an in-depth look at what will make you truly happy in your work. Although you have already made the decision to pursue nursing, knowing your strengths and weaknesses can help you select the work setting that will be personally satisfying (Ellis, 1999). Your SWOT analysis may include the following factors (Pratt, 1994).

Strengths

- Relevant work experience
- Advanced education
- Additional product knowledge
- Good communication and people skills
- Computer skills
- Self-managed learning skills
- Flexibility

Weaknesses

- Poor communication and people skills
- Inflexibility
- Lack of interest in further training
- Difficulty adapting to change
- Inability to see health care as a business

Opportunities

- Expanding markets in health care

- New applications of technology

- New products and diversification

- Increasing at-risk populations

Threats

- Increased competition among health care facilities

- Changes in government regulation

Take some time to personalize the preceding SWOT analysis. What are your strengths? What are the things that you are not so good at? What weaknesses do you need to minimize or which strengths do you need to develop as you begin your job search? What opportunities and threats exist in the health care community you are considering? Doing a SWOT analysis will help you make an initial assessment of the job market. It can be used again after you narrow down your search for that first nursing position.

Beginning the Search

It is no longer true for many nursing graduates that once they have a degree, they can get a job anywhere. As this book goes to press, we are in the midst of a nationwide nursing shortage that is predicted to last for at least 10 years. However, even with a nursing shortage, hospital mergers, emphasis on increased staff productivity, budget crises, staffing shifts, and changes in job market availability affect the numbers and types of nurses employed in various facilities and agencies. Instead of focusing on long-term job security, the career-secure employee focuses on becoming a career survivalist. A career survivalist focuses on the person, not the position. Consider the following career survivalist strategies (Waymon & Baber, 1999):

- **Be psychologically self-employed.** Your career belongs to you, not to the person who signs your paycheck. Security and advancement on the job are up to you.

Security may be elusive, but opportunities for nurses are growing every day.

- **Learn for employability.** Take personal responsibility for your career success. Learn not only for your current position but also for your next position. Employability in health care today means learning technology tools, job-specific technical skills, and people skills such as the ability to negotiate, coach, work in teams and make presentations.

- **Plan for your financial future.** Ask yourself, "How can I spend less, earn more, and manage better?" Often people make job decisions based on financial decisions, which makes them feel trapped instead of secure.

- **Develop multiple options.** The career survivalist looks at multiple options constantly. Moving up is only one option. Being aware of emerging trends in nursing, adjacent fields, lateral moves, and special projects presents other options.

- **Build a safety net.** Networking is extremely important to the career survivalist. Joining professional organizations, taking time to build long-term nursing relationships, and getting to know other career survivalists will make your career path more enjoyable and successful.

What do employers think you need to be ready to work for them? Besides passing the NCLEX examination, employers cite the following skills as desirable in job candidates (Shingleton, 1994).

Oral and Written Communication Skills

- Ability to assume responsibility

- Interpersonal skills

- Proficiency in field of study/technical competence

- Teamwork ability

- Willingness to work hard

- Leadership abilities

- Motivation, initiative, and flexibility
- Critical thinking and analytical skills
- Computer knowledge
- Problem-solving and decision-making abilities
- Self-discipline
- Organizational skills

Active job searches may include looking in a variety of places (Beatty, 1991; Hunsaker, 2001):

- Public employment agencies
- Private employment agencies
- Human resource departments
- Information from friends or relatives
- Newspapers, professional journals
- College and university career centers
- Career and job fairs
- Internet websites
- Other professionals (networking)

In recent years, three trends have emerged related to recruiting. First, employers are using more creativity by using alternative sources to increase diversity of employees. They are commonly running advertisements in minority newspapers and magazines and recruiting nurses at minority organizations. Second, employers are using more temporary help as a way to "look at" potential employees. Nursing staffing agencies are common in most areas of the county. Third, the Internet is being used more frequently for advertising and recruitment (Hunsaker, 2001).

Regardless of where you begin your search, explore the market vigorously and thoroughly. Looking only in the classified ads on Sunday morning is a limited search. Instead, speak to everyone you know about your job search. Encourage classmates and colleagues to share contacts with you, and do the same with them. Also, when possible, try to speak directly with the person who is looking for a nurse when you hear of a pos-

sible opening. The people in human resources offices (personnel) may reject a candidate on a technicality that a nurse manager would realize does not affect that person's ability to handle the job if he or she is otherwise a good match for the position. For example, experience in day surgery prepares a person to work in other surgery-related settings, but a human resources interviewer may not know this.

Try to obtain as much information as you can about the available position. Is there a match between your skills and interests and the position available? Ask yourself whether you are applying for this position because you really want it or just to gain interview experience. Be careful about going through the interview process and receiving job offers only to turn them down. Employers may share information with one another, and you could end up being denied the position you really want.

Researching Your Potential Employer

You have spent time taking a look at yourself and the climate of the health care job market. You have narrowed your choices to the organizations that really interest you. Now is the time to find out as much as possible about these organizations.

Ownership of the company may be public or private and foreign-owned or American-owned. The company may be local or regional, a small corporation or a division of a much larger corporation. Depending on the size and ownership of the company, information may be obtained from the public library, chamber of commerce, government offices, or company website. A telephone call or letter to the corporate office or local human resources department may also furnish you with valuable information on organizations of interest (Crowther, 1994). Has the organization recently gone through a merger, a reorganization, downsizing? Information from current and past employees is valuable and may provide you with more details about whether or not the organization might be suitable for you. Be wary of gossip and half-truths that may emerge, however, because they may discourage you from applying to an excellent health care facility. In other words, if you hear something negative about an organization, check it out for yourself.

You may want to obtain the mission statement of organizations that interest you. The mission statement reflects what the institution sees as important to its public image. A look at the department of nursing philosophy and objectives indicates how the nursing department defines nursing and outlines the objectives for the department; in other words, it identifies what the important goals are for nursing. The nursing philosophy and goals should reflect the mission of the organization. Where is nursing administration on the organizational chart of the institution? To whom does the chief nursing administrator report? Although much of this information may not be obtained until an interview, a preview of how the institution views itself and the value it places on nursing will help you to decide if your philosophy of health care and nursing is compatible with that of a particular organization. To find out more about a specific health care facility, you can (Zedlitz, 2003):

- Talk to nurses currently employed at the facility.

- Access the Internet website for information on the mission, philosophy, and services.

- Check out the library for newspaper and magazine articles related to the facility.

◘ Writing a Résumé

Your résumé is your personal data sheet and self-advertisement. It is the first impression the recruiter or your potential employer will have of you. Through the résumé you are selling yourself: your skills, talents, and abilities. You may decide to prepare your own résumé or have it prepared by a professional service. Regardless of who prepares it, the purpose of a résumé is clear: to get a job interview. Many people dislike the idea of

writing a résumé. After all, how can you sum up your entire career in a single page? We want to scream out at the printed page, "Hey, I am bigger than that! Look at all I have to offer!" Ultimately, this one-page summary has to work well enough to get you the position you want. Chestnut (1999) summarized résumé writing by stating, "Lighten up. Although a very important piece to the puzzle in your job search, a résumé is not the only ammunition. What's between your ears is what will ultimately lead you to your next career" (p. 28). Box 15–1 summarizes reasons for preparing a well-thought-out, up-to-date résumé.

Although we labor intensively over preparing our résumé, the truth is that most job applications live or die within 10 to 30 seconds as the receptionist or applications examiner decides whether your résumé should be forwarded to the next step or rejected. The initial screening is usually done by non-nursing personnel. Some beginning helpful tips include: (Marino, 2000 :

- Keep the résumé to one or two pages. Don't use smaller fonts to cram more information on the page.

- Your educational background goes at

BOX 15–1
Reasons for Preparing a Résumé

- Assists in completing an employment application quickly and accurately
- Demonstrates your potential
- Focuses on your strongest points
- Gives you credit for all your achievements
- Identifies you as organized, prepared, and serious about the job search
- Serves as a reminder and adds to your self-confidence during the interview
- Provides initial introduction to potential employers in seeking the interview
- Serves as a guide for the interviewer
- Functions as a tool to distribute to others who are willing to assist you in a job search

Source: Adapted from Marino, K. (2000). *Resumes for the Health Care Professional.* New York: John Wiley & Sons; and Zedlitz, R. (2003). *How to Get a Job in Health Care.* New York: Delmar Learning.

the end of the résumé unless either you are a recent graduate and your degree is stronger than your experience or you are applying for a job at an educational institution.

• State your objective. Although you know very well what position you are seeking, the receptionist doing the initial screening does not want to take the time to determine this.

• Employers care about what you can do for them and your potential future success with their company. Your résumé must answer that question.

Essentials of a Résumé

Résumés most frequently follow one of four formats: standard, chronological order, functional, or a combination. Regardless of the type of résumé, basic elements of personal information, education, work experience, qualifications for the position, and references should be included (Marino, 2000; Zedlitz, 2003):

• **Standard résumé.** The standard résumé is organized by categories. By clearly stating your personal information, job objective, work experience, education, and work skills, memberships, honors, and special skills, the employer can easily have a "snapshot" of the person requesting entrance into the workforce. This is a useful résumé for first-time employees or recent graduates.

• **Chronological résumé.** The chronological résumé lists experiences in order of time with the most recent experience listed first. This style is useful in showing stable employment without gaps or many job changes. The objective and qualifications are listed at the top.

• **Functional résumé**. The functional résumé also lists work experience but in order of importance to your job objective. List the most important work-related experience first. This is a useful format when you have gaps in employment or lack direct experience related to your ob-

jective. Figure 15–1 demonstrates a functional résumé that could be used for seeking initial employment as a registered nurse (RN)

• **Combination**. The combination résumé is a popular format, listing work experience directly related to the position but in a chronological order.

Most professional recruiters and placement services agree on the following tips in preparing a résumé (Anderson, 1992; Rodriquez & Robertson, 1992):

• *Make sure your résumé is readable.* Is the type large enough for easy reading? Are paragraphs indented or bullets used to set off information, or does the entire page look like a gray blur? Using bold headings and appropriate spacing can offer relief from lines of gray type, but be careful not to get so carried away with graphics that your résumé becomes a new art form. The paper should be an appropriate color such as cream, white, or off-white. Use easily readable fonts and a laser printer. If a good computer and printer are not available, most printing services prepare résumés at a reasonable cost.

• *Make sure the important facts are easy to spot.* Education, current employment, responsibilities, and facts to support the experience you have gained from previous positions are important. Put the strongest statements at the beginning. Avoid excessive use of the word I. If you are a new nursing graduate and have little or no job experience, list your educational background first. Remember that positions you held before you entered nursing can frequently support experience that will be relevant in your nursing career. Do let your prospective employer know how you can be contacted.

• *Do a spelling and grammar check.* Use simple terms, action verbs, and descriptive words. Check your finished résumé for spelling, style, and grammar errors. If you are not sure how something sounds, get another opinion.

Delores Wheatley
5734 Foster Road
Middleton, Indiana 46204
(907) 123-4567

Objective: Position as staff registered nurse on medical-surgical unit

HIGHLGHTS OF QUALIFICATIONS

High School Diploma, 2001
Coral Ridge High School
Dolphin Beach, Florida

Associate of Science Degree in Nursing, 2004
Howard Community College (HCC)
Middleton, Indiana
Currently enrolled in the following courses at HCC:
30-hour IV certification course
8-hour phlebotomy course
16-hour 12-lead EKG course

EXPERIENCE

Volunteer, Association for the Blind, 1998–2001
Nursing Assistant, Howard Community Hospital, 2001–2004
       (summer employment)
Special Olympics Committee, 2003–2004

QUALIFICATIONS

Experience with blind and disabled children
Pediatric inpatient experience
Ability to work as part of an interdisciplinary team
Experience with families in crisis

Figure 15–1 Sample résumé.

- *Follow the don'ts.* Don't include pictures, fancy binders, salary information, or hobbies (unless they have contributed to your work experience). Don't include personal information such as weight, marital status, and number of children. Don't repeat yourself just to make the résumé longer. A good résumé is lean and to the point and focuses on your strengths and accomplishments.

No matter which format you use, it is essential to include the following (Parker, 1989):

- A clearly stated job objective

- Highlighted qualifications

- Directly relevant skills experience

- Chronological work history

- Relevant education and training

How to Begin

Start by writing down every applicable point you can think of in the preceding five categories. Work history is usually the easiest place to begin. Arrange your work history in reverse chronological order, listing your current job first. Account for all your employable years. Short lapses in employment are acceptable, but give a brief explanation for longer periods (e.g., "maternity leave"). Include employer, dates worked (years only, e.g., 2001–2002), city, and state for each employer you list. Briefly describe the duties and responsibilities of each position. Emphasize your accomplishments, any special techniques you learned, or changes you implemented. Use action verbs, such as those listed in Table 15–1, to describe your accomplishments. Also cite any special awards or committee chairmanships. If a previous position was not in the health field, try to relate your duties and accomplishments to the position you are seeking.

Education

Next, focus on your education. Include the name and location of every educational institution you attended, the dates you attended, and the degree, diploma, or certification attained. Start with your most recent degree. It is not necessary to include your license number because you will give a copy of the license when you begin employment. If you are still waiting to sit for the NCLEX you need to indicate when you are scheduled to sit for the exam. If you are seeking additional training, such as for intravenous certification, include only what is relevant to your job objective.

Your Objective

It is now time to write your job objective. Write a clear, brief job objective. To accomplish this, ask yourself: What do I want to do? For whom or with whom? When? At what level of responsibility? For example (Parker, 1989):

- **What.** RN

- **For whom.** Pediatric patients

- **Where.** Large metropolitan hospital

- **At what level.** Staff

A new graduate's objective might read: "Position as staff nurse on a pediatric unit" or "Graduate nurse position on a pediatric unit." Do not include phrases such as "advancing to neonatal intensive care unit." Employers are trying to fill current openings and do not want be considered a stepping stone in your career.

Skills and Experience

Relevant skills and experience are included in your résumé not to describe your past but to present a "word picture of you in your proposed new job, created out of the best of your past experience" (Parker, 1989, p. 13). Begin by jotting down the major skills required for the position you are seeking. Include five or six major skills such as:

- Administration/management

- Teamwork/problem-solving

- Patient relations

- Specialty proficiency

- Technical skills

What if you were "just a housewife" for many years? First, let's do an attitude adjust-

TABLE 15–1
Action Verbs

Management Skills	*Accomplishments*
Attained	Achieved
Developed	Adapted
Improved	Coordinated
Increased	Developed
Organized	Expanded
Planned	Facilitated
Recommended	Implemented
Strengthened	Improved
Supervised	Instructed
	Reduced (losses)
	Resolved (problems)
Communication Skills	Restored
Collaborated	*Helping Skills*
Convinced	
Developed	Assessed
Enlisted	Assisted
Formulated	Clarified
Negotiated	Demonstrated
Promoted	Diagnosed
Reconciled	Expedited
Recruited	Facilitated
	Motivated
	Represented

Source: Adapted from Parker, Y. (1989). *The Damn Good Resume Guide*. Berkeley, Calif.: Ten Speed Press.

ment: you were not "just a housewife" but a family manager. Explore your role in work-related terms such as *community volunteerism, personal relations, fund-raising, counseling,* and *teaching.* A college career office, women's center, or professional résumé service can offer you assistance with analyzing the skills and talents you shared with your family and community. A student who lacks work experience has options as well. Examples of non-work experience that show marketable skills include (Eubanks, 1991; Parker, 1989):

- Working on school paper or yearbook

- Serving in student government

- Leadership positions in clubs, bands, church activities

- Community volunteerism

- Coaching sports or tutoring children in academic areas

Now that you have jotted down everything relevant about yourself, it is time to develop the highlights of your qualifications. This area could also be called the summary of qualifications or just summary. These are immodest one-liners designed to let your prospective employer know that you are qualified and talented and absolutely the best choice for the position. A typical group of highlights might include (Parker, 1989):

- Relevant experience

- Formal training and credentials, if relevant

- Significant accomplishments, very briefly stated

- One or two outstanding skills or abilities

- A reference to your values, commitment, or philosophy, if appropriate

A new graduate's highlights could read:

- Five years of experience as a licensed practical nurse in a large nursing home

- Excellent client/family relationship skills

- Experience with chronic psychiatric patients

- Strong teamwork and communication skills

- Special certification in rehabilitation and re-ambulation strategies

Tailor the résumé to the job you are seeking. Include only relevant information, such as internships, summer jobs, inter-semester experiences, and volunteer work. Even if your previous experience is not directly related to nursing, your previous work experience can show transferable skills, motivation, and your potential to be a great employee.

Regardless of how wonderful you sound on paper, if the paper itself is not quality your résumé may end up in trashcan. Do let your perspective employer know whether you have an answering machine or fax for leaving messages.

Job Search Letters

The most common job search letters are the cover letter, thank-you letter, and acceptance letter. Job search letters should be linked to the SWOT analysis you prepared earlier. Regardless of their specific purpose, letters should follow basic writing principles (Banis, 1994):

- State the purpose of your letter.

- State the most important items first and support them with facts.

- Keep the letter organized.

- Group similar items together in a paragraph, and then organize the paragraphs to flow logically.

- Business letters are formal, but they can also be personal and warm but professional.

- Avoid sending an identical form letter to everyone. Instead, personalize each letter to fit each individual situation.

- As you write the letter, keep it work-centered and employment-centered, not self-centered.

- Be direct and brief. Keep your letter to one page.

- Use the active voice and action verbs with a positive, optimistic tone.

- If possible, address your letters to a specific individual, using the correct title and business address. Letters addressed to "To Whom It May Concern" do not indicate much research or interest in your prospective employer.

- A timely (rapid) response demonstrates your knowledge of how to do business.

- Be honest. Use specific examples and evidence from your experience to support your claims.

Cover Letter

You have spent time carefully preparing the résumé that best sells you to your prospective employer. What about your cover letter? The cover letter is your introduction. If it is true that first impressions are lasting ones, the cover letter will have a significant impact on your prospective employer. The purposes of the cover letter include (Beatty, 1989):

- Acting as a transmittal letter for your résumé

- Presenting you and your credentials to the prospective employer

- Generating interest in interviewing you

Regardless of whether your cover letter will first be read by human resources personnel or by the individual nurse manager, the effectiveness of your cover letter cannot be overemphasized. A poor cover letter can eliminate you from the selection process before you even have an opportunity to compete. A sloppy, unorganized cover letter and résumé may suggest that you are sloppy and unorganized at work. A lengthy, wordy cover letter may suggest a verbose, unfocused individual (Beatty, 1991). The cover letter should include the following (Anderson, 1992):

- **State your purpose in applying and your interest in a specific position.** Identify how you learned about the position.

- **Emphasize your strongest qualifications, those that match the requirements for the position.** Provide evidence of experience and accomplishments that relate to the available position and refer to your enclosed résumé.

- **Sell yourself!** Convince this employer that you have the qualifications and motivation to perform in this position.

- **Express appreciation to the reader for consideration.**

If possible, address your cover letter to a specific person. If you do not have a name, call the health care facility and obtain the name of the human resources supervisor. If you do not have a name, create a greeting by adding the word "manager" so that your greeting reads: Dear Human Resource Manager or Dear Personnel Manager (Zedlitz, 2003, p. 19).

Figure 15–2 is an example of a cover letter.

Thank-You Letter

Thank-you letters are important but seldom used tools in a job search. You should send a thank-you letter to everyone who has helped in any way in your job search. As stated earlier, promptness is important. Thank-you letters should be sent out within 24 hours to anyone who has interviewed you. The thank-you letter (Banis, 1994, p. 4a) should be used to:

- Express appreciation

- Reemphasize your qualifications and the match between your qualifications and the available position

- Restate your interest in the position

- Provide any supplemental information not previously stated

Figure 15–3 is a sample thank-you letter.

Acceptance Letter

Write an acceptance letter to accept an offered position; confirm the terms of employment, such as salary and starting date; and

5734 Foster Road
Middleton, Indiana 46204

April 15, 2004

Ms. Joan Smith
Human Resources Manager
All Care Nursing Center
4431 Lakeside Drive
Middleton, Indiana 46204

Dear Ms. Smith:

I am applying for the registered nurse position that was advertised in the *Fort Lauderdale News* on April 14. The position seems to fit very well with my education, experience, and career interests.

Your position requires interest and experience in caring for the elderly and in IV certification. In addition to my clinical experience in the nursing program at Howard Community College (HCC), I worked as a certified nursing assistant at St. Mary's Nursing Home 25 hours/week during the 2 years I was enrolled in the HCC nursing program. My responsibilities included assisting the elderly clients with activities of daily living, including special range-of-motion and reambulation exercises. The experience of serving as a team member under the supervision of the registered nurse and physical therapist has been invaluable. I am currently enrolled in several continuing education courses at HCC. My enclosed resume provides more details about my qualifications and education.

My background and career goals seem to match your job requirements. I am confident that I can perform the duties of a registered nurse at All Care Nursing Center. I am genuinely interested in pursuing a nursing career in care of the aging. Your agency has an excellent reputation in the community, and your parent company is likewise highly respected.

I am requesting a personal interview to discuss the possibilities of employment. I will call you during the week of April 21 to request an appointment. Should you need to reach me, please call 907-123-4567 or email me at dwheatley@bellspot.com. My telephone has an answering machine. I will return your call or email promptly.

Thank you for your consideration. I look forward to talking with you.

Sincerely yours,

Delores Wheatley

Delores Wheatley

Figure 15–2 Sample cover letter.

5734 Foster Road
Middleton, Indiana 46204

April 27, 2004

Ms. Martha Berrero
Nurse Manager, 3 East
All Care Nursing Center
4431 Lakeside Drive
Middleton, Indiana 46204

Dear Ms. Berrero:

Thank you very much for interviewing me yesterday for the registered
nurse position at All Care Nursing Center. I enjoyed meeting you and
learning more about the role of the registered nurse in long-term care with
Jefferson Corporation.

My enthusiasm for the position and my interest in working with the elderly
have increased as a result of the interview. I believe that my education and
experience in long-term care fit with the job requirements. I know that
currently I can make a contribution to the care of the residents and over time
I hope to qualify as a nursing team leader.

I wish to reiterate my strong interest in working with you and your staff. I
know that All Care Nursing Center can provide the kind of opportunities I
am seeking. Please call me at 907-123-4567 if I can provide you with any
additional information.

Again, thank you for the interview and for considering me for the registered
nurse position.

Sincerely,

Delores Wheatley

Delores Wheatley

Figure 15–3 Sample thank-you letter.

reiterate the employer's decision to hire you.
The acceptance letter often follows a telephone conversation in which the terms of
employment are discussed. Figure 15–4 is a
sample acceptance letter.

Rejection Letter

Although not as common as the first three
job search letters, you should send a rejection
letter if you are declining an employment

5734 Foster Road
Middleton, Indiana 46204

May 2, 2004

Ms. Martha Berrero
Nurse Manager, 3 East
All Care Nursing Center
4431 Lakeside Drive
Middleton, Indiana 46204

Dear Ms. Berrero:

I am writing to confirm my acceptance of your employment offer of
May 1. I am delighted to be joining All Care Nursing Center. I feel
confident that I can make a significant contribution to your team, and
I appreciate the opportunity you have offered me.

As we discussed, I will report to the Personnel Office at 8 a.m. on
May 15 for new employee orientation. I will have the medical
examination, employee, and insurance forms completed when I
arrive. I understand that the starting salary will be $33.10/hour with
full benefits beginning May 15. Overtime salary in excess of 40
hours/week will be paid if you request overtime hours.

I appreciate your confidence in me and look forward to joining your
team.

Sincerely,

Delores Wheatley

Delores Wheatley

Figure 15–4 Sample acceptance letter.

offer. When rejecting an employment offer, indicate that you have given the offer careful consideration but have decided that the position does not fit your career objectives and interests at this time. As with your other letters, thank the employer for his or her consideration and offer. Figure 15–5 is a sample rejection letter.

Using the Internet

It is not uncommon to search the Internet for positions. Numerous sites either post positions or assist potential employees in matching their skills with available employment. More and more corporations are using the Internet to reach wider audiences. If you use

5734 Foster Road
Middleton, Indiana 46204

May 2, 2004

Ms. Martha Berrero
Nurse Manager, 3 East
All Care Nursing Center
4431 Lakeside Drive
Middleton, Indiana 46204

Dear Ms. Berrero:

Thank you for offering me the position of staff nurse with All Care Nursing Center. I appreciate your taking the time to give me such extensive information about the position.

There are many aspects of the position that appeal to me. Jefferson Corporation is an excellent provider of health care services throughout this area and nationwide. However, after giving it much thought, I have decided to accept another position and must therefore decline your offer.

Again, thank you for your consideration and the courtesy extended to me. I enjoyed meeting you and your staff.

Sincerely yours,

Delores Wheatley

Delores Wheatley

Figure 15–5 Sample rejection letter.

the Internet in your search, it is always wise to follow up with a hard copy of your résumé if an address is listed. Mention in your cover letter that you sent your résumé via the Internet and the date you did so. If you are using an Internet-based service, follow up with an email to ensure that your résumé was received.

◼ The Interview Process

Initial Interview

Congratulations! Your superb résumé got you (and perhaps 10 others) through the door for an interview. Your first interview may be with the nurse manager, someone in the human resources office, or an interviewer at a job fair or even over the telephone. Regardless of with whom or where you interview, preparation is the key to success.

You began the first step in the preparation process with your SWOT analysis. If you did not obtain any of the following information regarding your prospective employer at that time, it is imperative that you do it now:

- Key people in the organization

- Number of clients and employees

- Types of services provided

- Reputation in the community

You also need to review your qualifications for the position. What does your interviewer want to know about you? Consider the following:

- Why should I hire you?

- What kind of employee will you be?

- Will you get things done?

- How much will you cost the company?

- How long will you stay?

- What haven't you told us about yourself or your weaknesses?

Answering Questions

The interviewer may ask background questions, professional questions, and personal questions. If you are especially nervous about interviewing, role-play your interview with a friend or family member acting as the interviewer. Have this person help you evaluate not just what you say, but also how you say it. Voice inflection, eye contact, and friendliness are demonstrations of your enthusiasm for the position (Costlow, 1999).

Whatever the questions, know your key points and be able to explain in the interview why the company will be glad they hired you, say, 4 years from now. Never burn bridges or badmouth the former company before you leave. Personal and professional integrity will follow you from position to position. Many companies count on personal references when hiring, including those of

faculty and administrators from your nursing program. When leaving positions you held during school or on graduating from your program, it is wise not to take parting shots at someone. Doing a professional program evaluation is fine, but taking cheap shots at faculty or other employees is unacceptable (Costlow, 1999).

Background Questions

Background questions usually relate to information on your résumé. If you have no nursing experience, relate your prior school and work experience and other accomplishments in relevant ways to the position you are seeking without going through your entire autobiography with the interviewer. You may be asked to expand on the information in your résumé about your formal nursing education. Here is your opportunity to relate specific courses or clinical experiences you enjoyed, academic honors you received, and extracurricular activities or research projects you pursued.

Professional Questions

Many recruiters are looking for specifics, especially those related to skills and knowledge needed in the position available. They may start with questions related to your education, career goals, strengths, weaknesses, nursing philosophy, style, and abilities. Interviewers often open their questioning with words such as "review," "tell me," "explain," and "describe," followed by such phrases as "How did you do it?" or "Why did you do it that way?" (Mascolini & Supnick, 1993). How will you be successful with these types of questions?

When answering "what if" questions, it is especially important that you remain specific. Cite your own experiences and relate these behaviors to a demonstrated skill or strength. Examples of questions in this area include the following (Bischof, 1993):

- **What is your philosophy of nursing?** This is a frequently asked question, so you may want to think about how you would answer it. Your response should relate to the position you are seeking.

- **What is your greatest weakness?** Your greatest strength? Don't be afraid to present a weakness, but present it to your best advantage, making it sound like a desirable characteristic. Even better, discuss a weakness that is already apparent such as lack of nursing experience, stating that you recognize your lack of nursing experience but that your prior work or management experience has taught you skills that will assist you in this position. These skills might include organization, time management, team spirit, and communication. If you are asked for both strengths and weaknesses, start with your weakness, and end on a positive note with your strengths. Don't be too modest, but don't exaggerate. Relate your strengths to the prospective position. Skills such as interpersonal relationships, organization, and leadership are usually broad enough to fit most positions.

- **Where do you see yourself in 5 years?** Most interviewers want to gain insight into your long-term goals, as well as a feel for whether you are likely to use this position as a brief stop on the path to another job. It is helpful for you to have some history regarding the position in question. How long have others usually remained in this position? Your answer should reflect a career plan in tune with the organization's needs.

- **What are your educational goals?** Be honest and specific. Include both professional education such as RN or bachelor of science in nursing and continuing education courses. If you want to pursue further education in related areas, such as a foreign language or computers, include this as a goal. Indicate schools to which you have applied or in which you are already enrolled.

- **Describe your leadership style.** Be prepared to discuss your style in terms of how effectively you work with others, and give examples of how you have implemented your leadership in the past.

- **What can you contribute to this posi-**

tion? Review your SWOT analysis as well as the job description for the position before the interview. Be specific in relating your contributions to the position.

- **What are your salary requirements?** You may be asked about minimum salary range. Try to find out the prospective employer's salary range before this question comes up. Be honest about your expectations, but make it clear that you are willing to negotiate.

- **"What if" questions.** Prospective employers are increasingly using competency-based interview questions to determine people's preparation for a job. There is often no single correct answer to these questions. The interviewer may be assessing your clinical decision-making and leadership skills. Again, be concise, focusing your answer in line with the organizational philosophy and goals. If you do not know the answer, tell the interviewer how you would go about finding the answer. You cannot be expected to have all the answers before you begin a job, but you can be expected to know how to obtain the answers once you are in the position.

Personal Questions

Personal questions deal with your personality and motivation. Common questions include the following:

- How would you describe yourself? This is a standard question. Most people find it helpful to think about an answer in advance. You can repeat some of what you said in your résumé and cover letter. You do not have to provide an in-depth analysis of your personality. In fact, you should not do this.

- How would your peers describe you? Ask them! Again, be brief, describing several strengths. Forget about your weaknesses unless you are asked about them.

- What would make you happy with this position? Be prepared to discuss your needs related to your work environment.

Do you enjoy self-direction, flexible hours, and strong leadership support? Now is the time to cite specifics related to your ideal work environment.

• Describe your ideal work environment. Give this question some thought before the interview. Be specific but realistic. If the norm in your community is two RNs to a floor with licensed practical nurses and other ancillary support, do not say that you feel a total RN staff is needed for good client care.

• Describe hobbies, community activities, and recreation. Again, brevity is important. Many times this question is used to further observe the interviewee's communication and interpersonal skills.

Never pretend to be someone or something other than who or what you are. If doing this is necessary to obtain the position, then the position is not right for you.

Additional Points About the Interview

Federal, state, and local laws govern employment-related questions. Questions asked on the job application and in the interview must be related to the position advertised. Questions or statements that may lead to discrimination on the basis of age, gender, race, color, religion, or ethnicity are illegal. If you are asked a question that appears to be illegal, you may wish to take one of several approaches:

• You may answer the question, realizing that it is not a job-related question. Make it clear to the interviewer that you will answer the question even though you know it is not job-related.

• You may refuse to answer. You are within your rights but may be seen as uncooperative or confrontational.

• Examine the intent of the question and relate it to the job.

Just as important as the verbal exchanges of the interview are the nonverbal aspects.

These include appearance, handshake, eye contact, posture, and listening skills.

Appearance

Dress in business attire. For women, a skirted suit or tailored jacket dress is appropriate. Men should wear a classic suit, light-colored shirt, and conservative tie. For both men and women, gray or navy is rarely wrong. Shoes should be polished, with appropriate heels. Nails and hair for both men and women should reflect cleanliness, good grooming, and willingness to work. The 2-inch red dagger nails worn on prom night will not support an image of the professional nurse. Paint stains on the hands from a weekend of house maintenance are equally unsuitable for presenting a professional image.

Handshake

Arrive at the interview 10 minutes before your scheduled time (allow yourself a little extra time to find the place if you have not previously been there). Introduce yourself courteously to the receptionist. Stand when your name is called, smile, and shake hands firmly. If you perspire easily, wipe your palms just before handshake time.

Eye Contact

During the interview, use the interviewer's title and last name as you speak. Never use the interviewer's first name unless specifically requested to do so. Use good listening skills (all those leadership skills you've just learned). Smile and nod occasionally, making frequent eye contact. Do not fold your arms across your chest, but keep your hands at your sides or in your lap. Pay attention, and sound sure of yourself.

Posture and Listening Skills

Phrase your questions appropriately, and relate them to yourself as a candidate: "What would be my responsibility?" instead of "What are the responsibilities of the job?" Use appropriate grammar and diction. Words like "yeah," "uh-huh," "uh," "you know," or "like" are too casual for an interview.

Don't say "I guess" or "I feel" about any-thing. These words make you sound indeci-sive and wishy-washy. Remember your action verbs—I analyzed, I organized, I de-veloped. Do not evaluate your achievements as mediocre or unimpressive. (Of course, that walkathon you organized was a huge success!)

Asking Questions

At some point in the interview, you will be asked if you have any questions. Knowing what questions you want to ask is just as im-portant as having prepared answers for the interviewer's questions. The interview is as much a time for you to learn the details of the job as it is for your potential employer to find out about you. You will need to obtain spe-cific information about the job itself, includ-ing the type of clients you would be caring for, the people with whom you would be working, the salary and benefits, and your potential employer's expectations of you. Be prepared for the interviewer to say, " Is there anything else I can tell you about the job?" Jot down a few questions on an index card before going for the interview. You may want to ask a few questions based on your re-search, demonstrating knowledge about and interest in the company. In addition, you may want to ask questions similar to the ones listed next. Above all, be honest and sincere (Bhasin, 1998; Bischof, 1993; Johnson, 1999):

- What is this position's key responsibil-ity?

- What kind of person are you looking for?

- What are the challenges of the position?

- Why is this position open?

- To whom would I report directly?

- Why did the previous person leave this position?

- What is the salary for this position?

- What are the opportunities for advance-ment?

- What kind of opportunities are there for continuing education?

- What are your expectations of me as an employee?

- How, when, and by whom are evalua-tions done?

- What other opportunities for profes-sional growth are available here?

- How are promotion and advancement handled within the organization?

The following are a few additional tips about asking questions during a job inter-view:

- *Do not* begin with questions about va-cations, benefits, or sick time. This gives the impression that these are the most im-portant part of the job to you, not the work itself.

- *Do* begin with questions about the em-ployer's expectations of you. This gives the impression that you want to know how you can contribute to the organiza-tion.

- *Do* be sure you know enough about the position to make a reasonable decision about accepting an offer if one is made.

- *Do* ask questions about the organiza-tion as a whole. The information is useful to you and demonstrates that you are able to see the big picture.

- *Do* bring a list of important points to discuss to help if you are nervous.

During the interview process, there are a few "red flags" to be alert for (Tyler, 1990):

- Lots of turnover in the position

- A newly created position without a clear purpose

- An organization in transition

- A position that is not feasible for a new graduate

- A gut feeling that things are not what they seem

The exchange of information between you

and the interviewer will go more smoothly if you review Box 15–2 before the interview.

After the Interview

If the interviewer does not offer the information, ask about the next step in the process. Thank the interviewer, shake hands, and exit. If the receptionist is still there, you may quickly smile and say thank you and goodbye. Don't linger and chat, and do not forget your follow-up thank-you letter.

The Second Interview

Being invited back for a second interview means that the first interview went well and you made a favorable impression. Second visits may include a tour of the facility and meetings with a higher-level executive or a supervisor in the department in which the job opening exists and perhaps several colleagues. In preparation for the second interview, review the information about the organization and your own strengths. It does not hurt to have a few résumés and potential references available. Pointers to make your second visit successful include the following (Muha & Orgiefsky, 1994):

- Dress professionally.

- Be professional and pleasant with everyone, including secretaries and housekeeping and maintenance personnel.

- Do not smoke.

- Remember your manners.

- Avoid controversial topics for small talk.

- Obtain answers to questions you might have thought of since your first visit.

In most instances, the personnel director or nurse manager will let you know how long it will be before you are contacted again. It is appropriate to get this information before you leave the second interview. If you do receive an offer during this visit, graciously say "thank you" and ask for a little time to consider the offer (even if this is the offer you have anxiously been awaiting).

If the organization does not contact you by the expected date, don't panic. It is appropriate to call your contact person and state your continued interest and tactfully express the need to know the status of your application so that you can respond to other deadlines.

BOX 15–2
Do's and Don'ts for Interviewing

DO:
- Shake the interviewer's hand firmly and introduce yourself.
- Know the interviewer's name in advance and use it in conversation.
- Remain standing until invited to sit.
- Use eye contact.
- Let the interviewer take the lead in the conversation.
- Talk in concrete terms, relating everything to the position.
- Be specific. Responses should be in behavioral terms supported by personal experience and specific examples.
- Make connections for the interviewer. Relate your responses to the needs of the individual organization.
- Show interest in the facility.
- Ask questions about the position and the facility.
- Come across as sincere in your goals and committed to the profession.
- Indicate a willingness to start at the bottom.
- Take any examinations requested.
- Express your appreciation for the time.

DON'T
- Place your purse, briefcase, papers etc. on the interviewer's desk. Keep them in your lap or on the floor.
- Slouch in the chair.
- Play with your clothing, jewelry, or hair.
- Chew gum or smoke even if the interviewer is.
- Be evasive, interrupt, brag, or mumble.
- Gossip or badmouth former agencies, schools, or employees.

Source: Adapted from Bischof (1993); Mascolini & Supnick (1993); Krannich & Krannich (1993); Zedlitz (2003).

◼ Making the Right Choice

You have interviewed well, and now you have to decide among several job offers. Your choice not only will affect your immediate work but will also influence your future career opportunities. There are several factors to consider.

Job Content

The immediate work you will be doing should be a good match with your skills and interests. Although your work may be personally challenging and satisfying this year, what are the opportunities for growth? How will your desire for continued growth and challenge be satisfied?

Development

You should have learned from your interviews whether the initial training and orientation seem sufficient and well organized. Don't forget to inquire regarding continuing education to keep you current in your field. Is tuition reimbursement available for further education? Is management training provided, or are supervisory skills learned on the job?

Direction

Good supervision and mentors are especially important in your first position. You may be able to judge prospective supervisors throughout the interview process, but you should also try to get a broader view of the overall philosophy of supervision. You may not be working for the same supervisor in a year, but the overall management philosophy is likely to remain consistent.

Work Climate

The day-to-day work climate must make you feel comfortable. Your preference may be formal or casual, structured or unstructured, complex or simple. It is easy to observe the way people dress, the layout of the unit, and lines of communication. It is more difficult to observe company values, factors that will affect your work comfort and satisfaction over the long-term. Try to look beyond the work environment to get a feel for values. What is the unwritten message? Is there an open-door policy sending a message that "everyone is equal and important," or does the nurse manager appear too busy to be concerned with the needs of the employees? Is your supervisor the kind of person for whom you could easily work?

Compensation

In evaluating the compensation package, starting salary should be less important than the organization's philosophy on future compensation. What is the potential for salary growth? How are individual increases? Can you live on the wages being offered?

◼ I Can't Find a Job (or I Moved)

It is often said that finding the first job is the hardest. Many employers prefer to hire seasoned nurses who do not require a long orientation and mentoring. Some require new graduates to do postgraduate internships. Changes in skill mix with the implementation of various types of care delivery influence the market for the professional nurse. The new graduate may need to be armed with a variety of skills such as intravenous certification, home assessment, advanced rehabilitation skills, and various respiratory modalities to even warrant an initial interview. Keep informed about the demands of the market in your area, and be prepared to be flexible in seeking your first position. Even with the continuing nursing shortage, hiring you as a new graduate will depend on you selling yourself!

Even after all this searching and hard work, you still may not have found the position you want. You may be focusing on work arrangements or benefits rather than on the job description. Your lack of direction may come through in your résumé, cover letter, and personal presentation. You may also have unrealistic expectations for a new graduate or be trying to cut corners, ignoring the basic rules of marketing yourself discussed in this chapter. Go back to your SWOT analysis. Take another look at your résumé and cover letter. Don't be afraid to become more assertive as you start again (Culp, 1999).

◼ The Critical First Year

Why a section on the "first year"? Don't you just get a nursing license and go to work? Aren't nurses always in demand? You have worked hard to succeed in college—won't those lessons help you to succeed in your new position? Of course they will, but some of the behaviors that were rewarded in school are not rewarded on the job. There are no syllabi, study questions, or extra credit points. Only "A's" are acceptable, and there do not appear to be many completely correct answers. Discovering this has been called "reality shock" (Kramer, 1974), which is discussed elsewhere in this book. Voluminous care plans and meticulous medication cards are out; multiple responsibilities and thinking on your feet are in. What is the new graduate to do?

Your first year will be a transition year. You are no longer a college student, but you are not yet a full-fledged professional. You are the new kid on the block, and people will respond to you differently and judge you differently than when you were a student. To be successful, you have to respond differently. You may be thinking, "Oh, they always need nurses—it doesn't matter." Yes, it does matter. Many of your career opportunities will be influenced by the early impressions you make. The following section addresses what you can do to help ensure first-year success.

Attitude and Expectations

Adopt the right attitudes and adjust your expectations. Now is the time to learn the art of being new. You felt like the most important, special person during the recruitment process. Now, in the real world, neither you nor the position may be as glamorous as you once thought. In addition, although you thought you learned a lot in school, your decisions and daily performance do not always warrant an "A." Above all, people shed the company manners that they displayed when you were interviewing, and organizational politics eventually surface. Your leadership skills and commitment to teamwork will get you through this transition period.

Impressions and Relationships

Manage a good impression and build effective relationships. Remember, you are being watched: by peers, subordinates, and superiors. Because you have no track record to fall back on, impressions are magnified. Although every organization is different, most are looking for someone with good judgment, a willingness to learn, a readiness to adapt, and a respect for the expertise of more experienced employees. Most people expect you to "pay your dues" to earn respect from them.

Organizational Savvy

Develop organizational savvy. An important person in this first year is your immediate supervisor. Support this person. Find out what is important to your supervisor and what he or she needs and expects from the team. Become a team player. Present solutions, not problems, as often as you can. You want to be a good leader someday; learn first to be a good follower. Finding a mentor is another important goal of your first year. Mentors are role models and guides who encourage, counsel, teach, and advocate for their mentee. In these relationships, both the mentor and mentee receive support and encouragement (Klein & Dickenson-Hazard, 2000). Mentoring is discussed further in Chapter 10.

The spark that ignites a mentoring relationship may come from either the protégé or the mentor. Protégés often view mentors as fonts of success, a bastion of life skills they wish to learn and emulate. Mentors often see the future that is hidden in another's personality and abilities. (Klein & Dickenson-Hazard, pp. 20–21)

Skills and Knowledge

Master the skills and knowledge of the position. Technology is constantly changing, and contrary to popular belief, you did not learn everything in school. Be prepared to seek out new knowledge and skills on your own. This may entail extra hours of preparation and study, but who said that learning stopped after graduation (Holton, 1994; Johnson, 1994)?

■ Advancing Your Career

Many of the ideas presented in this chapter will continue to be helpful as you advance in your nursing career. Continuing to develop your leadership and client care skills through practice and further education will be the key to your professional growth. RNs make up 77 percent of the nurse workforce with almost 60 percent employed in hospitals. The nationwide unemployment rate for RNs is only 1.0 percent nationwide. Even with this low unemployment rate, rising vacancy rates nationwide are reported, anywhere from 13 to 20 percent. (Florida Department of Labor, 1998). The RN will be expected to develop and provide leadership to other members of the health care team while providing competent care to clients. Landing your first job within the nursing shortage may not be so difficult, but moving forward in your career will be your responsibility.

■ Conclusion

Finding your first position is more than being in the right place at the right time. It is a complex combination of learning about yourself and the organizations you are interested in and presenting your strengths and weaknesses in the most positive manner possible. Keeping the first position and using the position to grow and learn are also a planning process. Recognize that the independence and the ability to "do your own thing" that you enjoyed through college may not be the skills you need to keep you in your first position. There is an important lesson to be learned: becoming a team player and being savvy about organizational politics are as important as becoming proficient in nursing skills. Take the first step toward finding a mentor—before you know it, you will be one yourself!

Study Questions

1. Using the SWOT analysis worksheet developed for this chapter, how will you articulate your strengths and weaknesses during an interview?

2. Design a one to two-page résumé to use in seeking your first position. Develop a cover letter, thank-you letter, acceptance letter, and rejection letter that you can use during the interview process.

3. Using the interview preparation worksheet developed for this chapter, formulate responses to the questions. How comfortable do you feel answering these questions? Share your responses with other classmates to get further ideas.

4. Evaluate the job prospects in the community where you now live. What areas could you explore in seeking your first position?

5. What plans do you have for advancing your career? What plans do you have for finding a mentor?

CHAPTER 15 SELF ASSESSMENT: SWOT Analysis Worksheet

Complete the following SWOT analysis

STRENGTHS	WEAKNESSES	OPPORTUNITIES	THREATS

Critical Thinking Exercise

Paul Delane is interviewing for his first nursing position after obtaining his RN license. He has been interviewed by the nurse recruiter and is now being interviewed by the nurse manager on the pediatric floor. After a few minutes of social conversation, the nurse manager begins to ask some specific nursing-oriented questions: How would you respond if a mother of a seriously ill child asks you if her child will die? What attempts do you make to understand different cultural beliefs and their importance in health care when planning nursing care? How does your philosophy of nursing affect your ability to deliver care to children whose mothers are HIV-positive?

Paul is very flustered by these questions and responds with "it depends on the situation," "it depends on the culture," and "I don't ever discriminate."

1 What responses would have been more appropriate in this interview?

2 How could Paul have used these questions to demonstrate his strengths, experiences, and skills?

CHAPTER 15 SELF ASSESSMENT: Interview Preparation Worksheet

Based upon the information presented in this chapter, formulate your responses to the following questions. Compare your responses with two peers. What suggestions did they make that would help you in the interview?

- How would you describe yourself?

- How would your peers describe you?

- What would make you happy with this position?

- Describe your ideal work environment.

- Describe your hobbies, community activities, and recreation.

- What will you do with your children if you have to work late?

- Your husband is a physician—do you really have to work?

REFERENCES

Anderson, J. (1992). Tips on résumé writing. *Imprint,* 39(1), 30–31.

Banis, W. (1994). The art of writing job-search letters. In College Placement Council, Inc. (ed.). *Planning Job Choices.* Philadelphia: College Placement Council, 44-51.

Beatty, R. (1989). *The Perfect Cover Letter.* New York: John Wiley & Sons.

Beatty, R. (1991). *Get the Right Job in 60 Days or Less.* New York: John Wiley & Sons.

Bhasin, R. (1998). Do's and don'ts of job interviews. *Pulp & Paper,* 72(2), 37.

Bischof, J. (1993). Preparing for job interview questions. *Critical Care Nurse,* 13(4), 97–100.

Chestnut, T. (1999). Some tips on taking the fear out of résumé writing. *Phoenix Business Journal,* 19(47), 28.

Costlow, T. (1999). How not to create a good first impression. *Fairfield County Business Journal,* 38(32), 17.

Crowther, K. (1994). How to research companies. In College Placement Council, Inc. (ed.). *Planning Job Choices.* Philadelphia: College Placement Council, 27–32.

Culp, M. (1999). Now's the time to turn the corner on your job search. *San Diego Business Journal,* 20(50), 35.

Ellis, M. (1999). Self-assessment: Discovering yourself and making the best choices for you! *Black Collegian,* 30(1), 30, 3p, 1c.

Eubanks, P (1991). Experts: Making your résumé an asset. *Hospitals,* 5(20), 74.

Florida Department of Labor. Office of Labor Market Statistics (1998). *http://www.nursingworld.org/pressrel/2000/oe0502.htm* Op-Ed: Ration Nursing Care—And Patients Pay. May 1, 2000. American Nurses Association.

Holton, E. (1994). The critical first year on the job. In College Placement Council, Inc. (ed.). *Planning Job Choices.* Philadelphia: College Placement Council, 68–71.

Hunsaker, P. (2001). *Training in Management Skills.* New Jersey: Prentice-Hall

Johnson, K. (1994). Choose your first job with your whole future in mind. In College Placement Council, Inc. (ed.). *Planning Job Choices.* Philadelphia: College Placement Council, 65–67.

Johnson, K. (1999). Interview success demands research, practice, preparation. *Houston Business Journal,* 30(23), 38.

Klein, E., & Dickenson-Hazard, N. (2000). The spirit of mentoring. *Reflections on Nursing Leadership,* 26(3), 18–22.

Kramer, M. (1974). *Reality Shock: Why Nurses Leave Nursing.* St. Louis, Mo.: C.V. Mosby.

Krannich, C., & Krannich, R. (1993). *Interview for Success.* New York: Impact Publications.

Marino, K. (2000). *Resumes for the Health Care Professional.* New York: John Wiley & Sons.

Mascolini, M., & Supnick, R. (1993). Preparing students for the behavioral job interview. *Journal of Business and Technical Communication,* 7(4), 482–488.

Muha, D., & Orgiefsky, R. (1994). The 2nd interview: The plant or office visit. In College Placement Council, Inc. (ed.). *Planning Job Choices.* Philadelphia: College Placement Council, 58–60.

Parker, Y. (1989). *The Damn Good Résumé Guide.* Berkeley, Calif.: Ten Speed Press.

Pratt, C. (1994). Successful job-search strategies for the 90's. In College Placement Council, Inc. (ed.). *Planning Job Choices.* Philadelphia: College Placement Council, 15–18.

Rodriquez, K., & Robertson, D. (1992). Selling your talents with a résumé. *American Nurse,* 24(10), 27.

Shingleton, J. (1994). The job market for '94 grads. In College Placement Council, Inc. (ed.). *Planning Job Choices.* Philadelphia: College Placement Council, 19–26.

Tyler, L. (1990). Watch out for "red flags" on a job interview. *Hospitals,* 64(14), 46.

Waymon, L., & Baber, A. (1999). Surviving career. *Balance,* 3(2), 10–13.

Zedlitz, R. (2003). *How to Get a Job in Health Care.* New York: Delmar Learning

CHAPTER 16

Nursing Today

OBJECTIVES

After reading this chapter, the student should be able to:

- Identify methods nurses can use to project a positive image.

- Compare and contrast historical and current definitions of nursing.

- Describe the characteristics considered indicative of a true profession.

- Evaluate nursing based on the criteria established for the profession.

- Evaluate strengths and weaknesses of self related to professional behaviors.

- Differentiate the roles of the American Nurses Association, the National League for Nursing, and the National Organization for Associate Degree Nursing.

- Identify ways to prepare for National Council Licensure Examination for Registered Nurses (NCLEX-RN), based on a test plan.

- Identify how differentiated practice models might work in institutions in which you have done clinical rotations.

- Differentiate between the various programs that offer nursing education.

- Identify technology issues in health care currently affecting the new graduate.

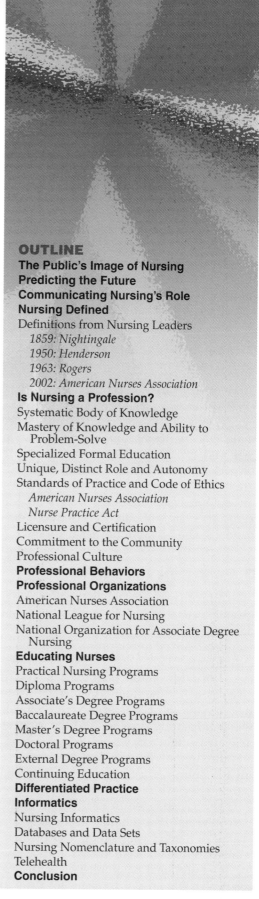

OUTLINE

The Public's Image of Nursing
Predicting the Future
Communicating Nursing's Role
Nursing Defined
Definitions from Nursing Leaders
  1859: Nightingale
  1950: Henderson
  1963: Rogers
  2002: American Nurses Association
Is Nursing a Profession?
Systematic Body of Knowledge
Mastery of Knowledge and Ability to
  Problem-Solve
Specialized Formal Education
Unique, Distinct Role and Autonomy
Standards of Practice and Code of Ethics
  American Nurses Association
  Nurse Practice Act
Licensure and Certification
Commitment to the Community
Professional Culture
Professional Behaviors
Professional Organizations
American Nurses Association
National League for Nursing
National Organization for Associate Degree
  Nursing
Educating Nurses
Practical Nursing Programs
Diploma Programs
Associate's Degree Programs
Baccalaureate Degree Programs
Master's Degree Programs
Doctoral Programs
External Degree Programs
Continuing Education
Differentiated Practice
Informatics
Nursing Informatics
Databases and Data Sets
Nursing Nomenclature and Taxonomies
Telehealth
Conclusion

What image comes to mind when the word *nurse* is mentioned? Why do most nurses continue to feel unappreciated by the public, physicians, administrators, and coworkers? Why is it still difficult to define what nursing really is?

Lack of a clear definition of the profession, control of nursing by institutions and physicians, roles of American women in society, and failure by nurses to take control of their own profession have all influenced nursing as it developed in the United States. Many of these influences continue today, as nursing moves toward achieving a clearer identity and acceptance as a true profession.

▪ The Public's Image of Nursing

More than a quarter century ago, Beletz (1974) wrote that society perceived nurses in gender-linked, task-oriented terms: "a female who performs unpleasant technical jobs and functions as an assistant to the physician" (p. 432). Although television programs and advertisements featuring nurses are more realistic than they were a decade ago, nurses are still often depicted as handmaidens who carry out physician orders.

▪ Predicting the Future

"It is difficult to predict the future of nursing, given the fact that we have not always taken advantage of opportunities. Nursing has always been forced to compromise and do the expeditious thing, or been subject to an external locus of control" (Joel, 2002, p. 11). To take charge for the future, Joel (2002) wrote that nursing must look at the environment within which nurses work and the services delivered within today's health care system, and through this examination we can identify what nurses must do and become for the future.

What has changed in health care in the past 10 years? Probably the most significant change is the growing strength of the consumer. Consumers have moved from allowing the traditional paternalistic health care establishment to make decisions for them to demanding information and participating in health care. Today, 37 million Americans "surf the Net" to find answers to health questions or to obtain information they need to help make informed decisions. Changes in the client-provider partnership are made more complex by our multicultural and multigenerational society. The silent generation of our grandparents, the huge generation of post-war baby boomers, the rising generations X and Y all bring different values, beliefs, and expectations. Table 16–1 identifies differences in the beliefs and values of the different generations (Joel, 2002).

The second significant change focuses on where health care is delivered. Over the past 20 years, the majority of health care services have migrated from the hospital to the community. All but the most intense and complicated services are provided through home care and other community-based agencies. As managed care grows, integrated services and the movement of patients across agencies have increased. The focus on the interdisciplinary team continues (Joel, 2002).

What does this have to do with nursing's future? First, it is imperative that nurses continue to build on the trust that already exists with the consumer, moving toward an even more equal relationship with the consumer. "This takes much more self-confidence than the authoritarian posture that has often been our mantra. Listen carefully to what people want, educate them to your way of thinking, accept when they knowledgeably reject your proposals, and make every attempt to get them where they ultimately want to be, even if their choices are not consistent with yours. This degree of confidence only comes with total comfort in your field of work, and that only comes with maturity and education" (Joel, 2002, p. 13). Second, nursing must be aware that the roles and activities that nurses practice today will shift, some will disappear, and others will be delegated to others. We must keep our minds open to new functions as atmosphere continues to move and change. The blending and blurring of roles demands that the practitioners have compatible educational backgrounds. Your initial nursing degree will probably be your first

TABLE 16–1
Values and Beliefs

Generation	Born Between	Beliefs, Values, and Expectations
Silent Generation	1925–1942	Is respectful of authority; holds one job until retirement; is loyal to the company; believes authority is all knowing
Baby Boomers	1943–1960	Sees authority as vulnerable, unreliable, and often just wrong; seeds of independence were planted in childhood; saw migration of women into workforce; maintains sense of autonomy; lived through the most dramatic wave of education in history
Generation X	1961–1981	Had dual-career parents; came from divorced families; majored in business and economics rather than political science and psychology; pragmatic and cynical realism have replaced the idealism of the boomers; desire balance in their lives; loyalty rests with yourself and your team, not your corporation
Generation Y	1982–present	Have values and attitudes more aligned with baby boomers; have an emerging sense of optimism and idealism; place renewed emphasis on family and religious values

Source: Adapted from Joel, L. (2002). Reflections and Projections on Nursing. *Nursing Administration Quarterly,* 26(5), 11–17.

step as you continue the lifelong learning process. The multicultural community and the specialization of health care will create roles for specialty nurses and markets for health care facilities that cater to specific ethnic groups to develop.

According to Joel (2002), the future of nursing also depends on how successful we are in resolving the current nursing shortage. Chapter 8 discussed current issues in the nursing labor market. According to the Bureau of Health Professionals, in 2000, 25% of registered nurses (RNs) did not use their licenses. More than 61% of nurses currently work part-time (Joel, 2002). Bringing these nurses back into full service to the profession and encouraging nursing as a viable profession for college-bound high school seniors continues to be a challenge. We need to continue to portray nursing as an exciting profession with status, good remuneration, and staffing adequate to provide safe, effective care.

◼ Communicating Nursing's Role

The TriCouncil (a joint effort of several professional nursing organizations) organized a campaign in 1993 designed specifically to communicate the significant contributions of nurses. Three areas in particular were emphasized (Swirsky, 1993):

1 Nurses as resource people available to interpret technical health information for consumers

2 Nurses as health care coordinators who assist consumers in identifying and using appropriate health care services

3 Nurses as expert practitioners in the provision of health care

Collectively, nurses have more potential power and influence than they currently exhibit. To be able to use this power, nurses need to become more aware of it and more skilled in its use. To improve their confidence, Hess (1993) suggested that nurses think of themselves as "special agents" who have the following responsibilities:

1 *Carry your license.* The strongest legitimate power that nurses have is the exclusive license to provide the kind of care that the public sees as vitally important. This license provides nurses with intimate access to those entrusted to their care. Your license should also be advertised in the professional appearance that you maintain. Although you may believe that people should not be judged by their appearance, they often are.

Think, for example, of how you would feel at a restaurant if the person serving you had dirty hair or fingernails.

2 *Use your special training and experience.* Only nurses know what they know. No one else in health care has their broad, specialized education and skills. Be both self-confident and respectful of others when sharing your knowledge and skills with them.

3 *Become a double agent.* Use your personal knowledge and experience to form professional and personal coalitions, both at work and elsewhere.

4 *Network and empower your colleagues.* Extend your knowledge of caring to other nurses. Nurses can help each other increase their skills and advance their careers. Empowerment is defined as "the enabling of people and groups of people to act and make decisions where an equitable distribution of power exists" (Mason, Backer, & Georges, 1993). Focusing on consensus building and group decision-making will help empower nurses.

5 *Eliminate the enemy within.* The greatest enemy is self-defeating thoughts and behaviors. Mobilize yourself and others to positively plan for change. Destructive attitudes, criticism, and manipulation of others do not foster a spirit of group collectivity and equality.

6 *Focus on operations.* No matter what level you are, participate. Instead of focusing on the problem, become part of the solution. For example, be a positive infiltrator of relevant hospital committees and professional associations.

RNs comprise the largest segment of the health care workforce. There are more than 2.5 million licensed RNs, and approximately 2 million are employed in the profession (ANA, 2002). The future of nursing depends on nurses' ability to organize as a group, recognize and accept their differences, and develop the skills necessary to negotiate and manage within the changing health care system.

◼ Nursing Defined

Definitions from Nursing Leaders

The changes that have occurred in nursing are reflected in the definitions of nursing that have been developed since the time of Florence Nightingale.

1859: Nightingale

Florence Nightingale defined the goal of nursing as putting the client "in the best possible condition for nature to act upon him" (Nightingale, 1959, p. 79).

1950: Henderson

Virginia Henderson focused her definition on the uniqueness of nursing: "The unique function of the nurse is to assist the individual, sick or well, in the performance of those activities contributing to health or its recovery (or to peaceful death) that he would perform unaided if he had the necessary strength, will or knowledge. And to do this in such a way as to help him gain independence as rapidly as possible" (Henderson, 1966, p. 21).

1963: Rogers

Martha Rogers defined nursing practice as "the process by which this body of knowledge, nursing science, is used for the purpose of assisting human beings to achieve maximum health within the potential of each person" (Rogers, 1988, p. 100). Rogers emphasized that nursing is concerned with *all* people, only a segment of whom are ill.

2002: American Nurses Association

The American Nurses Association (ANA) publishes a social policy statement on the nature and scope of nursing practice. The ANA House of Delegates periodically reviews the Code of Ethics and makes recommendations for changes. In 2001, the ANA Congress on Nursing Practice and Economics voted to accept the first full revisions in more than 25 years of the Code of Ethics (Appendix 1). The statement was intended to promote unity and allow members of the profession to develop a common approach to practice.

Is Nursing a Profession?

There is probably more agreement on what a profession is than about what occupations qualify as professions. The term *professional* is used to describe college professors, rock stars, and athletes, all with very different occupations. Several scholars have tried to identify the benchmarks of a profession (Box 16–1).

Many nursing experts talk about the "art and science of nursing." Martha Rogers (1988), for example, wrote that nursing was a science developed through scientific research and analysis and enhanced by the imagination and creativity used by nurses in applying this knowledge to client care. Can this unique service to humanity be defined as a profession? How similar is nursing to the more traditional professions of medicine, law, and the ministry? We will look at each of these characteristics of a profession in terms of the degree to which nursing has met them.

Systematic Body of Knowledge

Does nursing have its own unique, systematic body of knowledge? Those who say "no" to this question argue that nursing has

borrowed from other disciplines, such as the social sciences, biologic sciences, and medicine. These same critics believe that knowledge from these other disciplines, technical skills, intuition, and experience have been combined to become what we call nursing knowledge. Many disciplines use knowledge from other professions. Physicists use knowledge from mathematics, and pharmacists rely on their background in chemistry. Those who say "yes" argue that nursing theorists and nursing researchers have identified and described a unique body of knowledge. As the results of their work are used in practice, the unique body of knowledge will become more widely recognized.

Mastery of Knowledge and an Ability to Problem-Solve

In a true profession, members use their knowledge in a systematic, rational way. The nursing profession applies the nursing process to clinical situations. The nursing process is a systematic, problem-solving approach that involves assessment, diagnosis, planning, implementation, and evaluation.

In recent years, emphasis has also been placed on the use of critical thinking. According to Paul (1993), *critical thinking* is purposeful thinking in which the individual systematically and habitually does the following:

- Imposes the criteria of solid reasoning such as precision, relevance, depth, and accuracy

- Becomes aware of all assumptions and points of view in an argument

- Continually assesses the process of thinking

- Determines strengths and limitations and implications of the thinking

Critical thinking is an important aspect of the nursing process because the nurse must continually analyze assumptions; weigh evidence; discriminate among possible choices; evaluate conclusions; and verify beliefs, actions, and conclusions.

> **BOX 16–1**
> **Characteristics of a Profession**
>
> - Has a systematic body of knowledge
> - Requires a mastery of knowledge and an ability to problem-solve
> - Requires specialized, formal education based in colleges and universities
> - Maintains a unique, distinct role and autonomy
> - Upholds standards of practice and a code of ethics
> - Has legal enforcement and professional accountability
> - Is motivated by commitment to the community
> - Creates a professional culture
>
> Source: Adapted from Flexner, A. (1915). Is social work a profession? *Scholastic Society*, 1(20), 901; and Bixler, G.K., & Bixler, R.W. (1959). The professional status of nursing. *American Journal of Nursing*, 59, 1142–1147.

Specialized Formal Education

One of the biggest threats to the recognition of nursing as a profession is the multiple ways in which a person can prepare to become an RN. As far back as 1965, the ANA published a paper recommending the following:

The education for all of those who are licensed to practice nursing should take place in institutions of higher education; minimum preparation for beginning professional nursing practice should be a baccalaureate degree; minimum preparation for beginning technical nursing practice should be an associate degree in nursing; education for assistants in health service occupations should be short, intensive preservice programs in vocational education rather than on-the-job training. (ANA, 1965, p. 107)

Similar recommendations continue to emanate from the ANA. In 1978, the ANA House of Delegates adopted a resolution that "by 1985, the minimum preparation for entry into professional nursing practice would be the baccalaureate in nursing and ANA would work with state nurses associations to identify and define two categories of nursing practice by 1980" (ANA, 1987a, p. 2). As of this writing, graduates from all types of nursing programs—diploma, associate's degree, and baccalaureate degree—are still taking a common licensure examination, and associate's degree graduates make up the largest number entering nursing each year. With the nursing shortage projected to continue for at least a decade, any calls for changes to the education of nurses that might decrease or limit the workforce will fall on deaf ears.

In addition, many nurses who return to a university for an advanced degree are still encouraged by employers and even by fellow nurses to obtain a baccalaureate or master's degree in a field other than nursing. This is not a common practice in other professions. In fact, the ANA has also issued a statement about this practice:

Requirement of the baccalaureate for entry into professional practice, of advanced learning [master's degree] for specialty practice, administration, and teaching, and of doctoral education that includes focus on research capabilities emerges as necessary to fulfillment of nursing's social responsibility. (ANA, 1980, p. 22)

Unique, Distinct Role and Autonomy

Are nurses independent and autonomous in their implementation of nursing actions? In some institutions, nursing practice is heavily controlled by medicine or health service administration. A physician must still make simple decisions, such as whether a client can get out of bed to sit in a chair or go to the bathroom. Even in situations in which nurses are allowed to make independent decisions, the protocols may be written and approved by physicians or health care administrators. "The structure of a new delivery system presents many challenges. We can serve best when are independent thinkers and doers" (Joel, 2002, p. 17).

Standards of Practice and Code of Ethics

American Nurses Association

The ANA has provided the nursing profession with Standards of Clinical Nursing Practice. *Standards of clinical nursing practice* are "authoritative statements that describe a level of care or performance common to the profession of nursing by which the quality of nursing practice can be judged" (ANA, 1998, p. 3). More and more, these standards are used in regulatory, legislative, and legal arenas. These standards are competency based and reflect contemporary nursing practice. Written in measurable terms, standards define the nursing profession's accountability to the public and the nurses' responsibility for client outcomes.

Both the effectiveness and acceptability of professional practice standards are directly related to the extent to which they are perceived by decision-makers to be of high quality. Thus, the nursing profession must continually review and assess its standards through a rigorous, structured process that synthesizes information in the scientific literature, extends it through the knowledge of the expert, and expresses the information in statements that are clinically based, specific, precise, and comprehensive. (ANA, 1998, p. 5)

Standards of practice have been developed for all areas of nursing for use by nurses, students, faculty, health care providers, consumers, and health care policymakers. The standards may be purchased from the ANA (*www.nursingworld.org*). Appendix 2 lists the current published nursing standards.

The current Standards of Clinical Nursing Practice and the Code for Nurses enhance the ability of the profession to self-regulate and articulate the role of nursing to the public.

Nurse Practice Act

In the United States, each state is responsible for having a Nurse Practice Act that defines requirements for licensure, endorsement, exemptions, and revocation of licenses. The responsibility of boards of nursing is to protect the public through the regulation of individual licensed nurses: RNs, licensed practical nurses (LPNs), licensed vocational nurses (LVNs), and advanced registered nurse practitioners (ARNP). In some states, certified nursing assistants (CNAs) have come under regulation by the board of nursing. The practice act establishes a board of nursing and outlines the board's responsibilities. Practice acts usually contain a definition of nursing and penalties for practicing nursing without a license as well. Box 16–2 outlines the typical regulations within a Nurse Practice Act.

The State Board of Nursing is the authorized state entity with the legal authority to regulate nursing and nursing education within that state. Through legislation, the Nurse Practice Act is enacted in each state. Boards of nursing, through legislation, may

---

 BOX 16–2

The Nurse Practice Act typically:
- Defines the authority of the board of nursing
- Defines nursing boundaries and scope of practice
- Identifies types of licenses and titles
- States the requirements for licensure
- Identifies grounds for disciplinary action
- Protects titles

---

develop administrative rules and regulations to clarify or make the statutes more specific. These rules and regulations must be consistent with the Nurse Practice Act. Before any rule changes, nurses, students, and the public must be allowed to participate in open hearings to discuss changes or proposed new rules (*http://ncsbn.org/public/regulation/regulation_index.htm*). Collectively, the individual boards of nursing compose the National Council of State Boards of Nursing (*www.ncsbn.org*).

Unless a license is revoked for inappropriate behavior, licensure is permanent. Registration is usually renewed every 1 to 2 years by payment of fees to the state or states in which you desire to remain registered. Some states also require evidence of participation in continuing education for license renewal. The National Council for State Boards is currently looking into the possibility of multistate licensure. As the nursing shortage grows, the need for nurses to be mobile from state to state will increase.

Nurses with licenses from other countries must apply through the State Board of Nursing for review of their credentials before receiving permission to take the National Council Licensure Examination for Registered Nurses (NCLEX-RN) examination. Often, nurses who were educated in countries other than the United States have to return to an approved nursing program to complete additional nursing courses before receiving permission to take the examination.

The board of nursing is formed for the protection of the public, not for the protection of the licensed practitioner. Licensed nurses are responsible for providing safe and competent care. Nurses may be held legally liable for malpractice or for negligence as a result of unsafe or incompetent practice. State Boards of Nursing review all charges of misconduct and recommend disciplinary actions.

Licensure and Certification

Licensure. This is the process by which an agency of state government grants permission to an individual to engage in a given profession upon finding that the applicant has attained the essential degree of competency necessary to perform a unique scope of practice. Licensing requirements define what is necessary for the majority of individuals to be able to practice the profession safely and validate that the applicant has met those requirements. This regulatory method is used when regulated activities are complex and require specialized knowledge and skill and independent decision-making. The licensure process includes the predetermination of qualifications necessary to perform a legally defined scope of practice safely and an evaluation of licensure applications to determine that the qualifications are met. Licensure provides that a specified scope of practice may only be performed legally by licensed individuals. Licensure provides title protection for those roles. It also provides authority to take disciplinary action should the licensee violate provision of the law or rules in order to ensure that the public health, safety, and welfare will be reasonably well protected.

Certification. Certification is another type of credential that affords title protection and recognition of accomplishment, but that does not include a legal scope of practice. The federal government has used the term *certification* to define the credentialing process by which a nongovernmental agency or association recognizes individuals who have met specified requirements. Many State Boards of Nursing use such professional certification as requirements toward granting authority for advanced practice RNs. Some state government entities have also used the term *certification* for governmental credentialing. Potential for confusion exists because regulatory agencies and professional associations in different contexts may use the term certification differently (*http://www.ncsbn.org/public/regulation/licensure.htm*).

Graduates of nursing programs become licensed when they have successfully completed the NCLEX-RN examination. The National Council of State Boards of Nursing, develops a licensure examination, the (NCLEX-RN), which is used by state and territorial boards of nursing to assist in making licensure decisions. The NCLEX-RN examination is based on current entry-level nursing practice. The nursing behaviors tested are categorized within the nursing process: assessment, diagnosis, planning, implementation, and evaluation. Nurses licensed to practice in one state may request permission to practice in another state. This procedure is called *endorsement* and indicates that the state will accept the registered professional for licensure without additional requirements. To be eligible to sit for the NCLEX-RN, students must be graduates of a state-approved school of nursing.

In the past, the NCLEX-RN examination was given on the same day, at the same time, twice a year throughout the United States. However, with the computerized adaptive testing (CAT) used now, students may apply to sit for the examination within weeks of graduation from an approved nursing program by making individual appointments at testing centers approved by their State Board of Nursing. With CAT, each candidate's test is unique and is assembled interactively as the individual is tested. As the candidate responds to each question, the computer calculates a competence estimate based on previous responses. The process is repeated with each question, tailoring an exam to each measure of the individual's knowledge while meeting the NCLEX-RN test plan requirements. All RN candidates must answer a minimum of 75 questions. The maximum number of questions that an RN candidate may answer is 265 during a 5-hour maximum test. The Test Plan for the current NCLEX-RN exam may be found on the NCSBN website (*http://www.ncsbn.org/public/resources/resources_publication.htm #num2*). The four major categories of Client Needs and the subcategories that comprise the NCLEX-RN are listed in Table 16–2.

Commitment to the Community

Commitment to the community and *altruism* (service to others) have been apparent since the early days of nursing. Other professions

TABLE 16–2
Major Categories of Client Needs: NCLEX-RN Test Plan

Safe, Effective Care Environment

1 Management of care
2 Safety and infection control

Health Promotion and Maintenance

1 Growth and development through the life span
2 Prevention and early detection of disease

Psychosocial Integrity

1 Coping and adaptation
2 Psychosocial adaptation

Physiological Integrity

1 Basic care and comfort
2 Pharmacological and parenteral therapies
3 Reduction of risk potential
4 Physiological adaptation

Source: Adapted from http://www.ncsbn.org/public/testing/res/NCSBNRNTestPlanBooklet.pdf.

such as law and medicine have had the same commitment to the community and have received generous economic rewards for their services. These rewards have ensured the attractiveness of their professions to new generations of potential professionals. Unfortunately, when nurses seek pay increases, employers frequently accuse them of lacking altruism and a commitment to serve (Hess, 1993). It is important to separate these two issues. Competitive salaries and fair working conditions are not incongruent with commitment and service to the community. In fact, they increase the profession's ability to attract the best and the brightest students.

Some practitioners view nursing as a job instead of a career. Nurses who lack a lifelong commitment to nursing may never consider themselves members of a professional group.

Professional Culture

Professional organizations have several functions that contribute to the creation of a professional culture. These include establish-ing and enforcing the profession's code of ethics, developing standards of practice, and establishing continuing education for members of the profession. In addition, professional organizations may represent their members in collective bargaining, in establishment of national policies affecting the profession, and in protecting the membership's general welfare and providing service to the community.

There are more than 50 professional nursing organizations. Many are related to specialty areas, such as maternal/child health, community health, critical care, or rehabilitation. Others serve a special purpose, as does Sigma Theta Tau, nursing's national honor society, or the Transcultural Nursing Society. The ANA publishes an updated list of these organizations each April in the *American Journal of Nursing.* The ANA, National League for Nursing (NLN), and the National Organization for Associate Degree Nursing are discussed in the next section.

In what other ways can nursing promote its professional culture? The current emphasis on caring and feminist ideology may assist nursing in defining the characteristics of the professional culture. The focus of feminist theory in nursing is the promotion of an atmosphere of mutual respect, trust, and community. Shared leadership, cooperation, and group process are emphasized (Mason, Backer, & Georges, 1993).

Along with a renewed emphasis on feminism, nursing literature is experiencing a renewed interest in caring. Although caring has been viewed as central to nursing, human care and caring are now defined as a personal, social, moral, and spiritual engagement of the nurse with other humans (Moccia, 1993).

Finally, becoming involved in being a role model, being a mentor, providing emotional support, and sharing powerful lived experiences of nursing are examples of the means by which we can promote our professional culture. A current criticism of nursing is the lack of professional behaviors by the members of the profession.

◼ Professional Behaviors

We have looked at the criteria for nursing as a profession. We can apply the criteria to ourselves. Ask yourself:

- Am I committed to lifelong learning and continued competence in nursing knowledge?

- Will I adhere to the ANA Code of Ethics?

- Will I be a member of my professional organization?

- Am I committed to my community?

- Will I participate actively in the culture of nursing as a mentor, leader, and follower?

- Do I view nursing as more than just a paycheck or a job?

Even if you have answered "yes" to all these questions, your instructors, classmates, employer, and co-workers may still say you are not demonstrating "professional behaviors." What are they really talking about? "Professionalism in nursing is a term freely used, but its definition and interpretation lack uniformity"(Adams & Miller, 1996, p. 77). Perhaps what they are really asking is "Does this person have the personal character to participate in the profession of nursing? Does this person have the passion and commitment to nursing to support the profession in the 21st century? Some of the issues surrounding personal professional behaviors include:

Responsibility and Accountability. We continue to practice nursing in a climate full of unknowns with clients who are more knowledgeable and assertive than in the past. In the future, we will be supervising and delegating more than "doing." Responsibility and accountability are not the same. *Being responsible* means being obligated to accomplish a task, whereas being *accountable* is the acceptance of ownership. Being accountable means that you have both the authority and autonomy to act responsibly. The accountable professional is able and willing to anticipate the results of his or her actions, act accordingly, and be held accountable by one's peers. Accountability means being answerable for one's actions and being able to disclose and deal with the consequences of disclosure (Anderson, 2001). This is the number one complaint of nursing managers today—lack of responsibility and accountability—the focus on the "job" not the "profession."

Communicating with Others. Communication is addressed in Chapter 3. The ability to communicate with others and to be part of the team are integral in professional behaviors. "Working with others involves common sense and an understanding of the underlying principles of shared values, communication, trust, and an appreciation or valuing of the other person" (Anderson, 2001, p. 132). Professional behaviors include your ability to collaborate with others and work in teams. Pointing fingers, gossiping about team members, focusing on your own interests, and holding grudges will label you as a troublemaker, not as a team player. As a professional nurse, it is your responsibility to role model teamwork. Make sure that you are (Anderson, 2001):

1 Open by sharing information.

2 Share the credit for work well done.

3 Role model, recognize, and praise honesty and openness.

4 Encourage and acknowledge active partnering.

5 Critique, refresh, and renew relationships with the group on a routine basis.

Demonstrating Caring Behaviors. This sounds like common sense. You might be thinking "Of course I am caring, I am a nurse." Caring is an active process. Caring is not unique to nursing, it is a value that human beings possess. According to Boykin and Schoenhofer (Parker, 2001), our ability to care is challenged on a daily basis as we deal with clients and peers who are difficult. The active process of caring calls for us to explore our knowledge, intuition, ethical beliefs, and values as we understand the situation and actively demonstrate caring behaviors to everyone, including ourselves. Our mothers were right when they said, "It's not what you say but how you say it!"

Dressing the Part. Look around your current clinical site. Is there a nurse in a starched white uniform, with impeccably clean white clinic shoes and stockings and a nurse's cap perched on her pulled up hair? Probably not. What do you see? A variety of colors and styles, running shoes, printed socks, hair ribbons, and lots of jewelry—very difficult to identify who is who. Dressing the part is not about money. It is about the professional look that the public identifies with nursing. You do not have to dress in the starched pinafores of 25 years ago; however, clean scrubs or uniforms, white shoes and stockings, and hair that is pulled up and out of the face can go a long way in instilling confidence in you and the profession.

Attitude Is Everything. The dictionary defines attitude as "a way of thinking or behaving" (*http://www.m-w.com/cgi-bin/dictionary*). We certainly know people who have a "poor attitude." What kind of attitude do we need in order to demonstrate professional behaviors? Our attitudes help create our reality. When we believe that everyone is out to get us, that no one works as hard as we do, or that no one understands, we behave with hostility toward our coworkers, families, and organizations. In return, they reciprocate, and the vicious cycle begins. An honest appraisal of our attitude is the first step in developing personal professional behaviors (Cloke & Goldsmith, 2000).

"I believe professionalism is earned by behavior, not bestowed. It's earned by taking care of business in a manner that is commensurate with one's vocation. There are ethics and morals involved in professionalism. There's also a big dose of competence." (Koepfer, 2001, p. 10)

◼ Professional Organizations

American Nurses Association

In 1896, delegates from 10 nursing schools' alumnae associations met to organize a national professional association for nurses. The constitution and bylaws were completed

in 1907, and the Nurses Associated Alumnae of the United States and Canada was born. The name was changed in 1911 to the American Nurses Association (ANA), which in 1982 became a federation of constituent state nurses associations.

The purposes of the ANA are to: (*http://nursingworld.org/about/index.htm*)

1 Work for the improvement of health standards and the availability of health care services for all people.

2 Foster high standards for nursing.

3 Stimulate and promote the professional development of nurses.

4 Promote the economic and general welfare of nurses in the workplace.

5 Project a positive and realistic view of nursing.

6 Lobby Congress and regulatory agencies about health care issues affecting nursing and the public.

These purposes, reviewed in each biennial meeting by the House of Delegates, are unrestricted by consideration of age, color, creed, disability, gender, health status, lifestyle, nationality, religion, race, or sexual orientation (ANA, 2000c). The core issues identified by the ANA in 2000 were (*http://nursingworld.org/ana2000/core.pdf*)

• Workplace rights

• Appropriate staffing

• Workplace health and safety

• Continuing competence

• Patient safety and advocacy

Although more than 2 million people are members of the nursing profession in the United States, only about 10 percent of the nation's RNs are members of their professional organization. The many different subgroups and numerous specialty nursing organizations contribute to this fragmentation, which makes presenting a united front from which to bargain for nursing difficult. As the ANA works on the goal of preparing nurses during the 21st century, nurses must work together in their efforts to identify and promote their unique, autonomous role within the health care system.

Many advantages are available to nurses who join the ANA. Membership offers benefits such as informative publications, group life and health insurance, malpractice insurance, and continuing education courses. The ANA also helps state nurses associations to support their members regarding workplace and client care issues such as salaries, working conditions, and staffing.

As the major voice of nursing, the ANA lobbies the government to influence laws that affect the practice of nursing and the safety of consumers. The power of the ANA was apparent when nurses lobbied against the American Medical Association's (AMA) proposal to create a new category of health care worker, the registered care technician, as an answer to the nursing shortage of the 1980s. The registered care technician category was never established, despite the AMA's vigorous support. The ANA frequently publishes position statements outlining organization's position on particular topics important to the health and welfare of the public and/or the nurse. Table 16–3 summarizes some of the current position statements available from the ANA, which can easily be accessed on the ANA website (*http://nursingworld.org/readroom/position/index.htm*) or are available by mail on request.

Finally, the ANA offers certification in various specialty areas. Certification is a formal, voluntary process by which the professional demonstrates knowledge of and expertise in a specific area of practice. It is a way to establish the nurse's expertise beyond the basic requirements for licensure and is an important part of peer recognition for nurses. In many areas, certification entitles the nurse to salary increases and position advancement. Some specialty nursing organizations also have certification programs.

National League for Nursing

Another large nursing organization is the National League for Nursing (NLN). Unlike the ANA, NLN membership is open to other health professionals and interested con-

TABLE 16–3
Position Statements

American Nurses Association

Bloodborne and Airborne Diseases

- Education and Barrier Use for Sexually Transmitted Diseases and HIV Infection
- The Health Care Service System and Linkage of Primary Care, Substance Abuse, Mental Health, and HIV/AIDS Related Services
- AIDS/HIV Disease and Socio-Culturally Diverse Populations
- Availability of Equipment and Safety Procedures to Prevent Transmission of Bloodborne Diseases
- Guidelines for Disclosure to a Known Third Party About Possible HIV Infection
- HIV Infected Nurse, Ethical Obligations and Disclosure
- Tuberculosis and HIV
- HIV Disease and Correctional Inmates
- Needle Exchange and HIV
- Support for Confidential Notification Services and a Limited Privilege to Disclose
- Personnel Policies and HIV in the Workplace
- Post-Exposure Programs in the Event of Occupational Exposure to HIV/HBV
- HIV Exposure from Rape/Sexual Assault
- HIV Infection and Nursing Students
- Tuberculosis and Public Health Nursing
- HIV Infection and U.S. Teenagers
- HIV Testing
- Travel Restrictions for Persons with HIV/AIDS
- HIV Disease and Women

Ethics and Human Rights

- Human Cloning by Means of Blastomere Splitting and Nuclear Transplantation
- Privacy and Confidentiality
- Assisted Suicide
- Nurses' Participation in Capital Punishment
- The Non-Negotiable Nature of the Code for Nurses

NOTE: This is NOT the Code for Nurses.
To order the Code for Nurses, go the Publications Catalog.
- Promotion of Comfort and Relief of Pain in Dying Patients
- Cultural Diversity in Nursing Practice
- Discrimination and Racism in Health Care
- Nursing Care and Do-Not-Resuscitate Decisions
- Ethics and Human Rights
- Active Euthanasia
- Foregoing Nutrition and Hydration
- Mechanisms Through Which SNAs Consider Ethical/Human Rights Issues
- Nursing and the Patient Self-Determination Acts
- Risk Versus Responsibility in Providing Nursing Care
- Reduction of Patient Restraint and Seclusion in Health Care Settings

TABLE 16–3

Position Statements *(Continued)*

American Nurses Association

Social Causes and Health Care

- Adult Immunization
- Cessation of Tobacco Use
- Childhood Immunizations
- Environmental Tobacco Smoke
- Home Care for Mother, Infant and Family Following Birth
- Informal Caregiving
- Lead Poisoning and Screening
- Long Term Care
- Nutrition Screening for the Elderly
- Physical Violence Against Women
- Prevention of Tobacco Use in Youth
- Health Promotion and Disease Prevention
- Reproductive Health
- Use of Placebos for Pain Management in Patients with Cancer

Drug and Alcohol Abuse

- Abuse of Prescription Drugs
- Polypharmacy and the Older Adult
- Opposition to Criminal Prosecution of Women for Use of Drugs While Pregnant
- Support for Treatment Services for Alcohol and Drug Dependent Women of Childbearing Age
- Drug Testing for Health Care Workers

Nursing Education

- Guideline for Commercial Support for Continuing Nursing Education

Nursing Practice

- A National Nursing Database to Support Clinical Nursing Practice
- Nurse-Midwifery
- Privatization and For-profit Conversion
- Psychiatric Mental Health Nursing and Managed Care

Nursing Research

- Education for Participation in Nursing Research

Consumer Advocacy

- Referrals to the Most Appropriate Provider

Workplace Advocacy

- Latex Allergy
- The Right to Accept or Reject an Assignment
- Restructuring, Work Redesign, and the Job and Career Security of Registered Nurses
- Sexual Harassment
- Polygraph Testing of Health Care Workers
- Opposition to Mandatory Overtime

TABLE 16–3

Position Statements *(Continued)*

American Nurses Association

Unlicensed Assistive Personnel

NOTE: ANA work on the UAP issue has been ongoing.
- Registered Nurse Utilization of Unlicensed Assistive Personnel
- Registered Nurse Education Relating to the Utilization of Unlicensed Assistive Personnel

Joint Statements

- AORN Official Statement on RN First Assistants
- Role of the Registered Nurse (RN) in the Management of Analgesia by Catheter Techniques
- Paper on Computer-based Patient Record Standards
- Paper on Authentication in a Computer-based Patient Record
- On Access to Patient Data
- Role of the Registered Nurse (RN) in the Management of Patients Receiving IV Conscious Sedation
- Maintaining Professional and Legal Standards During a Shortage of Nursing Personnel
- Services to Families Following a SIDS (Sudden Infant Death Syndrome)

Source: http://nursingworld.org/readroom/position/index.htm

sumers, not just nurses. Over 1500 nursing schools and health care agencies and more than 5000 nurses, educators, administrators, consumers, and students are members of the NLN (NLN, 2000b).

The NLN participates in test services, research, and publication. It also lobbies actively for nursing issues and is currently working cooperatively with the ANA and other nursing organizations on health care reform. To do such things more effectively, the ANA, NLN, American Association of Colleges of Nursing, and American Organization of Nurse Executives have formed a coalition called the TriCouncil for the purpose of dealing with issues that are important to all nurses. The NLN formed a separate accrediting agency, the National League for Nursing Accrediting Agency (NLNAC). The NLNAC is responsible for the specialized accreditation of nursing education schools and programs, both postsecondary and higher degree (master's degree, baccalaureate degree, associate degree, diploma, and practical nursing program).

National Organization for Associate Degree Nursing

Associate degree nursing programs prepare the largest number of new graduates for RN licensure. Many of these individuals would never have had the opportunity to become RNs without the access afforded by the community college system. The move to begin a national organization that would only address associate degree nursing began in 1986. The organization identified two major goals: (1) to maintain eligibility for licensure for associate degree graduates; and (2) to interact with other nursing organizations. Today, the mission of NOADN includes supporting the associate degree graduate through (*http://www.noadn.org conventionstate .htm*):

- Strong educational programs

- Dynamic curricula education of students in a variety of settings

- Emphasis on lifelong learning

- Continued articulation with colleges and universities

◼ Educating Nurses

As the controversy regarding whether nursing is or is not a profession continues, so does the controversy over the amount and type of education that should be required for entry into the profession. Today, there are more than 1600 basic programs that prepare beginning RNs (NLN, 2000a). Programs are offered in the traditional face-to-face format or online. Students may complete their program entirely on the Internet or through two-way audio two-way video technology. In 2002, students enrolled in programs for their initial nursing education were broken into the following categories: 32 percent in associate's degree programs, 31 percent in baccalaureate programs, and 27 percent in diploma programs (*http://www.nlnac.org/*). Although the majority of nurses begin their career with an associate's degree or diploma in nursing, many nurses continue their education and eventually obtain a BSN or higher degree in nursing.

Practical Nursing Programs

Practical nurses (LPNs or LVNs) are licensed separately and are not considered professional nurses (although they are sometimes called "nurses" in long-term care facilities). Their training is usually 9 months to 1 year in length, after which they are eligible to take the NCLEX-PN examination.

Many practical nurses find employment in long-term care facilities or private-duty home care. In any setting, they are expected to work under the supervision of an RN, even if the RN is not onsite. Increasing numbers of practical nurses are returning to community colleges to attend LPN-to-RN programs to obtain an associate's degree and become eligible to take the NCLEX-RN examination for RNs. It is important that the professional nurse identify himself or herself as the "RN" to assist the consumer in understanding that "a nurse is not a nurse is not a nurse."

Diploma Programs

Diploma nursing programs have existed in the United States since the late 1800s, when nursing education began as apprenticeship training in hospitals. The number of diploma programs has gradually declined; today there are fewer than 160 in the United States. The programs are clustered in the northeast, and half the remaining states have none at all (ANA, 2000a).

In the past, students in diploma programs were the primary workforce of the hospital. Most of the instructors were either graduates of the same program or members of the hospital's medical staff. Although they were well versed in nursing or medical skills, they were not necessarily well prepared to teach nursing theory and had no background in other important elements of a professional education: language, mathematics, psychology, sociology, microbiology, and so forth.

Diploma programs have continued to be valuable to hospitals because they generate a pool of new graduates who are easily assimilated into their existing nursing staff. Many have aligned themselves with local colleges or universities so that their students can obtain the necessary general education requirements and earn either an associate's or baccalaureate degree on completion of the program.

Associate's Degree Programs

Mildred Montag first proposed the establishment of nursing programs in community colleges in 1951. Her doctoral dissertation, "The Education of Nursing Technicians," proposed an approach that would produce nurses more quickly than the 3-year diploma or 4- to 5-year baccalaureate programs of that time. The graduates would be "technical nurses" who worked at the bedside. They would have less autonomy than the baccalaureate graduate but more than the LPN.

Montag envisioned the associate's degree as a terminal degree that students could complete in 2 years and then enter the job market. Approximately half of the coursework would be related to nursing; the other half would be related to general education courses.

Associate's degree nursing programs grew rapidly. However, some of Montag's original concepts have been abandoned. The degree is no longer considered a terminal one but a step toward a baccalaureate degree. Many of the programs also have had difficulty meeting the NLN's recommendation of a maximum of 72 credit hours in the nursing program.

Fueled by the high birth rates of the 1940s (the early "baby boomers"), the community college movement of the 1960s flourished, and their nursing programs flourished along with them. Community colleges promoted equal opportunity, provided flexible schedules, and improved accessibility to higher education. Married women, men, minorities, and students seeking career changes who were attracted to the associate's degree programs in nursing were quite different from the traditional 18- to 25-year-old white women who constituted the majority of nursing students until then.

There are more than 800 associate's degree programs in the United States today, and the number continues to increase.

Baccalaureate Degree Programs

Nursing leaders in the early 1900s felt strongly that nursing education should move from the hospitals into the universities with other professional programs. By this time, nursing education had become firmly entrenched within hospitals, despite Nightingale's early opposition to such an arrangement. Universities at first were reluctant to accept nursing as a profession worthy of a university education. However, as nursing leaders such as Nutting continued to press for an equal place in the university, the barriers slowly crumbled, and nursing is now an accepted member of the university community.

Nursing's leaders have continued to emphasize the importance of a solid foundation in sciences and humanities as a prerequisite to learning nursing. The debate about the differences between levels of nursing education continues today, 35 years after the ANA's initial position paper recommending baccalaureate education as entry into practice.

Baccalaureate programs today provide nursing education for beginning (generic) students and for RNs who have associate's degrees or diplomas and wish to earn the bachelor of science in nursing (BSN) degree. Basic programs combine general education and nursing courses in a 4-year curriculum.

In the past, many associate's degree and diploma program graduates sought baccalaureate level degrees in non-nursing fields, such as health education or business, primarily because they did not require any additional clinical courses and so could be completed more quickly. Non-nursing degrees do not provide advanced education in the discipline of nursing. Also, they offer little for the graduate in terms of job promotion or qualification for admission into a master's degree program in nursing.

Recently, many community colleges and universities established articulation agreements, whereby students from community colleges receive credit for their associate's degree nursing courses so that they do not have to repeat coursework unnecessarily. These cooperative arrangements have made it much easier for graduates of associate's degree programs to continue their education and earn a baccalaureate degree.

Master's Degree Program

There are currently more than 350 master's degree in nursing programs in the United States (NLN, 2000c). The demand for ARNPs has caused an increase in the growth of MSN programs. Entrance into a master's degree program usually requires a baccalaureate degree in nursing, a minimum grade point average of 3.0 on a 4-point scale, and a satisfactory score on the Graduate Record Examination (GRE) or a similar test. Some programs currently admit RNs with a bachelor's degree in another field into the MSN program. Some programs still require a year of experience in nursing practice as well.

Graduate programs prepare students for advanced clinical practice, teaching, and nursing administration. The most common specialty areas are adult health, child health, community/public health, gerontology, neonatal nursing, nurse anesthesia, nursing administration, nursing education, nurse midwifery, nursing information systems, oncology, and psychiatric/mental health (NLN, 1993). Students receive a master of science (MS) or master of science in nursing (MSN) degree after 1 or 2 additional years of study beyond the baccalaureate level.

As with the baccalaureate degree, students seeking advanced degrees should be encouraged to pursue a degree in nursing rather than in another discipline. Many times, a master's degree in a related field does not allow for the advancement that a nursing degree provides.

Doctoral Programs

Doctoral programs in nursing are comparatively new. As late as the 1970s, many nurses were still pursuing doctoral degrees in fields other than nursing. There currently are about 75 doctoral programs in nursing in the United States (NLN, 2000c). Most offer either a doctor of philosophy (PhD) or doctor of science in nursing (DNSc) degree. The DNSc degree is a practice-oriented degree that emphasizes clinical research. The PhD degree is considered to be more academically oriented, preparing scholars for the pursuit of research and theory development. Doctorally prepared nurses are in great demand in both university and community settings.

External Degree Programs

External degree programs grant credit to students for their knowledge and experience, regardless of where they were obtained. Students may obtain credit for life experience, for courses taken at other institutions, or through testing and receive a degree without the traditional coursework required by most institutions.

The best-known external degree program in nursing is the New York State Regents External Degree Program, established in 1972. Students in this program are expected to achieve the same competencies as a graduate from an associate's degree program in New York and to pass college-level tests in both nursing and general education. The program is accredited by the NLN.

External degree programs have advantages for the nontraditional student:

- Reduced commuting time to and from campus

- Reduced child care difficulties

- Freedom to work at your own pace and on your own time

- Reduced stress of returning to a classroom

On the other hand, the external degree student must be motivated and self-directed because there are few deadlines and few reminders that studying must be done. Although some places arrange for meetings of people pursuing an external degree (somewhat like a support group), it can be a lonely process in comparison to having a group of classmates with whom to share scholastic victories and defeats.

Continuing Education

In some states, participation in continuing education is required for licensure renewal. In other states, it is required only for ARNPs. Licensed nurses need to be aware of the requirements of the board of nursing in their own state. Continuing education programs provide an avenue for nurses to update and expand their knowledge and skills, and the time spent in obtaining continuing education should be viewed as valuable to professional growth.

◼ Differentiated Practice

You can see by the preceding discussions that nurses obtain their education in a variety of ways. Instead of continuing the discussion of how we should educate an RN for initial entry into practice, the discussion is moving toward asking the question, "How can we best utilize the different educations levels in the current health care environment?" The answer is differentiated practice (*http://www.nlnac.org/Manual%20&%20IG/interpretive_guidelines.htm#Differentiated%20Education*):

Differentiated practice describes the system of sorting roles, functions, and work of nurses according to education, clinical experience, and defined competence and decision-making skills required by different client needs and settings in which nursing is practiced. What this means is identifying the skills and core competencies needed, the best educational experiences and care that reflect those skills and core competencies, and accreditation policies that demand active participation in developing, measuring, and promoting educational outcomes for different practice domains and core competencies for nursing practice.

The National Organization for Associate Degree Nursing published a resolution on differentiated nursing practice in 1997. The use of differentiated nursing practice models continue to be explored. The idea that "a nurse is a nurse is a nurse" is no longer acceptable to nurses regardless of their entry into practice. See Appendix 3 for the N-OADN Resolution on Differentiated Nursing Practice.

◼ Informatics

Regardless of your basic nursing education, one thing is certain: you will be expected to have computer skills and knowledge in the workplace. Into the 21st century, computerized information systems, electronic monitoring devices, microprocessor implants, automated imaging systems, telehealth, and robotics have already permeated the health care system (Travis & Brennan, 1998). You may be expected to be familiar with:

- Accessing medical records in real-time online

- Using a bedside or portable computer to document patient data and nursing care while accessing information from other team members

- Holding conferences with other health care providers via the Internet

- Accessing information via the world wide web (Bachman & Panzarine, 1998)

Two examples of using technology to access and disseminate information quickly and accurately are the electronic medical record and decision support software. Several benefits of using an electronic medical record are:

- Accessing the medical record from several different locations simultaneously and by different levels of providers

- Allowing for quick access of records for use in research

- Decreasing error potential while improving communication

- Decreasing documentation time and thereby increasing time for client care

Decision support software is written into many computerized patient records. These decision support tools notify the clinician of possible concerns or omissions with the use of a variety of alerts and reminders. For example, when a drug is ordered an alert notifies the primary care provider of any known allergies or even potential interactions with other drug orders for that client.

The term *informatics* was defined in 1983 as "computer science plus information science." Adding the name of the discipline, informatics denotes the application of computer and information sciences to the data management, information, and knowledge of that discipline (Graves & Corcoran, 1989, p. 227).

The idea of "medical informatics" began in the 1970s as technologic advances made it possible to enter data about patient care into computers. The term *health informatics* was later applied to information encompassing medicine, nursing, dentistry, pharmacy, and other health care disciplines. As members of each discipline identified the distinct information needed for professional practice, multiple informatics systems were developed (Graves & Corcoran, 1989). In the late 1960s, nurses began to use electronic tools to assist in the collection and management of nursing information. Although slow to develop initially, the field is now advancing rapidly (NINR, 1999).

Nursing Informatics

Nursing informatics is defined as the "combination of computer science, information science, and nursing science designed to assist in management and processing of nursing data, information, and knowledge to support the practice of nursing and the delivery of nursing care" (Graves & Corcoran, 1989, p. 227). As outlined by the ANA (1994), nursing informatics includes identifying, acquiring, preserving, managing, retrieving, aggregating, analyzing, and transmitting data; information; and knowledge to make it meaningful and useful to nurses. Effective application requires (1) use of computers and understanding of computer technology, (2) identification of conceptual issues and key concepts related to nursing knowledge, and (3) development of computerized information management systems to enhance nursing practice through the entering, organizing, and retrieval of information. The interaction of these three requirements constitutes the core of nursing informatics (Turley, 1996).

Economics and the knowledge explosion continue to drive the need to advance nurs-

ing informatics. The major economic concerns are the need to maximize nursing productivity, achieve efficiency, and ensure satisfactory patient outcomes. In addition, informatics supports nursing research, which continues to expand nursing's knowledge base, while the increasing complexity of patient care forces nurses to use increasing amounts of information when making decisions (Zielstorff, Hudgings, & Grobe, 1993).

Using an integrated information system, patient-specific data, collected only once, could be used in many different situations (Fig. 16–1). For example, when the patient is admitted to the hospital, a computerized medical record can be initiated. With the use of an integrated information system, the insurance company is billed electronically. It now becomes unnecessary to incur costs for printing and mailing statements. Staff of the quality improvement department can collect data on all patients and look for trends in cost and patient outcomes. Also, there is no need to copy and mail client records or referral forms to other agencies or for an individual to be designated as the person to code and enter data from each paper chart. The software used to access the computerized patient record can automatically search for identified information.

Databases and Data Sets

The development of computer systems to handle nursing data may well be the easy part. Historically, nurses have had difficulty articulating what nurses actually do and what impact nurses have on outcomes. The problem becomes more acute when the information is computerized. As early as 1986, the ANA supported the development of a national nursing database for clinical practice. In response, the Steering Committee on Databases to Support Clinical Nursing Practice was formed in 1989. This committee recommended adoption of the Nursing Minimum Data Set (NMDS), originally developed by 64 nursing experts during a 3-day invitational conference in 1985. The NMDS is a minimum set of essential informational items concerned with nursing care and supported by standardized definitions and categories. This

User	Data	Scope
Caregiver, insurer, individual agency	Patient-specific data: assessments, diagnoses, interventions, test results, procedures, treatments, patient care hours, outcome	Individual client data
Administrators, researchers, accrediting bodies, QA departments	Cost by patient categories; number of patients with specific diagnoses, tests, procedures; interventions by volumes; diagnostic group patient outcomes	Agency-wide data
Analysts, public health departments, researchers	Comparisons of treatments, outcomes, costs, incidences, and prevalences	Community and regional data
Policy makers, researchers, lawmakers, insurers	Trends related to incidence, prevalence, outcomes, costs, diagnosis	Nationwide data
World health officials, national policy makers and lawmakers, national research organizations	General health-related information of individual nations	Worldwide data

Figure 16–1 Multiple uses of patient data. Source: Adapted from Zielstorff, R., Hodgings, C., & Grobe, S. (1993). *Next Generation Nursing Information Systems.* Washington, D.C.: ANA.

information is entered into a computerized patient record. The NMDS provides a common language of nursing that can be used in health care information systems, provides a common language for nursing research and outcomes assessment, and assists nursing to move toward third-party reimbursement (ANA, 1995b). Using a common language facilitates sharing information across disciplines. The NMDS elements included are shown in Figure 16–2.

Nursing Nomenclature and Taxonomies

In addition to the NMDS, the ANA supports the development of scientifically based naming systems that address the uniqueness of nursing practice (ANA, 1994). The holistic nature of nursing phenomena and the use of multiple conceptual frameworks have contributed to difficulty in standardizing nursing data. The question arises not only as to what data to include, but also as to how one defines commonly held concepts. Descriptions such as "copious," "frail," or "weak,"

for example, are difficult to specify in a data set that will be produced by a "point and click" computer application. This fuzzi-

Nursing diagnosis/problem
Nursing intervention/treatment
Nursing-sensitive patient outcome
Intensity of nursing care
Patient personal identification
Patient date of birth
Patient sex
Patient race and ethnicity
Patient residence
Unique facility service number
Unique health record number of patient
Unique number of principal registered nurse provider
Episode admission or encounter date
Discharge date
Disposition of client
Expected payer for most of the bill

Figure 16–2 Nursing minimum data set. Source: American Nurses Association. (1995a). *Nursing's Social Policy Statement.* Washington, D.C.: ANA.

ness of clinical terms and the use of clinical judgments in nursing are critical nursing information issues (NINR, 1999). The development of a system to collate, integrate, compare, and monitor computerized patient data is essential. In 1994, the ANA Steering Committee published a set of policy statements related to developing a single, comprehensive system for classifying nursing practice. To date, there is not one universally accepted classification system. The predominant nursing classifications systems in use today are:

- North American Nursing Diagnosis Association (NANDA)
- The Omaha System
- The Home Healthcare Classification
- The Nursing Interventions Classification System

North American Nursing Diagnosis Association (NANDA). Work on the NANDA taxonomy began in the early 1970s as part of a demonstration project that required patient data to be computerized and discipline specific. The nurses involved in the project soon realized that they were unable to do either. They recognized what a difficult task they had undertaken and sought assistance and advice from other nurses. Their efforts at problem-solving soon led to the initial 1973 meeting of the National Conference Group for the Classification of Nursing Diagnoses. The initial group decided to hold more formalized meetings. After five yearly conferences, members of the group were still unable to agree on a classification scheme; a decision was made to list the nursing diagnoses alphabetically. During the fifth annual meeting, NANDA was formed. NANDA is recognized by the ANA as the group responsible for the maintenance and development of a standardized nursing taxonomy (ANA, 1995b).

The Omaha System. The Visiting Nurse Association of Omaha developed the Omaha System through a series of research projects. The system is a method of describing and measuring client problems, interventions, and outcomes. It has been found to be useful in home care, public and school health, correctional facilities, and outpatient facilities.

The Home Healthcare Classification. Development of the Home Healthcare Classification began as a project at Georgetown University in the early 1990s. The purpose of the original study was to determine the resources required to provide home care services to Medicare clients and to identify the expected outcomes of those services. Today, this system is used as the basis for measuring outcomes and effectiveness in many home health and community health agencies.

The Nursing Interventions Classification (NIC) (Iowa Intervention Project). Nurse researchers at the University of Iowa have been working since 1987 on developing the Nursing Interventions Classification (NIC) and the Nursing Outcomes Classification (NOC) (University of Iowa, 1999). In 1995, the Center for Nursing Classification was established at the University of Iowa to facilitate the research and development of NIC and NOC. The Center supports a web page, an active listserv, a newsletter, and several other publications. NIC includes 433 interventions and is linked to NOC.

A computer program that would link these different systems so that common meanings across terms can be identified is also being developed. This common language or Unified Nursing Language System (UNLS) is an important step in organizing and classifying nursing-related information. By using accepted terms, nurses can move toward a system for evaluating the quality and effectiveness of nursing care and services (ANA, 1995a). Guidelines and outcomes established by such agencies as the Healthcare Financing Administration (HCFA), Agency for Healthcare Policy and Research (AHCPR), and Centers for Disease Control and Prevention (CDC), as well as private insurance companies, can also be linked to the UNLS to further support the evaluation of nursing outcomes.

The computerized patient record (CPR) is an electronic file that stores patient information internally by a variety of health care providers. The data specified in the NMDS should be included. The Institute of

Medicine has identified the 12 major characteristics that they consider to be essential for an effective CPR system (Andrew & Dick, 1996):

1 Problem list that indicates the client's current clinical problems for each episode

2 Provision for evaluation of patient health status and functional level using standardized definitions of these outcomes

3 Documentation of the clinical reasoning/rationale for diagnoses and conclusions

4 Link to other client data and records

5 Confidentiality, privacy, and audit trails

6 Continuous and simultaneous access for authorized users

7 Links to local and remote information resources

8 Access to decision analysis tools to facilitate clinical problem-solving

9 Direct entry of client data by providers

10 Mechanisms for monitoring the cost and quality of care

11 Flexibility and expandability of the system

The gold standard is still a goal to be accomplished. Many health care systems have automated part or all of the patient record, but automation alone does not constitute a fully functional CPR as described. A truly longitudinal CPR that can be accessed by all providers, provides links to other client data and records, allows for documentation or outcomes, and allows for assistance with decision-making is now becoming a reality.

Benefits. A well-developed CPR used by staff who are adequately trained in the system can be of benefit to the entire health care team. On CPRs, information is more readable, is better organized, and should be more complete. Access to client information is available at multiple locations at any time of the day or night. Decision trees and other systems for decision analysis allow caregivers to logically plan care and identify appropriate interventions and outcomes. Use of CPRs can facilitate the automation of critical pathways and allows easy access to current and historical data. Less space is needed for record storage, and the chance of losing the record is decreased.

Acceptance. Resistance to implementation of a CPR is not uncommon. The end user, whether an RN, a physician, or another staff member, may feel totally overwhelmed by the need to learn an entirely new system. Some health care providers still do not use a computer in their personal life. Their unwillingness to use the CPR may be due to lack of familiarity with computers, complexity of the software, availability of computer terminals, disruptive effect on their preferred work flow pattern, or even an inability to type (Simpson, 1997). Being a role model in accepting new ideas and learning new skills is one of the responsibilities of being a professional. Make sure you are not one of the complainers in the group. Your support and enthusiasm will go a long way in helping others accept change.

Security Issues. As a rule, upper-level managers and information systems department personnel work together to develop policies and procedures related to security functions. As a professional nurse, you can set a positive example related to protection of client privacy and confidentiality. Make sure you have knowledge of the following:

• Policies and procedures related to levels of access to patient and administrative databases

• User authentication

• Secure data entry guidelines

• Training and service support available to staff

• Procedure for handling incorrect data entries, data tampering, and system failures

• Procedure for reporting security concerns or breaks in security

Audit Trails. An audit trail is a record of all who have accessed the computer system. Audit software records access to any part of the system by user name or password to identify unauthorized entry into client records or other organizational information. The software searches for unusual activity of any kind. In many organizations, employees are asked to sign a document stating they understand they will be terminated for inappropriate system use. Users must also be made aware of the danger of giving their password and/or user ID to others.

Telehealth

Telehealth is the use of electronic information and telecommunications technologies to support long-distance clinical health care, patient and professional health-related education, public health and health administration (*http://telehealth.hrsa.gov/*). The largest users of telehealth in the United States are NASA and the military. The federal government has a dedicated office telehealth, The Office for the Advancement of Telehealth (OAT), which coordinates the telehealth activities (*http://telehealth.hrsa.gov/*). As cost containment and access to health care services issues continue to increase, telehealth has become an attractive instrument to save health care dollars. Savings are achieved by (1) allowing earlier access to care, (2) decreasing travel expenses, (3) providing easier access to specialists and experts, and (4) providing easier access to continuing education for both consumers and professionals (Chaffee, 1999). As of 1997, the Balanced Budget Act allowed for Medicare reimbursement for telemedicine services. Although the laws were expanded in 2000, not all telehealth services are covered.

Telehome care is largely a nursing industry. Nurses play a key role in all telemedicine systems, often being the lead coordinators and managers of the programs. Nurses have been at the forefront in adapting video teleconferencing for preventive services and in advocating for effective telehealth policies at the national, state, and institutional levels; also, nurses often are the key providers of preventive services, many of which would be enhanced by access to telemedicine services. As the opportunities grow to adapt technologies to better meet the health care needs of this nation, we need our foremost care givers, especially nurses, at the table to provide, critique, assess, and strengthen our ability to use these technologies for improving access to care for all people (Puskin, 2001, *http://www.nursingworld.org/ojin/topic16/ tpc16_1.htm*).

◼ Conclusion

The public image of nursing has not always done justice to the unique combination of art and science that is truly nursing. Nurses need to take the lead in the movement toward defining a clearer identity and delineating a clearer role of the profession. Paramount to achieving these goals is the recognition of the value of nursing and acceptance of its professional status. The importance of viewing nursing as a profession with a systematic body of knowledge, formal college-based education, unique roles, standards of practice, professional accountability, professional culture, and community commitment continue to move nursing through the 21st century. Working toward a universal language for nursing practice and a unified nursing language system assists nurses in developing a system for evaluating the quality and effectiveness of nursing care and services.

Dr. Maryann Fralic, professor at Johns Hopkins University School of Nursing, gave a plenary session at the NLN 24th biennial convention in Miami Beach in 1999 (NLN, 2000). In discussing nursing for the new millennium, she closed with the following advice:

- Set and maintain high standards, both personally and professionally.

- Seek out a mentor.

- There is no substitute for competence. Cultivate your personal and professional competency as an active, lifelong learner.

- Be professionally productive. Add to the science and knowledge bases of nursing.

- Always respect the privilege to be part of a profession that intervenes intimately and meaningfully with people to truly make a difference.

Student Activity Worksheet 1

Review the following characteristics of a profession. Develop personal objectives that will assist you in maintaining your status as a professional nurse.

Systematic body of knowledge

Mastery of knowledge and an ability to problem-solve

Specialized, formal education based in colleges and universities

Unique, distinct role and autonomy

Standards of practice and a code of ethics

Legal enforcement and professional accountability

Motivated by commitment to the community

Creation of a professional culture

Student Activity Worksheet 2

Review the ANA website at *www.nursingworld.org*

1. Select the link Online Journal of Issues in Nursing. Review the articles posted. Which one(s) might be of most benefit to you as you begin your nursing career? Why?

_____

_____

_____

_____

2. Select the link Workplace Advocacy. Select the link WPA Programs and review the program(s) related to your state. What information did you learn that will be useful to you as a new RN? Why?

_____

_____

_____

_____

3. Select one other link of your choice. Why did you select this particular site? What will you do with the information?

_____

_____

_____

_____

Overall, evaluate the services and information available through ANA. Develop a plan to become a member of your professional organization.

Study Questions

1 How can you portray the profession of nursing in a positive manner in the workplace?

2 Discuss the characteristics of nursing that indicate that nursing is a profession.

3 Discuss the Code of Ethics with an experienced nurse. How does the Code of Ethics affect his or her daily practice?

4 What are the advantages to a nurse belonging to the ANA? Disadvantages? Would you persuade another RN to join the ANA and attend meetings with you? If so, how?

5 What is the purpose of the board of nursing? What impact do the ANA Standards of Clinical Nursing Practice have on decisions made by the board of nursing?

6 Explore your strengths and weaknesses related to the discussion of professional behaviors in this chapter. How might you develop your strengths and minimize your weaknesses?

7 Would a differentiated practice model work in your community? Why or why not?

8 Evaluate your technology strengths and weaknesses. Develop a 1-year plan to increase your technology knowledge and skills.

Critical Thinking Exercise

Ms. P. recently graduated from the local community college and received an associate's degree in nursing. On obtaining her RN license, she was hired to work on a busy pediatric floor of a large local hospital. She was responsible for delegating patient assignments to the LPN and nursing assistant who were assigned with her. She often felt uneasy about her decisions because of her inexperience in this area. When she joined the ANA, she received a copy of the Code for Nurses and Standards of Clinical Nursing Practice.

After a few weeks, Ms. P. told her nurse manager that she had seen Ms. A., the LPN, discontinuing IVs and hanging IV medications, even though the board of nursing in their state does not allow it. The nurse manager replied, "Oh, she's just like an RN. Don't worry, I'll cover for her."

1 Why should Ms. P. feel uneasy about that response?

2 What might happen to the nurse manager, the LPN, and Ms. P. if there is a problem with a patient regarding these IVs?

3 What can Ms. P. do about this situation?

4 How might these two documents guide her in making decisions about delegating patient assignments?

REFERENCES

Adams, D., & Miller, B. (1996). Professionalism behaviors of hospital nurse executives and middle managers in 10 western states. *Western Journal of Nursing Research*, 18(1), 77.

American Nurses Association (ANA). (1965). ANAs just position on education for nursing. *American Journal of Nursing*, 65, 106–111.

American Nurses Association. (1980). *Nursing: A Social Policy Statement*. Kansas City, Mo.: ANA.

American Nurses Association. (2001). *Code for Nurses*. Washington, D.C.: ANA.

American Nurses Association. (1994). *The Scope of Practice for Nursing Informatics*. Washington, D.C.: ANA.

American Nurses Association. (1995a). *Nursing's Social Policy Statement*. Washington, D.C.: ANA.

American Nurses Association. (1995b). *American Nurses Association Bylaws as Amended July 2, 1995*. Washington, D.C.: ANA.

American Nurses Association. (1998). *Aspects of Standards and Guidelines for Clinical Nursing Practice*. Washington, D.C.: ANA.

American Nurses Association. (1997). [Online]. Available: *http://www.nursingworld.org/readroom/position/uap/uapclass.htm*.

American Nurses Association. (April 27, 2000a). [Online]. Available: *http://www.nursingworld.org/readroom/fsdemogr.htm*.

American Nurses Association. (April 27, 2000b). [Online]. Available: *http://www.nursingworld.org/readroom/rwjpaper.htm*.

American Nurses Association. (April 27, 2000c). [Online]. Available: *http://www.nursingworld.org/readroom/position/index/htm*

Anderson, C. (2001). *Nursing Student to Nursing Leader: The Critical Path to Leadership Development*, 2nd ed.. New York: Delmar.

Andrew, W, & Dick, R. (1996). On the road to the CPR: Where are we now? *Healthcare Informatics*, 13(5), 48–52.

Bachman, J.A., & Panzarine, S. (1998). Enabling student nurses to use the information superhighway. *Journal of Nursing Education*, 37(4), 155–160.

Beletz, E. (1974). Is nursing's public image up-to-date? *Nursing Outlook*, 22, 432–435.

Bixler, G.K., & Bixler, R.W. (1959). The professional status of nursing. *American Journal of Nursing*, 59, 1142–1147.

Chaffee, M. (1999). A telehealth odyssey. *American Journal of Nursing*, 99(7), 27–33.

Cloke, K., & Goldsmith, J. (2000). *Resolving Conflicts at Work*. San Francisco. Jossey-Bass.

Ehrlich, E., Flexner, S., Carruth, G., & Hawkins, J. (1980). *Oxford American Dictionary*. New York: Oxford University Press.

Flexner, A. (1915). Is social work a profession? *Scholastic Society*, 1(20), 901.

Graves J.R., & Corcoran, S. (1989). The study of nursing informatics. *Image: Journal of Nursing Scholarship*, 21, 237–231.

Health and Human Services. [On-line] *http://telehealth.hrsa.gov/*

Henderson, V. (1966). *The Nature of Nursing*. New York: Macmillan.

Hess, R. (1993). In nursing as in life—No risks, no rewards. *Revolution: The Journal of Nurse Empowerment*, 3(1), 84–86, 111–112.

Joel, L. (2002). Reflections and projections on nursing. *Nursing Administration Quarterly*, 26(5), 11–17.

Koepfer, G.C. (2001). What makes people professionals? *Modern Machine Shop*, 74(3), 10.

Mason, D., Backer, B., & Georges, A. (1993). Toward a feminist model for the political empowerment of nurses. *Revolution: Journal of Nurse Empowerment*, 3(1), 63–71, 106–108.

Merriam-Webster Online Dictionary. (2002). [Online]. Available at *http://www.m-w.com/cgi-bin/dictionary.*

Moccia, P. (1993). Nursing education in the public's trust. *Nursing and Health Care*, 14(9), 472–474.

National Organization for Associate Degree Nursing. (2002). [Online]. Available: http://www.noadn.org/

National Council State Boards of Nursing. (2002). [Online]. Available: *http://www.ncsbn.org*

National Council State Boards of Nursing. (2002). [Online]. Available: *http://www.ncsbn.org/public/regulation/regulation_index.htm*

National Council State Boards of Nursing. (2002). [Online]. Available: *http://www.ncsbn.org/public/regulation/licensure.htm*

National Council State Boards of Nursing. (2002). [Online]. Available: *http://www.ncsbn.org/public/resources/resources_publication.htm#num2*

National Institute of Nursing Research. (1999). [Online]. Available: *http://www.nih.gov/ninr/vol4/Intro. html*

National League for Nursing. (1993). *A Vision for Nursing Education* (Publication No. 14-2581). New York: NLN.

National League for Nursing. (2000a). [Online]. Available: *http://www.nln.org/info-default.htm*

National League for Nursing. (2000c). [Online]. Available: *http://www.nln.org/fratic.htm*

Nightingale, E. (1959). *Notes on Nursing* (Facsimile of the First Edition). Philadelphia: J.B. Lippincott.

Parker, M. (2001). *Nursing Theories and Nursing Practice.* Philadelphia: F.A. Davis.

Paul, R. (1993). *Critical Thinking*. San Jose, Calif.: Foundations for Critical Thinking.

Puskin, D. (2001). Telemedicine: Follow the money. Online Journal of Issues in Nursing, 6(3). [Online] *http://www.nursingworld.org/ojin/topic16/tpc16_1.htm*

Rogers, M.E. (1988). Nursing science and art: A prospective. *Nursing Science Quarterly*, 1, 99–102.

Simpson, R. (Winter 1997). Are staff nurses prepared for the new information-based hospital enterprise? *Nursing Administration Quarterly*, 21(2), 85–88.

Swirsky, J. (1993). Exclusive interview with Virginia Trotter Betts, President of the American Nurses Association. *Revolution: The Journal of Nurse Empowerment,* 3(1), 41–48.

Travis, L., & Brennan, P. (1998). Information science for the future: An innovative nursing informatics curriculum. *Journal of Nursing Education,* 37(4), 162–167.

Turley, J. (1996). Toward a model for nursing informat-

ics. *Image: Journal of Nursing Scholarship,* 28(4), 309–313.

University of Iowa. (1999). [On-line]. Available: *http://www.nursing.uiowa.edu/cnc*

Zielstorff, R., Hodgings, C., & Grobe, S. (1993). *Next Generation Nursing Information Systems.* Washington, D.C.: ANA.

CHAPTER 17

Looking to the Future

OBJECTIVES

After reading this chapter, the student should be able to:

- Understand the impact of technology on the delivery of nursing care.

- Make some predictions about the delivery of health care in the 21st century.

- Describe characteristics of today's nursing workforce.

- Describe the changes occurring in the delivery of health care and their effects on client outcomes and on nursing.

- Discuss the effects of cost-containment efforts.

OUTLINE

Current Trends
Effects of Technology
Consumerism
Survival of Vulnerable Individuals
Emphasis on Economics

Changes in the Health Care System
Historical Perspective
Managed Care
Subacute Care
Community-Based Care

Effect on Nursing
Elimination of Positions
Changes in Practice Environment
Nursing Shortage
Preventing Patient Care Errors
Emphasis on Outcomes
Changing Competencies
Responding to Changes in the Health Care
    System

The Future

CHAPTER 17 SELF ASSESSMENT

Do you know what is happening within the nursing profession and our health care system? Try this quiz to find out how well informed you are.

1. The proportion of nurses age 30 and younger in the workforce has increased over the past 5 years.   True _____ False _____

2. The average age of working RNs today is approximately 35 years old.
   True _____ False _____

3. An Institute of Medicine report on the quality of health care estimates that as many as 98,000 people a year die from causes related to medical error.
   True _____ False _____

4. In general, for-profit managed care organizations provide poorer quality care than do not-for-profit organizations.   True _____ False _____

5. Everyone in the United States has some form of health insurance, either through their employer or through a government-supported program.
   True _____ False _____

6. Alternative and complementary treatments are gradually becoming integrated into mainstream health care.   True _____ False _____

7. The abbreviation HIPAA stands for the Health Insurance Payment Authorization Act.   True _____ False _____

8. For legal reasons, computer-based patient records and electronic ordering of prescriptions will never replace the paper versions.   True _____ False _____

9. The existence of a caring relationship between patient and provider may reduce stress, encourage freer exchange of information, and facilitate treatment.
   True _____ False _____

Answers: 1. F, 2. F, 3. T, 4. T, 5. F, 6. T, 7. F, 8. F, 9. T

How will health care be delivered in the future? How will nurses' roles change? The following story is one version of how health care may be delivered in the future:

Arriving at the surgical center of the future, a robot "nurse" greets the client and instructs him or her to proceed to the sign-in counter, which resembles an automatic teller machine. The screen instructs the client to place the appropriate health insurance card into the slot. A computer-generated voice offers the client several selections:

"Press 1 if you are having surgery. Press 2 if you are having diagnostic tests. Press 3 if you are here to have a postoperative evaluation. Press 4 if you need further assistance. A qualified health care person will be with you shortly."

The voice continues to direct the client, who requires surgery, to choose the appropriate surgical procedure from those listed on the screen. After the procedure is verified and approved, the client receives directions from the electronic voice:

"You may now enter through the double doors to your right. The doors will open automatically. Please step carefully onto the moving platform. The platform is traveling at the same speed as the treatment vehicle. Kindly enter the first treatment vehicle as it approaches. Place the second finger of your left hand on the yellow circle for a blood test. A blood pressure cuff will encircle your left upper arm. Do not pull on the bar or belts. The safety bars and seat belts will lock automatically as the back of your vehicle reclines and the footrest rises to the forward position. Your vital signs and other appropriate information will be monitored by highly sophisticated computer technology throughout your entire stay with us.

"As you pass through Station 1, please place your right arm through the designated opening for the placement of your intravenous line. An automated sensor robot will insert this. Through the use of infrared sensors and sonography, the sensor robot locates an appropriate vessel with greater skill than a human nurse. You may feel a slight burning at this time. Do not pull your arm away. Repeat; do not pull your arm away.

"You are now approaching Station 2. Please place your right hand through the designated opening to receive the appropriate medication. The computerized vehicle in which you are traveling has automatically calculated the accurate dosage of medication based on your body weight and metabolism. The medication you will receive has been determined by an analysis of your blood drawn at Station 1. This eliminates the possibility of human error. However, if at any time you feel any itching, tingling, or tightness in your throat or have difficulty breathing, please press the red button on the left side of your vehicle. Our computers will automatically institute emergency measures for your health and safety. This action precludes the possible delays that can occur in the human decision-making process.

"You have reached Station 3, your assigned surgical suite. Please observe the screen in front of the vehicle. Meet your surgeon, Dr. I.M. Yourfuture, from Houston, Texas. Through the use of computer technology and robotics, she will perform seven of these procedures simultaneously in different geographic locations. Anesthesia will be administered through the mask moving toward your face. Please remain still while the robot arm securely fastens the straps around your shoulders. Take several slow, deep breaths when the blue light on the console begins to flash. Your anesthetic dose has been predetermined through a highly sophisticated mathematical formula. Pleasant dreams. We hope you enjoy your surgery while at 21st Century Surgical Center, saving health care dollars for a better tomorrow."

Compare the experience of the 21st Century Surgical Center to this alternative view of the future of health care:

Arriving at the New Age Health Center, the client walks into a central atrium, is offered a cool drink, and is encouraged to "choose either a comfortable seat in the center where you can enjoy the musical fountain or meditate in one of our quiet corners, whichever you prefer." After relaxing for a while in the atrium, the client walks down the hall to the consultation rooms. The client notices that one of the center's animal healers (a big, friendly Labrador) has joined him and is accompanying him down the hall.

Guides along the walkway ask the client whether he knows the way or if he would like some assistance in choosing a healer to consult. "I'm feeling very stressed at work lately," answers the client. "Having trouble sleeping, which is unusual for me."

"We have several ways to approach your concerns," says the guide. "You could try our stress-reducing exercise path, our yoga path, the medicinal consultation, the sleep consultation, or all four if you'd like. We also have a group of traditional healers you can consult. For example, one is a licensed physician who spent several years studying with a Hopi medicine man."

"I already have a good exercise program and prefer not to use medicinal therapies unless they're necessary, so I think I'll try that sleep consultation. I really need to get more sleep than I have lately."

The guide nods and directs the client toward the sleep center. "Ralph (the Labrador) would be happy to go with you, if you'd like." Ralph wags his tail in agreement.

At the end of the consultation, the client walks to the door with his sleep tapes and a video explaining how to use them, the same directions given by the sleep consultant. His sleep consultant bids him "a good night's rest tonight," and Ralph walks him back to the atrium, leaving him with a quiet "woof."

What is your preferred view of future health care delivery: the high-tech approach of the 21st Century Surgical Center or the high-touch approach of the New Age Health Center? Which would your clients choose? Neither of these scenarios is far-fetched. Robots are used in surgery today (Sloan, 2003) and complementary medicine is often combined with orthodox medical treatment. Which one do you think will prevail in the future? Is there a way to combine the best of both approaches?

We don't know for sure how health care will be delivered in the future or what nurses' roles will be in the health care system of the future. However, we can look at the current trends in our society, their effect on today's health care system, and what they may tell us about the future. By doing this, we may find some clues to the future of health care and of the nursing profession.

◼ Current Trends

Many trends in our society appear to be influencing the direction of health care. Among the most important of these trends are the effects of technology, the culture of consumerism, the survival of greater numbers of people with high-risk conditions, and an increasing tendency to evaluate outcomes primarily in economic terms.

Effects of Technology

On the whole, Americans love technology (Mechanic, 2002). In seconds, computers can complete highly complex calculations that would take days or weeks if done by hand. Sophisticated computer programs, microsurgery, laser treatments, cellular phones, satellite transmission, and a wonderful array of technical advances have made it possible to do things faster, easier, and more accurately. For example, patients with computer access can now see their lab results, make appointments, refill routine prescriptions, ask questions, and review instructions online (Landro, 2002). Nurses may one day be able to lift heavy patients by themselves, with the help of a robotic "power suit" (Kunii, 2003). All health-related information, such as all the prescription drugs a person is taking, can

be brought together in one place, available to all who need to access it:

A 61-year-old man was admitted for surgery to a hospital that utilized a database that combined patient information from various sources. Imagine the surprise of the surgical team when it was discovered that he had been seeing three different primary care providers and was taking 20 different medications. (Wysocki, 2002)

Computerized medication order entry can alert care providers to patient allergies, duplications, potential drug interactions, and excessive dosages, reducing error and saving many steps in the process of ordering, checking, and dispensing medication.

Laptop computers, wireless communication, fax, email, video conferencing, and interactive television have all found places in health care. Consultations between professionals, staff education, patient diagnosis, patient monitoring, and patient education can all occur across long distances now (Larson-Dahn, 2002). Diabetics, for example, can transmit their glucose levels to their nurse specialist and immediately receive guidance on altering diet or medication in response. For those who live a long distance from their care provider or those who cannot travel easily, this makes careful monitoring, once an impossible goal, a reality.

Yet, there may be some downside to these technological advances. Technology should facilitate care, not dictate it or place restrictions on it. McNutt and Abrams (2002) recounted the story of a patient admitted to the intensive care unit (ICU) from the emergency room who was in immediate need of a particular medication. The doctor in the ICU could not find this new patient in the computer database, which meant that he was unable to order the medication; he decided to wait instead of trying to override the electronic order system. (The system had been very tightly designed so that no order could be received until the patient was in the database and the insurance company had authorized care). The patient died as a result of the delay.

Some are worried too, about threats to privacy and confidentiality when so much personal information is available in one place online. The Health Information Portability and Accountability Act addresses the importance of preventing unauthorized access to this information and provides for penalties for those who violate confidentiality (Follansbee, 2002). Others are concerned about the considerable cost of these high tech approaches to health care. "New medical technologies, too attractive to forbid and too expensive to be made generally available, will exacerbate the inequalities that now exist within and between societies" (Freeman, 1997, p. 88).

Another concern about the increasing influence (if not dominance) of technology on our lives is that it may be dehumanizing. It may lead us to neglect the emotional and spiritual aspects of the human experience, which are "invisible" when not included in the computerized databases used to guide patient assessment (Liaschenko, 2002). Postman (1992), for example, commented on the "chilling" use of computer-related metaphors to describe human behavior, especially thinking. He used the story of the introduction of the stethoscope to illustrate how a piece of equipment can come between the client and the physician. Before the stethoscope was developed, a physician placed his or her ear against the client's chest or relied on the client's description of symptoms to understand the problem. When stethoscopes became available, this was no longer necessary.

Diagnosis can be done through biopsies, radiographs, laboratory tests, electrocardiograms, computed tomography scans, magnetic resonance imaging, positron emission tomography, and so forth. An electrocardiogram or scan can be reviewed by a practitioner hundreds or thousands of miles away. We now have the ability to "view the insides" of the individual, allowing physicians and nurses to identify not only internal structures but also function. This has shifted our focus from attempting to understand the client's response to the problem to finding the cause and fixing it. The importance of the client's experience seems to diminish each time another piece of equipment is put into use. Each device or instrument is thought to supply more "objective" information than the words of the client or the eyes, ears, and hands of the care provider can supply. Specialists can direct surgery across the globe. Before long, it may be possible to monitor our clients without seeing or touching them at all.

In a technology-oriented health care environment, talking with a client and family could eventually become superfluous. In a caring environment, however, it is a priority (Locsin, 1995). The scenarios at the beginning of the chapter illustrate the differences between these two futures.

Most of our clients define quality of nursing care as a combination of both technical competence and caring behaviors. Although they want the health care provider to listen and provide the personal touch, they also expect the use of technology. Many feel that if the health care provider does not perform a scan or use the newest laser procedure, they are not receiving the highest quality health care. This creates some dilemmas for the health care provider. However, even in this difficult time when cost saving and efficiency are heavily emphasized, nurses can retain their commitment to caring and quality of care for the clients we serve. Miller (1996) suggested ways to keep caring in nursing practice (Box 17–1.)

Consumerism

Home pregnancy tests, personal HIV tests, whole body scans, and stool tests for occult blood are already available to the consumer. Personal computers allow individuals to access medical information previously available only to health care providers. As technology advances, consumers may someday have the ability to purchase more complicated tests and tools that allow self-diagnosis. Some are concerned that most consumers are not prepared to sort out all the information available to them or to accurately interpret the meaning of a positive laboratory test, such as a prostate-specific antigen (PSA) test (Wojner, 2001). Others are concerned about liability for advice provided online, especially if the patient has not been seen by his or her health care provider recently (Landro, 2002).

> ### BOX 17–1
> ### Keeping Caring in Your Nursing Practice
>
> - Analyze your own caring skills. Become more aware of your caring abilities throughout the work-day.
> - Understand that caring is an important part of all types of nursing practice: clinical, advanced practice, administration, education, and research. Learn to appreciate how other nurses use caring skills in their unique practices.
> - Think of caring as a set of skills that can be improved: showing kindness, preserving dignity, explaining with empathy, being patient, staying emotionally present, enabling another's life transitions, sustaining faith in another's life transitions, recognizing another's humanity weakness and strength, doing for another as you yourself would want. Practice these—become expert.
> - Be a role model for caring. If caring skills can be enhanced, they can be taught. Be a teacher to all around you.
> - Do not let anyone diminish the importance of the caring actions that you direct toward nurses and others in your organization. Support caring actions of clinical nurses toward patients and families, even when caregiving is focused on the technological tasks of nursing.
> - Patients do not equate time with caring. Make sure nurses understand the value of their caring actions to patients and families.
> - Let caring "civilize" the not-so-civilized current health care industry. Remind yourself every day that without caring, we would be like every other business. Patients, families, and colleagues need us and our caring skills.
> - Lastly, and importantly, use your caring skills on each other. Especially when stress is high, we all need to be cared for.
>
> Source: From Miller, K.L. (1996), Keeping the care in nursing care: Our biggest challenge. *Journal of Nursing Administration*, 25(11), 29–32. Used with permission of Lippincott-Raven Publishers, Philadelphia.

With the passage of time, this will probably shift the health care professional's role to that of counselor, most likely including an interpretation of the diagnostic testing.

Another trend spurred by the proactive, self-directed consumer is the great increase in the use of alternative and complementary treatments. From taking herbs such as gingko biloba to improve memory to doing yoga to reduce stress, consumers have embraced the idea that there is something they can do to improve their own health. At first skeptical of either the efficacy or influence of these treatments, health care professionals are now taking them seriously, learning how to use them, asking their patients if they use them, and recommending them as adjuncts to the usual medical care (Porter-O'Grady, 2001).

Survival of Vulnerable Individuals

Continued advances in technology will not only provide more treatment options but also keep people alive longer. From high-risk newborns to accident victims to the critically ill elderly, advances in health care have made it possible for many to survive who would not have survived in years past. The result is that we have both very high expectations of our health care system and larger numbers of people in need of care, especially of rehabilitation, long-term care, and home health care. The "baby boomers" are entering their sixties. As they move into their later years, their need for health care will increase. Longer life expectancy, more individuals with chronic problems, and diversity of the older population will challenge our present system (Roy, 2000; U.S. Census Bureau, 2000). Much concern has been expressed that the current health care system is not equipped to respond to these coming demands.

Emphasis on Economics

Concern about cost has driven the quest for the highest level of efficiency possible in the delivery of health care. The result is a whole range of changes designed to minimize the time and money spent on a patient and to maximize the profit gained. There is evidence, however, that the drive for profit has resulted in lower quality of health care, especially for the most vulnerable members of our society, people with mental illnesses and people with serious chronic diseases (Mechanic, 2002).

The drive for cost saving originated with large employers, who were concerned about the rising cost of health insurance. Insurance companies responded with a variety of plans that shifted more cost to employees and encouraged them to select less costly managed care plans (O'Connor, 2002).

In the past, patients, insurers, and the government rarely questioned a doctor's recommendations for a patient or the cost of implementing that decision. Today, the final decision may rest with a representative of an insurance company or health maintenance organization who does not have a health care background, unless the client is able to pay out of his or her own pocket. In some cases, the decision is made primarily on the basis of cost rather than the need of the client, and accusations of unnecessary harm and even death resulting from cost-based decisions have been made. There is evidence that health care consumers are rebelling against these cost-driven decisions, often by taking the issue to the courts (Felsenthal, 1996). In addition, some states are adopting laws to better define a client's rights in instances in which needed care is denied. In the next section, we describe some of these changes in more detail.

■ Changes in the Health Care System

What has been the response to these attempts to improve the efficiency and cost-effectiveness of health care? Curtin (1996, p. 7) described the response eloquently:

Administrators fear loss of influence, status, and income. Physicians fear loss of autonomy, control, and income. Nurses fear loss of professional standing, job, and income. And just about everyone with two live brain cells and a functioning conscience fears for the safety of patient care.

O'Connor (2002) added that hospital care "is stretched so thin that patients fear for their lives" now. It is important that we clearly separate fact from fiction as we respond to the current trends in health care. Let's begin with some background information.

Historical Perspective

Before 1965, the year Medicare (a federal program that pays a substantial portion of the health care costs of people over 65) was enacted, nurse vacancy rates in hospitals ran between 20 and 25 percent. Once Medicare was enacted, hospitals were able to shift much of the cost of nursing salaries onto Medicare, and the nursing shortages decreased.

When the diagnosis-related groups (DRGs), through which hospitals receive payment based on average cost per diagnosis, not on their cost, were introduced in the 1980s, the number of hospital admissions and average length of stay were reduced. Clients admitted to hospitals were more acutely ill and were discharged more quickly (the "quicker and sicker" phenomenon) to stay within the DRG guidelines. Hospitals realized that registered nurses (RNs) were best able to provide the care needed to move these clients safely and quickly through the hospital stay. They began questioning physicians about practice patterns that led to longer stays, but the use of RNs to provide most of the client care was not questioned. By the 1990s, however, hospitals were unable to reduce their costs any further and managed care emerged as another way to squeeze more out of every health care dollar.

Managed Care

In a managed care system, consumers select a primary care physician provider from an approved list generated by their plan. Each provider is paid a predetermined (capitation) rate for each client, usually on a monthly basis. The primary care provider is the "gatekeeper" because the client must obtain a referral from the primary care physician before seeing a specialist. Those who want to see an out-of-plan provider usually have to pay for new services out-of-pocket.

The original idea behind managed care was that emphasizing preventive health care, including yearly physicals, immunizations, and health education, is an effective way to avoid illness and future hospitalizations, thereby reducing costs (Richards, 1996). It was based on evidence that eight of the nine leading causes of death in the United States can be reduced by attention to lifestyle changes: smoking, lack of exercise, unsafe sex, unsafe driving, and poor diets (Hayes, 2000). If clients do become ill, the physicians within the plan are often given powerful incentives to control costs (Buerhaus, 1996) by limiting the number of diagnostic tests done, for example, or by avoiding a hospital stay altogether, if possible.

Among the industrialized countries around the world, the United States is the only one that does not provide basic health care coverage to every citizen (Lieberman, 2003). In fact, one in seven people in the United States does not have health insurance (Pear, 2002). The United States does have technologically advanced, highly sophisticated health care and spends more per capita (per person) than most countries. This amount is increasing. Yet our health care system has been described as a "shipwreck" (O'Connor, 2002), a system with "growing cracks" in it that are serious enough to raise high levels of concern (McGinley & Lueck, 2002). One recent study of medical errors estimated that 36% of all patients admitted to a teaching hospital can expect to encounter some iatrogenic event during their stay (Yourstone & Smith, 2002). An Institute of Medicine report estimated that somewhere between 44,000 and 98,000 hospital patients in a year die as a consequence of medical error (Mechanic, 2002). This is equivalent to having a jumbo jet crash every day (Yourstone & Smith, 2002). Would we tolerate such a risk in our transportation system? Of course not. Then why do we tolerate it in health care?

You may be asking, if we have the most advanced knowledge and equipment and are spending a great deal of money on our health care, why the cause for alarm? What is wrong? Why doesn't everyone have health care insurance? Why are people so worried about the quality of care? The answer is complex. Let's look at some of the reasons why our system is developing serious cracks:

- For most of us, our health insurance comes through our place of employment. One problem with this is that many employers are motivated to keep the cost as low as possible or transfer much of the cost to the employee. Another problem is that if you lose your job, you also lose your health insurance.

- Managed care is designed to limit the amount spent on health care. Some have said that it has become a way to limit choices and ration care (Mechanic, 2002) rather than prevent illness.

- As managed care plans grow and spread across the country, these companies become powerful enough to be able to negotiate reduced rates (discounts) from local hospitals (Trinh & O'Connor, 2002). They can, in effect, say, "We can get an appendectomy for $2300 at hospital A, why should we pay you $2700?" If hospital B doesn't agree, they may lose all the patients enrolled in that managed care plan. This pressures hospitals to reduce costs and spread their staff even thinner than before.

- Similar price pressures come from Medicare, Medicaid, and other health insurance companies. To keep costs under control, some states have cut benefits for people receiving Medicaid (state supported health benefits for low income people) (Pear, 2002).

- Although always an important issue, health care took a back seat to national security after the September 11th attacks and conflict in the Middle East (Pear, 2002). We need now to renew the national debate on how to fix our health care system.

• With the upsurge in for-profit health plans and the purchase of not-for-profit hospitals by for-profit companies, our health care has become increasingly "corporatized." It had been thought that this would give us a highly efficient, responsive system ("the customer is always right") but it has not because the "customer" who pays for insurance coverage is actually the employer, not the individual patient. The care provided by the for-profits appears to be of lesser quality than the old not-for-profit or fee-for service plans (Mechanic, 2002).

• There is a limit to the extent to which cost cutting can increase efficiency without endangering patients. A series of important research studies has shown that increasing the number of RNs providing care in a hospital has a direct effect on improving the outcomes of patient care. The opposite is also true: each additional patient assigned to a nurse increases the odds of the patient dying within 30 days of admission by 7% (Aiken et al., 2002).

For many years, we have been trying to fix our system by applying patches over its worst cracks but this has apparently not worked very well. Does our system need a major overhaul? Probably, but first, as a group, we need to agree on a vision of what it should be and what it should do (O'Connor, 2002). Whatever way that vision develops, it is certain that nurses will have an important role in our future health care system. As Aiken and colleagues (2002) wrote, "nurses contribute importantly to surveillance, early detection and timely interventions that save lives" (p.18).

Subacute Care

One way to reduce cost is to shift people out of expensive acute care hospitals as quickly as possible into less costly settings, such as subacute care units. Subacute units can offer round-the-clock nursing care to stable clients with a variety of diagnoses. Subacute care may be found in a variety of settings: free-standing skilled nursing facilities, hospital-based skilled nursing units, swing bed units, and rehabilitation hospitals or units.

Many subacute care providers have developed programs for specific populations, such as people on ventilators or in need of wound care, oncology treatment, or rehabilitation. Staffing them with nurses skilled in these areas can significantly decrease the cost of providing care. Many believe that the subacute setting will continue to grow as a viable alternative to more costly acute care (Masso, 1995). Nurses with associate's degrees are in great demand in subacute units. Their expertise in the essentials of nursing care for the relatively stable client will contribute to offering cost-effective, quality care (Browne & Biancolillo, 1996, p. 23).

Community-Based Care

Another alternative to the acute care setting is to provide care in ambulatory settings and in the home. Many types of surgery can be done on an outpatient basis, and many therapies once considered too complex to do at home (intravenous therapies and dialysis, for example) are now being done safely and effectively in clients' homes. The specialization common in acute facilities is entering home care: wound care, dialysis care, perinatal care, and congestive heart failure management are a few examples (McClure, 2000). Buerhaus (1996) listed characteristics of the past and future health care delivery systems (Table 17–1).

▣ Effect on Nursing

The past decade has seen pronounced changes in the organization and delivery of health care services. Several related to nursing were identified in both North America and Europe:

1 Decentralization of allied health services such as physical and respiratory therapy. In some cases, much of the responsibility was

TABLE 17–1

Comparison of the Past and Future Health Care Delivery Systems

Past/Traditional	Future Managed Health Care System
Episodic illness-focused	Wellness and prevention-oriented
Insurance-based payment	Managed care
Inpatient care	Ambulatory and community-based
Hospitals as profit centers	Hospitals as cost centers
Specialist providers	Primary care providers
Independent solo physicians	Multispecialty group practices
Fee for service payments	Predetermined capitated fee
Heavily regulated environment	Highly competitive environment
Provider-driven system	Cost-driven system
Presumption of high quality	Systematic evaluation of quality indicators

Source: Adapted from Buerhaus, P.I. (1996). A heads up on capitation. *Nursing Policy Forum*, 2(3), 21.

moved back to nursing; in others, the therapists were asked to supervise ancillary personnel (techs, aides) so that more patients could be treated at a lower cost

2 Cross-training of workers with varying education and expertise to assume tasks traditionally outside their scope of work so that workers can do interchangeable tasks and therefore be substituted for each other

3 Assignment of ancillary personnel, such as housekeeping, to patient units

4 Skill mix reductions with a decreasing percentage of RNs on patient units (Aiken, Clarke & Sloan, 2000)

Nurses have moved into other settings, as predicted, but concern about shortage is increasing again (Bleich, Santos, & Cox, 2003). Today, the greatest impact to nursing appears to be in the following areas.

Elimination of Positions

Forced to reduce costs, hospitals have merged and eliminated duplicative departments and units such as psychiatry or positron emission tomography scans (Baz-

zoli et al., 2002). This has resulted in the loss of some nursing positions. Nurse managers may be responsible for two or three units instead of just one. Staffing levels were reduced to the minimum necessary to provide safe care. These practices continue to result in too few nurses for too many clients, often causing long hours, complex demands, information overload, and stress for the staff (Yourstone & Smith, 2002).

Changes in Practice Environment

It was claimed that the changes in skill mix were made to relieve RNs from non-nursing duties. In reality, this strategy decreased RN staffing but not RN responsibilities. Nurses are still responsible for supervising the decentralized staff, a task that is extremely time-consuming and raises concerns for patient safety. As early as 1990, nurses voiced their concerns about safety for patient care related to inadequate RN-to-patient ratios. In 1999, California became the first state to mandate minimum nurse-to-patient ratios in response to these concerns (Aiken, Clarke, & Sloan, 2000).

Nursing Shortage

Another concern is the "aging" of the nursing workforce. The statistics seem to support this notion: the average age of an RN today is 45 years (Stevenson, 2003). Even more surprising is the proportion of RNs who are younger than 30: this has dropped from 30% to 12%. In 2010, 40% of the nursing workforce will be over the age of 50 if the trends continue (*Advances*, 2000).

We're also going to see a decrease in the number of RNs per capita if the trends do not change. The number per capita will peak in 2007 and then decline just at the time when demand for nursing care is expected to explode because it coincides with the time that the baby boomer generation begins to enroll in Medicare (*Advances*, 2000). Ten years from now, we will not have enough RNs to staff nursing homes at their current levels, much less increase the level of professional staff (*http://www.AHCA.org*). Employers of nurses need to work with educators of new nurses to find betters ways to engage, challenge, and nurture new nurses (Wieck, Prydun, & Walsh, 2002).

Ensuring an adequate RN workforce is not as simple as the "a nurse is a nurse is a nurse" mentality implies, either. Experienced nurses specialize in various fields: surgery, long-term care, home health, and so on. The question becomes which types of RNs, in terms of educational achievement and experience, will be needed. The National Advisory Council on Nurse Education has recommended that at least two-thirds of the basic nurse workforce hold bachelor of science in nursing (BSN) degrees by 2010, with a projected deficit of more than 200,000 BSN nurses. Entry-level baccalaureate enrollments and RN-BSN completion enrollments are dropping. Approximately 15 percent of nurses with associate's degrees nationwide eventually pursue the BSN (Blouin & Brent, 2000; Rapson & Rice, 2000).

Preventing Patient Care Errors

The committee that prepared the report on deaths from medical errors for the Institute of Medicine indicated that the majority of errors result from basic flaws in the way health care organizations are run. As a member of the health care team, you have a responsibility to identify system and personnel issues that may potentially cause patient care errors (Blouin & Brent, 2000).

Emphasis on Outcomes

Outcomes measurement is the process of collecting and analyzing data using predetermined outcomes indicators to make decisions about health care. Each specific indicator must be defined very precisely so that consistent data is collected. Outcomes measurement is required by most accrediting organizations as a method of evaluating quality on the basis of objective evidence about the results of the health care process. Many outcomes measures currently are used to evaluate health care, but few of them rep-

resent nursing's specific and unique contribution to patient care.

To address this issue, the American Nurses Association (ANA) instituted the Nursing Care Report Card for Acute Care in which 10 specific quality indicators of nursing were developed and defined. The ANA felt that these indicators had a strong connection to quality nursing care. Table 17–2 outlines the indicators and their operational definitions (ANA, 2000).

You may be thinking that collecting "numbers" is too time-consuming for you, the new staff nurse, and certainly does not rank high on your list of priority nursing activities. However, without evidence that nursing is having an impact on the quality of care, decisions will be made in health care that may be detrimental to patients and to the nursing profession. Being able to link these outcomes to staffing levels is one way in which nursing can impact health and institutional policies. As a staff nurse, your ability to focus on evidence-based practice instead of a collection of tasks is of the utmost importance.

> The contribution that nursing makes to health care is well known, but it has not been clearly demonstrated. Little objective evidence presently exists establishing linkages between nursing and health outcomes. Most present day nursing care is still based on intuition or trial and error practices. Although it presents challenges, the profession of nursing must join its medical colleagues in the routine investigation of its practices for the purpose of generating evidence. (*http://www.nursingworld.org/mods/Working/QY/ceomfull.htm*, 12/7/00).

Leadership in the Future

Management visionaries predict that the leaders of the future are more likely to be women and/or members of a minority group than has been the case in the past. They will also be more empowering and less directive (Bennis, Spreitzer, & Cummings, 2001). This is important for nurses, many of whom fit this new profile. Joel and Kelly (2002) urged nurses to manage their futures actively. This includes developing the skills needed to function in a changing environment. Competencies identified by nurse

TABLE 17–2
ANA Nursing Quality Indicators and Their Operational Definitions

Nursing Quality Indicators	Operational Definitions
Nosocomial infection rate	The rate per 1000 patient acute care days at which patients develop clinically active bacteremia (as defined by CDC) in whom there is no evidence to suggest that infection was present or incubating at admission (using CDC differential criteria) under development.
Patient fall rate	The rate at which patients fall during the course of their hospital stay per 1000 patient days.
Patient satisfaction with nursing care	Patient opinion of care received from nursing staff during the hospital stay as determined by scaled responses to a uniform series of questions designed to elicit patient views regarding key elements of nursing care services.
Patient satisfaction with pain management	Patient opinion of how well nursing staff managed their pain as determined by scaled responses to a uniform series of questions designed to elicit patient views regarding specific aspects of pain management.
Patient satisfaction with educational information	Patient opinion of nursing staff efforts to educate them regarding their condition and care requirements as determined by scaled responses to a uniform series of questions designed to elicit patient views regarding specific aspects of patient education activities.
Patient satisfaction with care	Patient opinion of the care received during the hospital stay as determined by scaled responses to a uniform series of questions designed to elicit patient views regarding global aspects of care.
Nursing job satisfaction	Job satisfaction expressed by nurses working in hospital settings as determined by scaled responses to a uniform series of questions designed to elicit nursing staff attitudes toward specific aspects of their employment situation.
Maintenance of skin integrity	Rate per 1000 patient days at which patients develop pressure ulcers (Grade 1 or greater) during the course of their hospital stay, but 72 hours or more following their admission.
	Mix of RNs, LPNs, unlicensed staff caring for patients in acute care settings: The ratios (expressed in FTEs) of registered nurses with direct patient care responsibilities to LPNs and unlicensed workers.
Total Nursing Care Hours Provided per Patient Day	Total number of hours worked by nursing staff with direct patient care responsibilities on acute care units per patient day.

Source: http://www.nursingworld.org/mods/working/QY/ceomfull.htm. Accessed 12/7/2000.

managers as essential for the workplace of the future include (Byers, 2000; Rapson & Rice, 2000):

- Critical thinking skills
- Understanding systems
- Case management
- Team-building and communication skills
- Interpersonal skills of negotiation, collaboration, conflict management
- Cultural competency
- Flexibility
- Technological competence
- Business skills

Evaluate your current strengths and weaknesses in these areas. Consider which areas you need to explore further at this time. As you continue to grow in your nursing career, refer to this list of competencies. Are you growing in these areas? Are the positions you desire requiring you to update these skills?

Responding to the Changes in the Health Care System

It is time to take stock of what nurses do, what they can do, and what they should do. Following are some suggestions for dealing with the ongoing changes in health care. They are based on a set of "rules for successful redesign" developed by Porter-O'Grady (1996):

1 Remember that everyone is affected in some way by these changes. No one is exempt. Don't be like the ostrich that buries its head in the sand. Look up; look around at what's happening, and prepare to respond effectively.

2 Watch for clues that indicate what trends are occurring. Use your own insight and experience to analyze these trends. Listen to what others are saying, especially the leaders of the profession; read the news reports and professional literature to keep abreast of what is expected to happen.

3 Follow your vision. What is it about nursing that is especially important to you? What are your values? Hold on to what is most meaningful, and continue to work toward accomplishing your vision.

4 Empower yourself and others. In reality, there is "precious little real empowerment" of employees in most health care organizations (Porter-O'Grady, 1996, p. 50). Some of the suggestions elsewhere in the text about power and organizations may help you develop your own sense of empowerment.

5 Understand how your own goals fit with your employer's goals. Your personal goals and vision for nursing may or may not agree with your employer's. It is important that you recognize whatever differences exist and decide how you can reconcile them, if necessary.

6 Look past today. When changes come at you fast and furiously, it is very difficult to step back and evaluate the effect of those changes and to decide how to respond to them. You need to keep in mind your own long-term career plan and to evaluate how you can accomplish your goals in a changing environment.

Although some of the changes discussed may be disturbing, there are positive aspects to what is happening in health care. These changes provide an opportunity for nursing to emerge as a positive force in the midst of a revolution. Nursing offers caring in a system that appears to have forgotten its importance to people and their well-being.

◘ The Future

Many predictions have been made about the directions in which our health care system will go in the future. Predicted trends include (Coughlin, 2000a, 2000b; Hayes, 2000; O'Leary & O'Leary, 1999; Porter-O'Grady, 2003):

- Increasing pressure from consumers for quality health care services

- Accelerating movement from inpatient to outpatient care

- Focus on family responsibilities, such as wellness, health promotion, safety, self-care management, advanced directives

- Hospital profitability continuing to drive change

- Demand for innovative nurse leadership with an ability to operate in the political arena

- Tracking of outcomes and profitability

- More collaborative partnerships between physicians and nurses

What does all this mean to the graduate nurse entering the health care system? Health care institutions will expect new nurses to be flexible and to use skills that may not have been included in their basic education. Graduate nurses will need to be open to learning new information and developing new skills. You should also consider your future education plans. The demands on the new graduate will be greater, and client outcomes will be observed more closely. Nurses will also find opportunities in a variety of health settings, particularly in the community (Lescavage, 1995).

Earlier chapters discussed client care management techniques, communication skills, and teamwork. Now is the time to put all these ideas together and develop your leadership role in the working environment. If you maintain a positive attitude as you gain experience, you will become more comfortable in this challenging environment.

This is the time for nursing to demonstrate what it has to offer. Consider these changes to be positive, and realize that to gain satisfaction from your chosen profession, you must be proactive within it. Anticipate the future with excitement and remember that "a nurse is never finished" (Nightingale, 1859).

Study Questions

1 What are the major forces affecting the health care system today? What kinds of changes have occurred in response to these changes?

2 Describe the current employment picture for nurses. What changes do you expect in the future?

3 Explore one of the health care agencies in your area. What quality indicators are they measuring at this time? Think back to clinical experiences you have had. What quality indicators would you suggest to be important to nursing?

4 Based on the competencies needed today and in the future, what educational goals do you have for the future? What competencies do you expect to develop and/or further expand as you obtain your BSN? MSN?

Critical Thinking Exercise

Read the two scenarios at the beginning of this chapter a second time. Then create your own futuristic scenario for an episode of client care. If you can, share your scenario with your classmates.

1 What do you think are the most promising characteristics of these imaginary health care systems?

2 What characteristics concern you the most?

3 Explain why you find some characteristics promising and others troublesome.

4 What is your vision of an ideal health care system?

REFERENCES

Aiken, L., Clarke, S.P., Sloane, D. Sochalski, J., & Silber, J.H. (2002). Hospital nurse staffing and patient mortality, nurse burnout and job dissatisfaction. *JAMA*, 288(16), 1987–1993.

Aiken, L., Clarke, S., & Sloane, D. (2000). Hospital restructuring: Does it adversely affect care and outcomes? *Journal of Nursing Administration*, 30(10), 457–465.

American Health Care Association. *http://www.ahca. org. Accessed 12/19/2002.*

American Nurses Association. *http://www.nursing-world.org/mods/working/QY/ceomfull.htm.* Accessed 12/7/2000.

Bazzoli, G.J., LoSasso, A., Arnould, R., & Schalowitz, M. (2002). Hospital reorganization and restructuring achieved through merger. *Health Care Management Review*, 27(1), 7–20

Bennis, W. Spreitzer, G.M., & Cummings, T.A. (2001). *The Future of Leadership*. San Francisco: Jossey-Bass.

Bleich, M.R., Santos, S.R., & Cox, K.S. (2003). Analysis of the nursing workforce crisis: A call to action. *American Journal of Nursing*, 103(4), 66–74.

Blouin, A., & Brent, N. (2000). Happy Y2K: New and old challenges for the nurse administrator. *Journal of Nursing Administration, 30*(6), 292–294.

Browne, R., & Biancolillo, K. (1996). The integral role of nursing in managed care. *Nursing Management, 27*(4), 22–24.

Buerhaus, P.I. (1996). A heads up on capitation. *Nursing Policy Forum, 2*(3), 21.

Bureau of Health Professions. *http://www.bhpr.hrsa. gov.* Accessed 12/19/2002.

Byers, J. (2000). Knowledge, skills, and attributes needed for nurse and non-nurse executives. *Journal of Nursing Administration, 30,* 354–356.

Coughlin, C. (2000a). Is now the time to design new care delivery models? *Journal of Nursing Administration, 30,* 403–404.

Coughlin, C. (2000b). Where will tomorrow's nurse managers come from? *Journal of Nursing Administration, 30*(4), 157–159.

Curtin, L. (1996). Editorial: Other people's lives. *Nursing Management, 27*(5), 7.

Follansbee, N.M. (2002). Implications of the health information portability and accountability act. *Journal of Nursing Administration, 32,* 42–47.

Felsenthal, E. (May 17, 1996). When HMOs say no to health coverage, more patients are taking them to court. *Wall Street Journal,* p. B1.

Freeman, D. (October 20, 1997). Science's great dreamspinner. *Business Week,* 84–89.

Hayes, P.G. (Fall 2000). Observations on apparent paradoxes: Health care markets in the new millennium. *The Forum,* 79–84.

Joel, L.A., & Kelly, L.Y. (2002). *The Nursing Experience: Trends, Challenges and Transitions.* New York: McGraw-Hill.

Kunii, I.M. (February 17, 2003). A muscle suit you can strap right on. *Business Week,* 13.

Landro, L. (February 11, 2002). Unhealthy communication. *Wall Street Journal,* PR12.

Larson-Dahn, M.L. (2002). Tele nursing practice: Setting standards for practice across the continuum of care. *Journal of Nursing Administration, 32,* 524–530.

Lescavage, N. (1995). Nurses, make your presences felt: Taking off the rose-colored glasses. *Nursing Policy Forum, 1*(1), 18–24.

Liaschenko, J. (2002). Thoughts on nursing work. *Journal of Nursing Administration, 32*(2), 69–70.

Lieberman, T. (2003). Bruised and broken: The US health system. *AARP Bulletin, 44*(3), 3–5.

Locsin, R. (1995). Machine technologies and caring in nursing. *Image, 27*(3), 201–203.

Masso, A. (1995). Managed care and alternative-site health care delivery. *Journal of Care Management, 1*(1), 45, 47–48, 50–51.

McClure, M.L. (2000). A look back and a look ahead. *Nursing Administration Quarterly, 25*(1), 107–114.

McGinley, L., & Lueck, S. (November 14, 2002). Gore's position on health care signals a sharp shift in mood. *Wall Street Journal,* A8.

McNutt, R.A., & Abrams, R.L. (2002). Model of medical error based on a model of disease: Interactions between adverse events, failures and their errors. *Quality Management in Health Care, 10*(2), 23–28.

Mechanic, D. (2002). Socio-cultural implications of changing organizational technologies in the provision of care. *Social Science and Medicine, 54,* 459–467.

Miller, K. (1996). Keeping the care in nursing care. *Journal of Nursing Administration, 25*(11), 29–38.

Nightingale, F. (1859). *Notes on Nursing.* Reprinted 1992. Philadelphia: J.B. Lippincott.

O'Connor, K. (April 8, 2002). Healthcare in need of a fix. *Modern Healthcare,* 27.

O'Leary, J., & O'Leary, P. (1999). What is the future for nurse executives? *Journal of Nursing Administration, 23*(3), 4–10.

Pear, R. (November 20, 2002). Report: Health System in crisis. *Sun Sentinel,* 3A.

Pew Health Professions Commission. (1995). *Critical Challenges: Revitalizing the Health Profession for the Twenty-First Century.* San Francisco: UCSF Center for the Health Professions.

Pew Health Professions Commission. (1995). Primary Care Workforce-2000—Federal Policy Paper. San Francisco: UCSF Center for the Health Professions.

Porter-O'Grady, T. (2003). A different age for readership, part I. *Journal of Nursing Administration, 33*(2), 105–110.

Porter-O'Grady, T. (2001). Profound change: 21st century nursing. *Nursing Outlook, 49*(4), 182–186.

Porter-O'Grady, T. (1996). The seven basic rules for successful redesign. *Journal of Nursing Administration, 26*(1), 46–53.

Postman, N. (1992). *Technopoly: The Surrender of Culture to Technology.* New York: Vintage Books.

Rapson, M., & Rice, R. (2000). Progress and outcomes of the colleagues in caring program: Phase one. *Journal of Nursing Administration, 29*(7/8), 4–8.

Richards, S. (1996). The pulse of managed care. Managed care 101. *Nursing Policy Forum, 2*(3), 13.

Roy, S.C. (2000). The visible and invisible fields that shape the future of the nursing care system. *Nursing Administration Quarterly, 25*(1), 119–131.

Sloane, M.M. (2003). Robotics in surgery. *Nursing Spectrum, 13*(5FL), 8, 21.

Stevenson, E.L. (2003). Future trends in nursing employment. *American Journal of Nursing: Career Guide 2003,* part 2 of 2, 19–25.

The US nursing workforce: Aging and shrinking. (2000). *Advances, 4,* 5–6.

Trinh, H.Q., & O'Connor, S.J. (2002). Helpful or harmful? The impact of strategic change on the performance of U.S. urban hospitals. *Health Services Research, 37*(1), 145–171.

U.S. Census Bureau. (2000). *April 12, 1999 Population Division Revisions to Standards for Classification of Federal Data in Race and Ethnicity.* Washington, D.C.: Department of Commerce.

Wieck, K.L., Prydum, M., & Walsh, T. (2002). What emerging workforce wants in its leaders. *Journal of Nursing Scholarship, 34,* 283–288.

Wojner, A.W. (2001). *Outcomes Management: Applications to Clinical Management.* St. Louis, Mo.: Mosby.

Wysocki, B. (November 11, 2002). Personal Health (A Special Report): Treatments–Medication makeover: Tallahassee Memorial Hospital is upending the way it prescribes and delivers drugs; It's a glimpse of even bigger changes to come. *Wall Street Journal*, p. R6.

Yourstone, S.A., & Smith, H.L. (2002). Managing system errors and failures in health care organizations: Suggestions for practice and research. *Health Care Management Review*, 27(1), 50–61.

APPENDIX 1

Code of Ethics for Nurses

American Nurses Association Code of Ethics for Nurses

1 The nurse, in all professional relationships, practices with compassion and respect for the inherent dignity, worth, and uniqueness of every individual, unrestricted by considerations of social or economic status, personal attributes, or the nature of health problems.

2 The nurse's primary commitment is to the patient, whether an individual, family, group, or community.

3 The nurse promotes, advocates for, and strives to protect the health, safety, and rights of the patient.

4 The nurse is responsible and accountable for individual nursing practice and determines the appropriate delegation of tasks consistent with the nurse's obligation to provide optimum patient care.

5 The nurse owes the same duties to self as to others, including the responsibility to preserve integrity and safety, to maintain competence, and to continue personal and professional growth.

6 The nurse participates in establishing, maintaining, and improving health care environments and conditions of employment conducive to the provision of quality health care and consistent with the values of the profession through individual and collective action.

7 The nurse participates in the advancement of the profession through contributions to practice, education, administration, and knowledge development.

8 The nurse collaborates with other health professionals and the public in promoting community, national, and international efforts to meet health needs.

9 The profession of nursing, as represented by associations and their members, is responsible for articulating nursing values, for maintaining the integrity of the profession and its practice, and for shaping social policy.[1]

Approved July 2001

http://www.nursingworld.org/ethics/ chcode.htm

---

[1]Source: Reprinted with permission from American Nurses Association, Code of Ethics for Nurses with Interpretive Statements, ©2001 American Nurses Publishing , American Nurses Foundation/American Nurses Association, Washington, DC.

■ Canadian Nurse Association Code of Ethics for Registered Nurses

Values

A value is something that is prized or held dear; something that is deeply cared about. This code is organized around eight primary values that are central to ethical nursing practice:

Safe, Competent, and Ethical Care

Nurses value the ability to provide safe, competent and ethical care that allows them to fulfill their ethical and professional obligations to the people they serve.

Health and Well-Being

Nurses value health promotion and well-being and assisting persons to achieve their optimum level of health in situations of normal health, illness, injury, disability or at the end of life.

Choice

Nurses respect and promote the autonomy of persons and help them to express their health needs and values, and also to obtain desired information and services so they can make informed decisions.

Dignity

Nurses recognize and respect the inherent worth of each person and advocate for respectful treatment of all persons.

Confidentiality

Nurses safeguard information learned in the context of a professional relationship, and ensure it is shared outside the health care team only with the person's informed consent, or as may be legally required, or where the failure to disclose would cause significant harm.

Justice

Nurses uphold principles of equity and fairness to assist persons in receiving a shar of health services and resources proportionate to their needs and in promoting social justice.

Accountability

Nurses are answerable for their practice, and they act in a manner consistent with their professional responsibilities and standards of practice.

Quality Practice Environments

Nurses value and advocate for practice environments that have the organizational structures and resources necessary to ensure safety, support and respect for all persons in the work setting.[2]

Approved September 2002

http://www.cna-nurses.ca/pages/ethics/ethicsframe.htm

---

[2]Source: Reprinted with permission from the Canadian Nurses Association, *http://www.can-nurses.ca/pages/ethics/ethicsframe.htm.* Accessed May 4, 2003.

■ The International Council of Nurses Code of Ethics for Nurses

Nurses and People

The nurse's primary professional responsibility is to people requiring nursing care.

In providing nursing care, the nurse promotes an environment in which the human rights, values, customs and spiritual beliefs of the individual, family and community are respected.

The nurse ensures that the individual receives sufficient information on which to base consent for care and related treatment.

The nurse holds in confidence personal information and uses judgement in sharing this information.

The nurse shares with society the responsibility for initiating and supporting action to meet the health and social needs of the public, in particular those of vulnerable populations.

The nurse also shares responsibility to sustain and protect the natural environment from depletion, pollution, degradation and destruction.

Nurses and Practice

The nurse carries personal responsibility and accountability for nursing practice, and for maintaining competence by continual learning.

The nurse maintains a standard personal health such that the ability to provide care is not compromised.

The nurse uses judgement regarding individual competence when accepting and delegating responsibility.

The nurse at all times maintains standards of personal conduct which reflect well on the profession and enhance public confidence.

The nurse, in providing care, ensures that use of technology and scientific advances are compatible with safety, dignity and rights of people.

Nurses and the Profession

The nurse assumes the major role in determining and implementing acceptable standards of clinical nursing practice, management, research and education.

The nurse is active in developing a core research-based professional knowledge.

The nurse, acting through professional organization, participates in creating and maintaining equitable social and economic working conditions in nursing.

Nurses and Co-workers

The nurse sustains a co-operative relationship with co-workers in nursing and other fields.

The nurse takes appropriate action to safeguard individuals when their care is endangered by a co-worker or any other person.[3]

Approved 2000
http://www.icn.ch/ethics.htm

---

[3]Source: Used with permission International Council of Nurses, Geneva Switzerland, copyright 2000.

APPENDIX 2

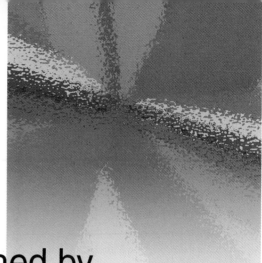

Standards Published by American Nurses Association

Standard	Year Published
Standards of Nursing Practice	1973
Standards of Psychiatric-Mental Health Nursing Practice	1973
Standards of Medical Surgical Nursing Practice	1974
Standards of Orthopedic Nursing Practice	1975
Standards of Neurological and Neurosurgical Nursing Practice	1977
Standards of Urological Nursing Practice	1977
Standards of Pediatric Oncology Nursing Practice	1978
Outcome Standards for Cancer Nursing Practice	1979
A Statement of the Scope of Medical-Surgical Nursing Practice	1980
Standards of Cardiovascular Nursing Practice	1981
Standards of Perioperative Nursing Practice	1981
Standards for Organized Nursing Services	1982
Outcome Standards for Rheumatology Nursing Practice	1983
Standards for Maternal-Child Health Nursing Practice	1983
Standards for Professional Nursing Education	1984
Standards for the Perinatal Nurse Specialist	1985
Standards of Child and Adolescent Psychiatric and Mental Health Nursing Practice	1985
Standards of Nursing Practice in Correctional Facilities	1985
Standards of Rehabilitation Nursing	1986
Orthopedic Nursing Process: Process and Outcome Criteria for Selected Diagnoses	1986
Standards of College Nursing Practice	1986
Standards of Community Health Nursing Practice	1986
Standards of Home Health Nursing Practice	1986
Standards and Scope of Gerontological Nursing Practice	1987
Scope and Standards of Hospice Nursing Practice	1987
Standards of Oncology Nursing Practice	1987

Standard	Year Published
Standards of Practice for the Primary Health Care Nurse Practitioner	1987
Standards of Addictions Nursing Practice with Selected Diagnoses and Criteria	1988
Standards for Organized Nursing Services (Revised)	1988
Standards of Clinical Nursing Practice	1991
Scope of Cardiac Rehabilitation Nursing Practice	1993
Standards for Nursing Professional Development: Continuing Education and Staff Development	1994
Standards of Nursing Informatics	1994
Scope of Practice for Nursing Informatics	1994
Statement on the Scope and Standards of Respiratory Nursing Practice	1994
Statement on the Scope and Standards of Psychiatric-Mental Health Clinical Nursing Practice	1994
Statement on the Scope and Standards of Otorhinolaryngology Clinical Nursing Practice	1994
Standards and Scope of Gerontological Nursing Practice	1995
Standards of Clinical Practice and Scope of Practice for the Acute Care Nurse Practitioner	1995
Scope and Standards of Nursing Practice in Correctional Facilities	1995
Statement on the Scope and Standards of Pediatric Clinical Nursing Practice	1996
Statement on the Scope and Standards of Oncology Nursing Practice	1996
Scope and Standards of Nurse Administrators	1996
Scope and Standards of Advanced Practice Registered Nursing	1996
Scope and Standards of College Health Nursing Practice	1997
Scope and Standards of Forensic Nursing Practice	1997

Source: http://nursingworld.org/books/pdescr.cfm?cnum=15.

APPENDIX 3

National Organization for Associate Degree Nursing (N-OADN) Resolution: Differentiated Nursing Practice

Whereas differentiated nursing practice is an approach to assuring quality nursing care through the appropriate utilization of nursing resources; and

Whereas the approach may include a variety of models for the roles and functions of registered nurses defined by criteria which include, but are not limited to experience, competence, and life long learning; and

Whereas differential nursing practice is a response to an environment challenged by changing health care trends as well as cost containment; and

Whereas the model for differentiated nursing practice is developed by the registered nurse employed within a practice environment and requires the identification of nursing competencies needed to provide quality nursing care; therefore

Be It Resolved
that N-OADN strongly support those practice models affording the registered nurse the opportunity to participate in the develop-

ment of competencies for roles in varied practice environments; and

Be It Further Resolved
that N-OADN advocates registered nurses to have the opportunity to assume roles appropriate to their capabilities and experience; and

Be It Further Resolved
that N-OADN strongly supports differentiated practice models that value the registered nurse and his/her practice; and

Be It Further Resolved
that this resolution be widely distributed to nursing and health care organizations.

(Adopted: N-OADN Convention, November 1997)

National Organization for Associate Degree Nursing
11250 Roger Bacon Drive, Suite 8
Reston, VA 20190
www.noadn.org

APPENDIX 4*

Guidelines for the Registered Nurse In Giving, Accepting or Rejecting A Work Assignment

Registered Nurses, as licensed professionals, share the responsibility and accountability along with their employer to ensure that safe, quality-nursing care is provided. The scope of professional nurses' accountability involves legal, ethical and professional guidelines for assuring safe, quality patient care. Legal responsibility for the provisions, delegation and supervision of patient care is specified in the Nurse Practice Act 464.001, and the Administrative Rules Chapter 59S. The American Nurses Association (ANA) Code for Nurses with Interpretive Statements (1985) guides ethical conduct and decision making of professional nurses. The ANA Standards and Scope of Practice (1997) provides a systematic application of nursing process for patient care management across patient care settings. In addition, the ANA Restructuring Survival Kit (1996) suggests common strategies to assist the professional nurse facing assignment and delegation issues during reassignment and reorganization, temporary or permanent. Lastly, the employer requirements for safe, competent staffing are outlined in facility policies and guidelines.

Within ethical and legal parameters the nurse exercises informed judgment and uses individual competence and qualifications as criteria in seeking consultation, accepting responsibilities, and delegating nursing activities to others. The nurse's decision regarding accepting or making work assignments is based on the legal, ethical and professional obligation to assume responsibility for nursing judgment and action.

The document offers strategies for problem solving as the staff nurse, nurse manager, chief nurse executive and administrator practice within the complex environment of the health care system.

Nursing Care Delivery

Only a Registered Nurse (RN) will assess, plan and evaluate a patient's or client's nursing care needs. No nurse shall be required or directed to delegate nursing activities to other personnel in a manner inconsistent with the Nurse Practice Act, the standards of the Joint Commission on Accreditation of Health Organizations, the ANA Standards of Practice or

*Reproduced with permission of Florida Nurses Association, 1999, Orlando, Florida.

Hospital Policy. Consistent with the preceding sentence, the individual RN has the autonomy to delegate (or not delegate) those aspects of nursing care the nurse determines appropriate based on the patient assessment.

When a nurse is floated to a unit or area where the nurse receives an assignment that is considered unsafe to perform independently, the RN has the right and obligation to request and receive a modified assignment, which reflects the RN's level of competence.

The Florida Nurses Association (FNA), the Florida Organization of Nurse Executives (FONE), and the FNA Labor Employee Relations Commission (LERC) recognize that changes in the health care delivery system have and will continue to occur, while emphasizing the common goal to provide safe quality patient care. The parties also recognize that RNs have a right and responsibility to participate in decisions affecting delivery of nursing care and related terms and conditions of employment. All parties have a mutual interest in developing systems, which will provide quality care on a cost efficient basis without jeopardizing patient outcomes. Thus, commitment to measuring the impact of staffing and assignments to patient outcomes is a shared commitment of all professional nurses irrespective of organizational structure.

◘ Assignment Despite Objection (ADO)/ Documentation of Practice Situation (DOPS)

Staff nurses today face often-untenable assignments that need to be documented as such. Critical, clinical judgment should be utilized when evaluating the appropriateness of an assignment. Refusal to accept an assignment without appropriate discussion within the chain of command can be defined as insubordinate behavior. Each Registered Nurse should become familiar with organizational policies, procedures and documentation regarding refusal to accept an unsafe assignment. ANA has recently adopted a position statement and model ADO form

available for use by SNA members. (Please contact Florida Nurses Association for further information).

Staffing

In the event a registered nurse determines in his/her professional opinion that he/she has been given an assignment that does not allow for appropriate patient care, he/she shall notify the Supervisor or designee who shall review the concerns of the nurse. If the nurse's concerns cannot be resolved by telephone, the Supervisor or designee, except in instances of compelling business reasons that preclude him/her from doing do, will then come to the unit within four (4) hours of being contacted by the nurse to assess the staffing. Such assessment shall be documented with a copy given to the nurse. Nothing herein shall prohibit a registered nurse from completing and submitting a protest of assignment form.

◘ Nurse Practice Act, 1994, Administrative Rules Chapt. 59S, 14.001 Definitions (4/29/96)

"Assignments" - are the normal daily functions of the UAP's based on institutional or agency job duties to which do not involve delegation of nursing functions or nursing judgment.

"Competency" - is the demonstrated ability to carry out specified tasks or activities with reasonable skill and safety that adheres to the prevailing standard of practice in the nursing community.

"Delegation" - is the transference to a competent individual the authority to perform a selected nursing task or activity in a selected situation by a nurse qualified by licensure and experience to perform the task or activity.

"Supervision" - is the provision of guidance by a qualified nurse and periodic inspection by the nurse for the accomplishment of a nursing task or activity, provided the nurse is qualified and legally entitled to perform such task or activity. The supervisor may be the delegator or a person of equal or greater licensure to the delegator.

Scenario

- Suppose you are asked to care for an unfamiliar patient population or to go to a unit for which you feel unqualified—what do you do?

- Suppose you are approached by your supervisor and asked to work an additional shift. Your immediate response is that you don't want to work another shift—what do you do?

Such situations are familiar and emphasize the rights and responsibilities of the RN to make informed decisions. Yet all members of the health care team, from staff nurses to administrator, share a joint responsibility to ensure that quality patient care is provided. At times though, difference in interpretation of legal or ethical principles may lead to conflict.

Guidelines for decision making are offered to assist RN problem-solve work assignment issues. Applications of these guidelines are presented in the form of scenarios, examples of unsafe assignments experienced by RNs.

Guidelines for Decision Making

The complexity of the delivery of nursing care is such that only professional nurses with appropriate education and experience can provide nursing care. Upon employment with a health care facility the nurse contracts or enters into an agreement with that facility to provide nursing services in a collaborative practice environment.

It is the Registered Nurse's responsibility to:

- provide competent nursing care to the patient

- exercise informed judgment and use individual competence and qualifications as criteria in seeking consultation, accepting responsibilities and delegating nursing activities to others

- clarify assignments, assess personal capabilities, jointly identify options for patient care assignments when he/she does not feel personally competent or adequately prepared to carry out a specific function.

- refuse an assignment that he/she does not feel prepared to assume after appropriate consultation with supervisor.

It is nursing management's responsibility to:

- ensure competent nursing care is provided to the patient

- evaluate the nurse's ability to provide specialized patient care

- organize resources to ensure that patients receive appropriate nursing care

- collaborate with the staff nurse to clarify assignments, assess personal capabilities, jointly identify options for patient care assignments when the nurse does not feel personally competent or adequately prepared to carry out a specific function.

- take appropriate disciplinary action according to facility policies

- communicate in written policies to the staff the process to make assignment and reassignment decisions

- provide education to staff and supervisory personnel in the decision making process regarding patient care assignments and reassignments, including patients placement and allocation of resources

- plan and budget for staffing patterns based upon patient's requirements and priorities for care

- provide a clearly defined written mechanism for immediate internal review of proposed assignments, that includes the participation of the staff involved, to help avoid conflict

Issues Central to Potential Dilemmas are:

- the right of the patient to receive safe professional nursing care at an acceptable level of quality

- the responsibility for an appropriate utilization and distribution of nursing care services when nursing becomes a scare resource

- the responsibility for providing a practice environment that assures adequate nursing resources for the facility, while meeting the current socioeconomic and political realities of shrinking health care dollars

◘ Legal Issues

Behaviors and activities relevant to giving, accepting, or rejecting a work assignment that could lead to the disciplinary action include:

- practicing or offering to practice beyond the scope permitted by law, or accepting and performing professional responsibilities which the licensee knows or has reason to know that he or she is not competent to perform

- performing, without adequate supervision, professional services which the licensee is authorized to perform only under the supervision of a licensed professional, except in an emergency situation where a person's life or health is in danger

- abandoning or neglecting a patient or client who is in need of nursing care without making reasonable arrangements for the continuation of such care

- failure to exercise supervision over persons who are authorized to practice only under the supervision of the licensed professional

Of the above, the issue of abandonment or neglect has thus far proven the most legally devastating. Abandonment or neglect has been legally defined to include such actions

as insufficient observation (frequency of contact), failure to assure competent intervention when the patient's condition changes (qualified physician not in attendance), and withdrawal of services without provision for qualified coverage. Since nurses at all levels most frequently act as agents of the employing facility, the facility shares the risk of liability with the nurse.

◘ Application of Guidelines for Decision Making

Two clinical scenarios are presented for the RN to demonstrate appropriate decision-making when faced with an unsafe assignment. Sometimes an example or two can help the RN objectively examine legal, ethical and professional issues prior to making a final decision. Additional resources are listed following the scenarios.

Scenario - A Question of Competence

An example of a potential dilemma is when an evening supervisor pulls a psychiatric nurse to the coronary care unit because of a lack of nursing staff. The CCU census has risen and there is not additional qualified staff available.

Suppose you are asked to care for an unfamiliar patient population or to go to a unit for which you feel unqualified—what do you do?

1 CLARIFY what it is you are being asked to do.
- How many patients will you be expected to care for?

- Does the care of these patients require you to have specialty knowledge and skills in order to deliver safe nursing care?

- Will there be qualified and experienced RNs on the unit?

- What procedures and/or medications will you be expected to administer?

- What kind of orientation do you need to function safely in the unfamiliar setting?

2 ASSESS yourself. Do you have the knowledge and skill to meet the expectations that have been outlined for you? Have you had experience with similar patient populations? Have you been oriented to this unit or a similar unit? Would the perceived discrepancies between your abilities and the expectations lead to an unsafe patient care situation?

3 IDENTIFY OPTIONS and implications of your decision.
   a) If you perceive that you can provide safe patient care, you should accept the assignment. You would now be ethically and legally responsible for the nursing care of these patients.
   b) If you perceive there is a discrepancy between abilities and the expectations of the assignment, further dialogue with the nurse supervisor is needed before you reach a decision. At this point it may be appropriate to consult the next level of management, such as the House Supervisor or the Chief Nurse Executive.

   In further dialogue, continue to assess whether you are qualified to accept either a portion or the whole of the requested assignment. Also point out options which might be mutually beneficial. For example, obviously it would be unsafe for you to administer chemotherapy without prior training. However, if someone else administered the chemotherapy, perhaps you could provide the remainder of the required nursing care for that patient. If you feel unqualified for the assignment in its entirety, the dilemma becomes more complex.

   At this point the RN must be aware of the legal rights of the facility. Even though the RN may have legitimate concern for patient safety and one's own legal accountability in providing safe care, the facility has legal precedent to initiate disciplinary action, including termination, if you refuse to accept an assignment. Therefore, it is important to continue to explore options in a positive manner, recognizing that both the RN and the facility have a responsibility for safe patient care.

4 POINT OF DECISION/IMPLICATIONS
   If none of the options are acceptable, you are at your final decision point.
   a) Accept the assignment, documenting carefully your concern for patient safety and the process you used to inform the facility (manager) of your concerns. Keep a personal copy of this documentation and send a copy to the manager(s) involved. Once you have reached this decision it is unwise to discuss the situation or your feelings with other staff or patients. Now you are legally accountable for these patients. From this point withdrawal from the agreed upon assignment may constitute abandonment.
   b) Refuse the assignment, being prepared for disciplinary action. Document your concern for patient safety and the process you used to inform the facility (manager) of your concerns. Keep a personal copy of this documentation and send a copy to the Nurse Executive. Courtesy suggests that you also send a copy to the manager(s) involved.
   c) Document the steps taken in making your decision. It may be necessary for you to use the facility's grievance procedure.

Scenario - A Question of an Additional Shift

An example of another potential dilemma is when a nurse who recognizes his/her fatigue and its potential for patient harm, is required to work an additional shift.

Suppose you are approached by your supervisor and asked to work an additional shift. Your immediate response is that you don't want to work another shift—what do you do?

1 CLARIFY what it is you are expected to do.

   For example, would the additional shift be with the same patients you are currently caring for, or would it involve a new patient assignment?

- Is your reluctance to work another shift because of a new patient assignment you do not feel competent to accept? (If the answer is yes, then refer to the previous example, "A Question of Competence.")

- Is your reluctance due to work fatigue, or do you have other plans?

- Is this a chronic request due to poor scheduling, inadequate staffing, or chronic absenteeism?

- Are you being asked to work because there is no relief nurse coming for your present patient assignment? Because your unit will be short of professional staff on the next shift? Because another unit will be short of professional staff on the next shift?

- How long are you being asked to work—the entire shift or a portion of the shift?

2 ASSESS yourself.

Are you really tired, or do you just not feel like working? Is your fatigue level such that your care may be unsafe? Remember, you are legally responsible for the care of your current patient assignment if relief is not available.

3 IDENTIFY OPTIONS and implications of your decision.

a) If you perceive that you can provide safe patient care and are willing to work the additional shift, accept the assignment.

b) If you perceive that you can provide safe patient care but are unwilling to stay due to other plans or the chronic nature of the request, inform the manager of your reasons for not wishing to accept the assignment.

c) If you perceive that your fatigue will interfere with your ability to safely care for patients, indicate this fact to the manager.

If you do not accept the assignment and the manager continues to attempt to persuade you it may be appropriate to consult the next level of management, such as the House Supervisor or the Nurse Executive.

In further dialogue continue to weigh your reasons for refusal versus the facility's need for an RN. If you have a strong alternate commitment, such as no child care, or if you seriously feel your fatigue will interfere with safe patient care, restate your reasons for refusal.

At this point, it is important for you to be aware of the legal rights of the facility. Even though you may have legitimate concern for patient safety and your own legal accountability in providing safe care, or legitimate concern for the safety of your children or other commitments, the facility has legal precedent to initiate disciplinary action, including termination, if you refuse to accept an assignment. Therefore, it is important to continue to explore options in a positive manner, recognizing both you and the facility have a responsibility for safe patient care.

4 POINT OF DECISION/IMPLICATIONS

a) Accept the assignment, documenting your professional concern for patient safety and the process you used to inform the facility (manager) of your concerns. Keep a personal copy of this documentation and send a copy to the Nurse Executive. Courtesy suggests that you also send a copy to the manager(s) involved. Once you have reached this decision it is unwise to discuss the situation of your feelings with other staff and/or patients.

b) Accept the assignment, documenting your professional concerns for the chronic nature of the request and possible long-term consequences in reducing the quality of care. Documentation should follow the procedures outlined in (a).

c) Accept the assignment, documenting your personal concerns regarding working conditions in which management decides the legitimacy of employee personal commitments. This documentation should go to your manager. You may wish to request a meeting with your manager to discuss the incident and your concerns regarding future requests.

d) Refuse the assignment, being prepared for disciplinary action. If your reasons for refusal were patient safety or an imperative personal commitment, document this carefully including the process you used to inform the facility (nurse manager) of your concerns. Keep a personal copy of this documentation and send a copy to the Chief Nurse Executive. Courtesy suggests that you also send a copy to the manager(s) involved.

e) Document the rationale for your decision. It may be necessary to use the facility's grievance procedure.

Summary

Two scenarios of how a RN may apply the guidelines for decision-making in the actual work situation have been presented. Staffing dilemmas will always be present and mandate that active communication between staff nurses and all levels of nursing management be maintained to assure patient safety. The likelihood of a satisfactory solution will increase if there is prior consideration of the choices available. This consideration of available alternatives should include recognition that professional nurses are intelligent adults who should be involved in the decision-making process. Professional nurses are accountable for nursing judgments and actions regardless of the personal consequences. Providing safe nursing care to the patient is the ultimate objective of the professional nurse and the health care facility.

The Florida Nurses Association Labor and Employment Relations Commission acknowledges:

- the Florida Organization of Nurse Executives for input and collaboration in this document the development of the previous 1989 edition of this document.

- the **Florida Nurses Association Labor and Employment Relations Commis-**

sion for final preparation of the revised 1999 edition of this document:

Michael Nilsson, CRRN, RN, Chairman
Patricia Quigley, Ph.D., ARNP, CRRN
Nancy Hartley
Mary Healy Smith, ARNP
Patricia Cox, R.N.
Dorothy Walsh, R.N.
O'dell Anderson, R.N.

Resources

To maintain current and accurate information on accountability of registered nurses for giving, accepting, or rejecting a work assignment, the following resources are suggested:

- **Health Care Facility**: Nurses are encouraged to seek consultation with their nurse manager/executives to discuss the facility's missions and goals as well as policies and procedures.

- The **Florida Nurses Association**, the largest statewide organization for registered nurses, represents nursing in the governmental, policy-making arena and maintains current information and publications relative to the nurse's practice environment. Contact FNA, P.O. Box 536985, Orlando, FL 32853-6985, (407) 896-3261 OR check out our website *http://www.floridanurse.org* for the benefits and services of membership, as well as priorities and activities of the Association.

- The **American Nurses Association** serves as the national clearing-house of information and offers publications on contemporary issues, including standards of practice, nursing ethics, as well as legal and regulatory issues. Contact ANA for a complimentary copy of the Publications Catalogue: ANA, 600 Maryland Avenue, SW, Suite 100 West, Washington, DC 20024-2571 or phone (202) 651-7000.

- ANA Survival Kit (1996) available through the American Nurses Association.

- ANA Basic Guide to Safe Delegate available through the American Nurses Association.

- ANA Code of Ethics for Nurses (1998) available through the American Nurses Association.

- ANA Standards and Scope of Practice (1997) available through the American Nurses Association.

- Nurse Practice Act (Florida Statutes 464, January 1994) and Administrative Rules (59S).

- Board of Nursing: 4080 Woodcock Drive, Jacksonville, FL 32207, or phone (904) 858-6940. A complimentary copy of the Nurse Practice Act is available to each registered nurse upon request.

Revised 08/99

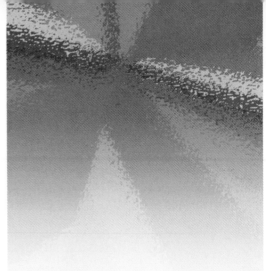

Index

A box is indicated by "b" following the page number; a figure by "f"; a table by "t."

A

Accountability, 230–231, 292
Adaptability, 9
Administrative law, 208, 209
Advance directives, 218–220
 do not resuscitate orders, 218b, 218–220
Alcohol abuse, by health care professionals, 189
Alexian Brothers, 252–253
Alternative treatment modalities, 110
Altruism, 290
American Association of Critical Care Nurses, delega-
  tion of client care and, 97, 99b
American Nurses Association, 84
 advantages of membership in, 294
 Code for Nurses, 192
 Code of Ethics of, 286, 289, 327
 Code of Ethics Project of, 231
 do not resuscitate orders and, 218
 education recommendations of, 288
 fighting sexual harassment and, 185
 history of, 253
 information for registered nurses and, 341–342
 mandatory overtime and, 191
 members of, 293
 Nursing Care Report Card for Acute Care, 321, 322t
 Nursing's Safety and Quality Initiative of, 118
 on delegation, 95–96, 97, 99
 origin of, 293
 position statements available from, 294–295t
 purposes of, 293
 quality indicators in acute care, 128
 reporting of questionable practices and, 192–193
 staffing ratios and, 191–192
 Standards of Clinical Nursing Practice of, 288–289,
   331–332
 standards of practice of, 213, 331–332
 standards published by, 331–332
 unlicensed assistive personnel and, 95, 102, 103t
 workplace safety and, 178–179
American Nurses Credentialing Center, certifications
  available from, 124t
Anxiety, personal, 152

Assault, 212
 placing blame on victim of, 182, 183t
Assertiveness, for time management, 144
 in communication, 23–24
Assignment sheets, 143
Assignments, coordinating of, 93, 94
Associate degree in nursing, 251
Associate's degree programs, 297
Attitude, for professional behavior, 293
Authoritarian leadership, 7–8
Authority, power and, 82, 83
Autonomy, 228–229

B

Baccalaureate degree programs, 297–298
Bachelor of science in nursing, 297
Back injuries, occupation-related, 188–189
Battery, 212
Behavior, alternative, suggestion of, 38
 questionable, reporting of, 192–193
 staff, recording of, 37
Behavioral theories, of leadership, 7t, 7–8
Belief systems, 226–227, 284, 285t
Beneficence, 229
Bill of Rights, Patient's, 213
Bioethics, definition of, 227
Biomedical ethics, 224
Bioterrorism, 193
Bloodborne pathogens, occupational exposure to,
  187–188
Body language, 22
Bolton, Frances Payne, 250
Brewster, Mary, 246
Bureaucracy, 80b
Burnout, 158–161
 awareness of, 161–162
 buffer against, 161
 causes of, 159–161
 conflicting demands and, 160
 consequences of, 161
 definition of, 158

Burnout (*Continued*)
  human service occupations and, 159–160
  job stress leading to, 159b
  personal factors influencing, 159
  risks for, assessment of, 162b
  stages of, 158–159
  stress and, 158–161
  stressors leading to, 159–161
  technological changes and, 160
  work-life balance and, 160–161
Business sense, of managers, 14
Byrne, Ethel, 248

C
Calendar-creator programs, computerized, 142
Canadian Nurse Association, Code of Ethics for
    Registered Nurses, 328
Cardiac resuscitation, 217
Career, advancement of, 278
Career survivalist strategies, 259
Caring behaviors, 292–293
Caring interventions, 291
Case management, 113–116
  external, 115
  internal, 115
  process of, and nursing process, compared, 114t
Case managers, functions of, 114, 115
Centers for Disease Control and Prevention, 177–178
Certificate of Need, 111
Certification(s), 290
  available from American Nurses Credentialing
      Center, 124t
Change, as natural phenomenon, 62–63
  designing of, 68
  implementation of, leading of, 67–69
    planning of, 68
  integration of, 69
  macro level vs. micro level, 63
  planned, 68, 68f
  process of, 63–64
  provision of catalyst for, 66
  resistance to, 64–67
    active vs. passive, 65, 65t
    position and power and, 65
    psychosocial needs and, 64f, 64–65
    recognition of, 65
    strategies to reduce, 66–67
    technical concerns and, 64
    use of command and, 67
Change-of-shift report, development of, 26–27
  information for, 27b
  presentation of, 27–29
Charting, by exception, 216
Chemical sensitivity dermatitis, 186
Civil law, 209–210
Client(s), care needs of, communication of, 26–29
  communication with, 30–31
  power of, 83
  safety of, 237
  teaching of, 30–31

Client care, assessment of needs for, 94
  coordination of, 94
  delegation of, 91–105. *See also* Delegation
  nurse as manager of, 30
  organization and time management schedule
      for, 28f
  personalized worksheets in, 94, 95
  prevention of errors in, 321
  priorities for, determination of, 99–100
  standards for, 134
Client care technicians. *See* Unlicensed assistive
    personnel
Client-focused care, 116
Clinical exterpise, of managers, 14
Code of ethics, 231
Collaboration, continuity of care through, 115
Collective bargaining, 56–58, 84
  pros and cons of, 58
Common law, 208
Communication, as core of leadership, 20
  assertiveness in, 23–24
  by new nurses, 157
  channels of, 21–22
  clarity in, 23
  contemporary model of, 20–21
  credibility and, 23
  cultural aspects of, 196
  direct channels of, 23
  effective, components of, 22–23, 23t
    in workplace, 24–25
  factors influencing, 21, 21f
  feedback in, 23
  gender barriers to, 25
  good, facilitation of, 25b
  historical view of, 20
  in nonthreatening manner, 38–39
  in professional behavior, 292
  lack of, 20
  need for, 20
  nonverbal, 21–22
  of client care needs, 26–29
  of vision for future, 12
  passive, 24
  passive-aggressive, 24
  physical barriers to, 24
  psychological barriers to, 24
  semantic barriers to, 24–25
  sharing of information in, 22–23
  skillful, 11–12
  skills desired by employers, 259–260
  verbal, 21
  with clients and families, 30–31
  with other disciplines, 30
  with physician, 30
Community, commitment to, 290
Community-based care, 319
Competence, question of, 338–339
Computerized adaptive testing, 290
Computerized Patient Record, 299, 302–303
  acceptance of, 303
  audit trails and, 303–304

benefits of, 303
  security issues in, 303
Computers, communication via, 25
  benefits of, 26b
Confidentiality, 211, 230
Conflict, 49–59
  benefits of, 49–50
  harmful effects of, 49
  inter-group, 49
  levels of, 51
  need for resolution of, 51b
  negotiation of, 14
  resolution of, 14, 51–58
    agreement on, 56
    by negotiation, 54–58
    by problem solving, 52f, 52–54
    myths concerning, 51–52
  sources of, 50b, 50–51
Constitutional law, 208–209
Constructive behavior, feedback and, 35
Continuing education, 299
Contraception, Sanger and, 248
Coronary heart disease, rotating shifts and, 190
Costs, health care decisions based on, 317
Creative selfishness, 165
Criminal law, 209
Critical pathways, of structured care, 119–120,
    121–123t
Critical thinking, 11, 287
  encouragement of, 195
Critical thinking exercise(s), 16–17, 31–32, 44, 59, 70, 88,
    104–105, 135, 148, 201, 221, 238, 255, 279, 307, 324
Cultural diversity, effective management of, 197, 197t
  fostering of, 195–196
  understanding of, 196–197
Cultural factors, in employee relations, 197

D

Danforth, Senator John, 218
Decision makers, 233
Decision-making, employee involvement in, 194
  participation in, 84–85
  sharing of, 85
Decision support software, 299
Decisional activities, 15
Deep breathing, in stress management, 163
Delegation, 91–105
  American Nursing Association on, 95–96, 97, 99
  barriers to, 102–103
  coordination of assignments in, 93, 94
  criteria for, 97–99, 99b
  decision-making for, 97, 97b, 98f, 100f
  definition(s) of, 92, 97
  difficulty of, reasons for, 103
  direct, 92
  experience issues and, 102
  fairness in, 101
  five rights of, 94, 94b
  increased efficiency from, 100–101
  indirect, 92

  knowledge of abilities and, 99
  liability and, 104
  licensure issues and, 102–103
  need for, 95–97
  nursing process and, 94–95
  permitted tasks and, 93
  quality-of-care issues and, 103
  regulations concerning, 99
  relationship-oriented concerns in, 101–102
  safety concerns in, 97
  setting priorities and, 99–100
  task-related concerns and, 99–101
  time management and, 144–145
  to licensed practical nurses, 93
  to unlicensed assistive personnel, 93, 97
  vs, supervision, 93
Deontological theories, 227
Dermatitis, chemical sensitivity, 186
Development skills, personal, 141
Diagnosis-related groups, 111, 317
Differentiated practice, 117–119, 299
  definition of, 117
  rationale for, 115
Diploma programs, 296–297
Directive leadership, 7–8
Dissemination of information, 15
Do not resuscitate orders, 218b, 218–220
Doctoral programs, 298
Documentation, appropriate, 215–216
  credible, 216
  guidelines for, 216
Drug abuse, by health care professionals, 189
Durable power of attorney for health care, 219–220

E

E-mail, communication via, 26
  rules of netiquette and, 26b
Economic Stabilization Program, 110
Economic trends, 316–317
  in health care, 110–112
Education, of nurses, 296
Educational opportunities, seeking of, 195
Efficiency, improvement of, 12–13
Einstein, Albert, 138
Electronic medical record, 299
Electronic medical record systems, 147
Emergency preparedness, 193
Emotional intelligence, 8, 9f
  leadership and, 8
Employee(s), efficient delegation of, 100
  floating of, 100, 101
  health needs of, recognition of, 101
  hiring and firing of, 15
  impaired, 189–192, 237
  incompetent, 237
  preferences of, consideration of, 102
  protection of, federal laws enacted for, 179b
  skills of, feedback and, 35
  supportive environment for, 194
Employee development, 15

Employee evaluation, 15
  formal, 37, 40
    performance appraisal in, 40–41
  informal, 37
  standards for, 40–41
  subjective, 37
Empowerment, 194
  definition of, 83, 286
  of nurses, 83–87, 194
End-of-life decisions, and law, 217–220
Environmental control, cultural aspects of, 196
Environmental modifications, for safety and
    efficiency, 197
Environmental stressors, 152
Ergonomic injuries, 188–189
Errors, medical, 318
Ethical codes, 231
Ethical dilemmas, 231–232
  assessment of, 232–233
  evaluation in, 234
  implementation in, 234
  planning and, 233–234
  resolving of, 232b, 232–237
Ethical issues, 235
  genetic technology and, 236
Ethical principles, 228
Ethical theories, 227–228
Ethics, definition of, 227
Ethics committees, 224
Evaluation, employee. *See* Employee evaluation
  informal, purpose of, 38
Evidence-based practice, 321
Exercise, in stress management, 164–165
Expectations, realistic, in stress management, 165
Expertise, enhancing of, 86–87
External degree programs, 298
Eye contact, in interview, 273
  listening and, 22

F
Fairness, in delegation, 101
False imprisonment, 211–212
Family(ies), communication with, 30–31
Feedback, acceptance of, 37–38
  as essential, 35
  based on observable behavior, 37
  evaluative, 35
    giving and receiving of, 34
    provision of, 35, 35b
    responding to, 39
    seeking of, 39
    situations with need for, 39, 39b
  frequent, 36
  immediate, 36
  in communication, 23
  negative, 38
    as learning experience, 36
    given privately, 36–37
    guidelines for providing, 38, 38b
  objectivity when giving, 37

  positive, to support colleagues, 36
  positive and negative, provision of, 35–36
  provision of, 12
    guidelines for, 35, 35t
  solicitation of, 39, 157
Filing systems, 143–144
Florida Nurses Association, information for registered
    nurse and, 341
Flow sheets, 143
Follower, becoming better, 5–6
  valuable, 5
Followership, definition of, 5
  effective, 5
Formal processes, 81
Fralic, Maryann, 304
Freudenberger, Herbert, 158
Future, communication of vision for, 12
  planning for, 15

G
General adaptation syndrome, 152
Genetic diagnosis, 235
Genetic engineering, 236
Genetic screening, 235–236
Genetics, limitations of technology and, 235–236
Goal setting, 12
Good Samaritan law, 210–211
Goodrich, Annie, 251
Growth, professional, rewarding of, 195
Growth and innovation, professional, 194–195

H
Hall, Doctor John, 244
Hampton, Isabel, 250
Hardiness, burnout and, 161
Health care, costs of, factors affecting, 111f
  decisions on, based on costs, 317
  delivery of, "corporatized," 319
    current trends in, 314–317
    directly to consumer, 315–316
    effects of technology on, 314–315
    historical perspective on, 317
    in future, 313–314
    in real world, 153–154
    past and future systems of, 320t
  economics of, 316–317
  evaluation of, 126–129
  indicators of, 130
  monitoring in, 130
  outcome of, 128–129
  preventive, managed care as, 318
  process(es) of, 127–128
  rationing of, 317
  structure of, 126–127
  system of, changes in, 317–320
    economic climate in, 110–112
    predicted trends in, 323–324
    resources and, 110
Health care insurance, 318

Health care organizations, functional divisions of, 81
goals of, 78–79
innovative, 80
learning about, 157
organic networks of, 80–81, 82f
power in, 82–83
processes of, 81–82
structure of, 79–81
traditional, hierarchial structure of, 79, 80b, 81f
types of, 77–78
understanding of, 76–82
Health care practices, laws governing, 192, 192b
Health care services, effect of nursing on, 319–320
Health care surrogate, 219, 233
Health care team, basic entitlements of members of, 102, 102b
working as, promotion of, 101–102
Health maintenance organizations, 77
Health-related information, access to, 314
Henderson, Virginia, 242, 251–252, 286
Henry Street Settlement House, 246–247
Herbert, Sir Sidney, 243
HMOs, 77
Home care, infection rates in, current research on, 133
Home Healthcare Classification, 302
Hospitals, potential hazards in, 178t
Human Genome Project, 236
Human immunodeficiency virus infection, employee assistance program and, 180–181
needlestick injuries and, 176–177
Human relations-oriented management, 13
Human service occupations, burnout and, 159–160
Hume, David, 228
Humor, in stress management, 165

I

Ideas, new, encouraging of, 195
Impaired workers, 189–192
Implementation, in ethical dilemmas, 234
Implied consent, 214
Incident report, 133
Infections, rates in home care, current research on, 133
Informal processes, 81
Informatics, 299–304
definition of, 300
nursing. *See* Nursing informatics
Information, client, presentation of, 27–29, 28f
dissemination of, 15
exchange of, 11–12
sharing of, in communication, 22–23
Information systems, communication via, 25
Informational activities, 15
Informed consent, 213–214
Insurance, health care, 318
liability, 217
malpractice, 217
Intensive care, 224
International Council of Nurses, Code of Ethics for Nurses, 328
Internet, in job search, 269–270

Interpersonal activities, 14
Interruptions, reduction of, 146
Interview, answering questions in, 271
appearance for, 273
asking questions in, 274–275
background questions in, 271
deciding on job following, 276
eye contact in, 273
follow-up after, 275
handshake and, 273
initial, 270–271
laws governing questions in, 273
listening skills for, 273–274
personal questions in, 272–273
posture for, 273
professional questions in, 271–272
second, 275
Iowa Intervention Project, 302–303

J

Job analysis and redesign, 15
Job descriptions, 41, 42b, 42–44
Job dissatisfaction, 112
Job search, career survivalist strategies for, 259
desirable skills and, 259–260
initiation of, 259–260
Internet in, 269–270
letters in, 265–270, 267f, 268f, 269f, 270f
places for, 260
researching employers in, 260–261
résumé in, 261–265
SWOT analysis in, 258–259
Joint Commission on Accreditation of Healthcare Organizations, 124
Justice, principle of, 229–230

K

Kevorkian, Jack, 235

L

Laissez-faire leadership, 8
Language, simple and exact, 23
Latex allergy, 185–187, 186t
Law(s), administrative, 208, 209
civil, 209–210
common, 208
constitutional, 208–209
criminal, 209
definition of, 208
end-of-life decisions and, 217–220
Good Samaritan, 210–211
governing health care practices, 192, 192b
nursing practice and, 207–222
sources of, 208–209
statutory, 208, 209
tort, 210
types of, 209–210
whistleblower, 192

Lawsuit, protection of self in, 217
Leader(s), effective, behavior of, 11–12
  qualities of, 10f, 10–11
  emotionally intelligent, 8, 9f
  qualities of, 7–12
  shared goals of, 5
  tasks of, 5
Leadership, and management, compared, 6, 6t
  assuming of, example of, 4–5
  authoritarian, 7–8
  autocratic, 7–8
  behavioral theories of, 7t, 7–8
  controlling, 7–8
  definition of, 5
  effective, definition of, 10
    keys to, 3–18
  emotional intelligence and, 8
  laissez-faire, 8
  nondirective, 8
  participative, 8
  permissive, 8
  situational theories of, 8–9
  task relationship of, 8
  theories of, 7–9
  trait theories of, 7
  transformational, theory of, 9–10
Learning, as continuous, 12
Legal issues, registered nurses and, 328
Legal problems, prevention of, 214–215, 215b
Letter(s), acceptance, 266–268, 269f
  cover, 266, 267f
  in job search, 265–270, 267f, 268f, 269f, 270f
  thank-you, 266, 268f
Liability, delegation and, 104
Liability insurance, 217
Libel, 211
License, nursing, 285–286, 288, 289
Licensed practical nurse(s), delegation to, 93
  skills of, 97
Licensure, 289–290
  delegation and, 102–103
  differentiated practice and, 117
Limit setting, time management and, 144–145
Listening, 11
  as communication skill, 22
  attentive body language and, 22
  awareness of vocal qualities and, 22
  eye contact and, 22
  to feedback, 38
  verbal tracking in, 22
Listening sequence, basic, 22, 22b
Listening skills, for interview, 273–274
Lists, time management and, 142
Living Will, 219
Long-term planning systems, 142–143

M

Mahoney, Mary Eliza, 242, 249
Malpractice, 210
Malpractice insurance, 217

Malpractice suits, actions leading to, 217
Managed care, 111, 317–319
  as preventive health care, 318
  efficiency of delivery and, 319
  price pressures on hospitals and, 318
Management, definition of, 6
  effective, keys to, 3–18
  human relations-oriented, 13
  scientific, 12–13
  theories of, 12
Manager(s), business sense of, 14
  clinical expertise of, 14
  effective, behaviors of, 14f, 14–15
    qualities of, 6, 13–14
  functions of, 6
  leadership by, 14
  power of, 83
Mechanical ventilation, 224
Medical errors, 318
Medicare, lengths of stay and, 115
  nurse shortages and, 317
Medicare Prospective Payment System, 111
Medication administration, 215
Medication errors, prevention of, 215
Medication order, computerized, 314
Mentor(s), 157, 158t
Mindell, Fania, 248
Modular nursing, 113
Monitoring, by nurse manager, 15
Montag, Mildred, 242, 250
MORAL model, 234, 235b
Morals, definition of, 227
Moynihan, Senator Daniel, 218

N

N-OADN Resolution on Differentiated Nursing
  Practice, 299, 333
National Council Licensure Examination for Retired
  Nurses, 289, 290, 291t, 296
National Council of State Boards of Nursing,
  delegation and, 94, 94b, 97
  delegation decision-making grid of, 97, 97b, 98f, 100f
National Institute for Occupational Safety and Health,
  178, 178t
National Organization for Associate Degree Nursing,
  296
  differentiated nursing practice, 299, 333
NCLEX examination, 289, 290, 291t, 296
Needlestick injuries, 176–177, 187–188
Negligence, 210
  causes of, 215t
Negotiation, 54–58
  assessment of situation for, 55
  conduction of, 55–56, 56b
  formal, 56–58
  in collective bargaining, 56–58
  informal, 54b, 54–56
  setting stage for, 55
Networking, 14
Newton, Isaac, 138

Nightingale, Florence, 83, 92, 110, 123, 242–245, 286
Nightingale Training School for Nurses, 244–245
Nixon, Richard, 110
Nonmaleficence, 229
North American Nursing Diagnosis Association, 302
Notes on Nursing: What It Is And What It Is Not,
    Nightingale, 244, 251
Nurse(s), as managers, 141
    associate degree, 117
    baccalaureate degree, 117
    distinct role of, 288
    empowerment of, 83–87, 194
    formal education of, 288
    impaired, 189–190
    increased demand for, 111–112
    initial concerns of, 154
    labor market for, 111–112
    learning by, as continuous, 154
    licensed, regulation of, 289
    master's degree, 117
    new, attitude and expectations of, 277
        communication by, 157
        communication of role of, 285–286
        development of professional identity by, 157
        expectations of, 155t, 155–156
        feedback and, 157
        impressions and relationships made by, 277
        mentor(s) for, 157, 158t
        objectives of, 40
        pressures on, 156
        reality shock for, 155
        support network for, 157
        testing of, 156
        use of energy by, 157
    power of, 83
    responding to changes in health care system, 320
    shortage of, 111, 320–321
        causes of, 111–112
    time management by, 139–141
Nurse manager(s), competencies necessary for, in
    future, 321–322
    monitoring by, 15
    responsibilities of, 337
Nurse Practice Act, 289, 289b
Nurse Practice Act of 1994, administrative rules,
    336–337
Nursing, areas of risk for, 133
    as profession, 287–291
    body of knowledge of, 287
    caring in, 316b
    definition(s) of, 286
    effect of health care services on, 319–320
    elimination of positions in, 320
    first year in, 277–278
    future of, 284–285
    mastery of knowledge by, 287
    men in, 252–253
    problem-solving in, 287
    public image of, 284–285
Nursing care, client-focused, 116
    contemporary models of, 113

delivery of, models of, 112–119
    whole-system approach to, 115–116
functional method of, 112–113
modular, 113
monitoring and evaluation of, 119–126
team method of, 113
total care method of, 112
Nursing care delivery systems, advantages and
    disadvantages of, 118, 118t
Nursing care management, goals of, 114–115
Nursing Care Report Card for Acute Care,
    321, 322t
Nursing education, 296–299
    American Nurses Association and, 288
    associate's degree programs in, 297
    baccalaureate degree programs in, 297–298
    bachelor of science in nursing, 297
    continuing, 299
    diploma programs in, 296–297
    doctural programs in, 298
    external degree programs in, 298
    practical nursing programs in, 296
    reduction in nursing faculty and, 112
Nursing informatics, databases and data sets in,
    300–301, 301f
    definition of, 300
    multiple uses of patient data, 300, 301f
    nomenclature in, 301–304
    taxonomies in, 301–304
Nursing Interventions Classification, 302–303
Nursing Minimum Data Set, 300–301
Nursing officers, chief, delegation by, 93
Nursing organizations, 291, 293
Nursing practice, and law, 207–222
    standards of, 213
Nursing process, delegation and, 94
Nursing programs, declining enrollments in, 111
Nursing research, 253–254
Nursing-sensitive quality indicators, 118, 119b
Nursing Studies Index, Henderson, 251
Nursing theory, 253–254
Nursing's Safety and Quality Initiative, of American
    Nurses Association, 118
Nutrition, in stress management, 164, 164b
Nutting, Adelaide, 242, 249–250

O

Observable behavior, feedback based on, 37
Occupational hazards, 176
Occupational Safety and Health Administration, 177
Omaha System, 302
Optimism, 10, 10f
Orders, physicians', verbal, 30
    written, 30
Organic networks, 81, 82f
Organization schedule, for client care, 28f
Organizational change, response to, factors influenc-
    ing, 9
Organizational cultures, 78
Organizational savvy, development of, 277

Organizations, health care. *See* Health care
    organizations
    professional nursing, 84, 293–296
Outcome measures, 128–129
Outcomes measurement, 321
Overtime, mandatory, 190–191

P
Paperwork, elimination of, 145
Paralanguage, 22
Patient Self-Determination Act, 218–219
    nursing implications of, 220
Patient worksheet, personalized, 130, 130t
Patient's Bill of Rights, 213
Peer review, 41–44, 42b, 43t
Peer support, 194
Performance appraisal, 40–41
Performance standards, 41, 42–44, 43t
Personal anxiety, 152
Personal digital assistants, 143
Personal space, cultural aspects of, 196
Personalized patient worksheet, 130, 130t
Physical health management, 163–165
Physician, communication with, 30
Physicians' orders, verbal, 30
    written, 30
Planned Parenthood, 248, 249
Posture, for interview, 273
    in stress management, 163
Power, and authority, 82, 83
    definition of, 82, 83
    expert, 86f, 86–87
    in health care organizations, 82–83
    of clients, 83
    of managers, 83
    of nurses, 83
    of technicians, 83
    sources of, 82–83
Power of attorney for health care, 219–220
Practical nursing programs, 296
Practice, standards of, 212–214
Preceptors, 157
Primary nursing, 113
Principalism, 228
Principles and Practice of Nursing, 251–252
Private health care organizations, for-profit, 77
    not-for-profit, 77
Problem solving, 11, 52f, 52–54
Product line management, 116–117
Profession, characterisitcs of, 287b
Professional behaviors, 292–293
Professional culture, 291
Professional identity, development of, 157
Professional look, 293
Professional nursing organizations, 84, 293–296
Professionalism, in nursing, 292
Progress reviews, 40
Psychological stressors, 152
Psychosocial needs, 64f, 64–65
Psychosocial Stages of Development, Erickson, 253

Public health nursing, origins of, 246
Publicly supported health care organizations, 77

Q
Quality improvement, 124
    at unit and organizational level, 129–131
    continuous, 125–126, 126f, 129
    guidelines for, 130, 131f
    in nursing examples, 127t
Quality improvement cycle, continuous, 130–131, 131f
Quality improvement programs, organization-wide,
    130
Quality management, total, 126–129
Quality management activities, 123–125
Quality-of-care issues, delegation and, 103
Quality performance, JCAHO dimensions of, 127t
Quasi-intentional tort, 210

R
Reality shock, 154, 277
    resolving of, 156–158
    stress and, 155
Record systems, electronic medical, 147
Reframing, in stress management, 165
Registered nurse(s), 111. *See also* Nurse(s)
    as case manager, 115
    assignment despite objection and, 336
    Canadian Nurse Association Code of Ethics
        for, 328
    changes in practice environment for, 320
    decision making by, guidelines for, 337, 338–341
    delegation by. *See* Delegation
    dilemma for, question of additional shift, 339–341
        question of competence, 338–339
    documentation of practice situation by, 336
    ensuring adequate number of, 321
    giving, accepting or rejecting work, guidelines for,
        335–342
    in health care, 286
    informed decisions by, 337
    legal issues and, 338
    licensure of, 117
    nursing care delivery by, 335–336
    resources for, 341–342
    responsibilities of, 337
Relaxation, in stress management, 163–164, 164b
Repetitive stress injuries, 189
Resource allocation, 15
Resources, health care system and, 110
Respect for individual, 11
Respondeat superior, 210
Responsibility, 292
Rest, in stress management, 163
Résumé, 261–265
    essentials of, 262
    formats for, 262
    guidelines for preparing, 262–264
    objectives stated on, 264
    reasons for preparing, 261b

sample, 263f
skills and experience on, 264–265
Rhythm Model for Time Management, 147, 147t
Risk events, 131–134
Risk management, 131–134
definition of, 131
goal of, 133
Rogers, Carl, 165
Rogers, Martha, 286
Russell, W.H., 243

S
Safety in workplace, 176–184
current research on, 199–200
federal laws enacted to protect worker, 179b
indoor pollution and, 176
latex allergy, 185–187, 186t
modification of physical environment for, 197–198
needlestick injuries, 187–188
range of threats to, 176–177
recognition of potential hazards and, 179–180
risk reduction and, 177–181
safety programs and, 179–181
sexual harassment, 184–185
terrorism, 193
violence and, 176, 181–184
actions to address, 182
protection from, 183b, 183–184
Safety plan, development of, 180
Sanger, Margaret, 242, 247–249
Schedules, time management and, 143
Schiff, Jacob, 246
School health nursing, origins of, 247
Scientific management, 12–13
Self-awareness, 11
Sexual harassment, 184t, 184–185
Seyle, Hans, 152, 153
Shared governance, 85–86
Shift(s), 143
additional, question of, 339–341
health effects of, 139
rotating, 190
time management and, 139, 143
Sick building syndrome, 176
Situational theories, of leadership, 8–9
Skills, employee, feedback and, 35
new, mastering of, 278
Slander, 211
Social environment, 194
Social organization, cultural aspects of, 196
Social stressors, 152
Social support, in stress management, 165
Socialization, in workplace, 145
Spokesperson, manager as, 15
Staffing, shortages of, coping with, 139
Staffing ratios, mandated, 191
Standards of care, 119
Standards of nursing practice, 213
Standards of practice, 212–214
State boards of nursing, 289, 290

State nurses' associations, 193
Statutory law, 208, 209
Stewart, Isabel, 250
Stress, 151–173
ability to handle, 11
and burnout, 158–161
awareness of, 161–162
coping with, 166b
current research on, 167
definition of, 152
differences in expectations and, 155t, 155–156
effects of, 152, 153t
good, adaptation to, 157
and bad, 153
in workplace, 154t
increase in, 153–154
initial, minimizing of, 154–155
job-related, 159
reality shock and, 155
repetitive, injuries related to, 189
responses to, 152–153
signs and symptoms of, 153t
Stress management, 161–165
ABCs of, 161b, 161–162
daily de-stress in, 166, 167b
mental health management in, 165, 166
physical health management in, 163–165, 166b
Structured care, algorithms for, 119
critical pathways of, 119–120, 121–123t
guidelines for, 119
protocols for, 119
standards of care for, 119
Structured care methodologies, 119–123, 123b
Subacute care, 319
Substance abuse, by health care professionals, 189
Supervision, requirements in, 93
vs. delegation, 93
Supervisors, support from, 194
SWOT analysis, 258–259

T
Task allocation, time management and, 140
Task relationship, of leadership, 8
Taylor, Frederick, 12
Teaching, of client, 30–31
Technicians, power of, 83
Technology, computerized patient record and, 314
downside of, 314–315
effects on health care delivery, 314–315
emphasis on economics and, 316–317
limitations of, genetics and, 235–236
patient monitoring and, 314
survival of vulnerable individuals and, 316
telehealth and, 304
Telehealth, 304
Teleological theories, 227–228
Telephone etiquette, 25
Terrorism, 193
Theory of Human Motivation, Maslow, 253
Theory of Psychosexual Development, Freud, 253

Theory X and theory Y of McGregor, 13, 13f
Time, cultural aspects of, 196
Time inventory, personal, 142, 142b
Time log, 140, 140f, 142, 145–146
Time management, 137–139
  assertiveness and determination for, 144
  automation and, 147
  blocks of time and, 143
  categorizing of activities and, 146
  definition of, 138, 142
  delegation and, 144–145
  energy levels and, 143
  filing systems and, 143–144
  finding fastest way and, 146–147
  goal setting and, 141–142
  interruptions and, 146
  limit setting and, 144–145
  lists and, 142
  long-term planning systems and, 142–143
  management responsibilities shift and, 140–141
  organization of work in, 141–144
  Rhythm Model for, 147, 147t
  schedules and, 143
  shifts and, 139, 143
  streamlining work and, 145–147
  task allocation and, 140
  time log and, 140, 140f, 142, 145–146
  worksheets for, 95
Time management schedule, for client care, 28f
Time-outs, in stress management, 164
Time perception, 138, 139b
Time saving strategies, 140–141
Tort, quasi-intentional, 210
Tort law, 210
Trait theories, of leadership, 7
Transformational leadership, 9–10
Treatment, alternative modalities for, 110
TriCouncil, 285
Trust, promotion of, communication and, 25

U
Unlicensed assistive personnel, American Nurses Association and, 95, 102, 103t
  definition of, 118

  delegation to, 93, 97
  direct and indirect client care activities of, 102, 103t
  need for services of, 95
  registered nurses and, 119
  tasks of, 116
Unproductive behavior, feedback and, 35
Utilitarianism, 227–228

V
Values, adoption of, 225
  behaviors motivated, 225
  belief systems and, 226–227
  definition of, 224
  development of, 225
  extrinsic, 225
  intrinsic, 225
  personal, 225
  professional, 225
  systems of, 224–225, 284, 285t
Values clarification, 225–226, 226t
Veracity, 230
Verbal tracking, 22
Violence, in workplace, 181–184
  protection from, 183b, 183–184
  potential for, behaviors indicating, 182b, 183
  safety in workplace and, 176
Voluntary Effort program, 111

W
Wald, Lillian, 242, 245–247
Walking rounds, to give "report," 27
Websites, 201–202
Whistleblower, 192
Whitman, Walt, 252
The Woman Rebel, 248
Work, unnecessary, elimination of, 144–145
Work life, quality of, enhancement of, 193
Workplace, physical environment of, 197–198
  safety in. *See* Safety in workplace
  working relationships and, 194
Worksheets, 143
  personalized patient, 94, 96f